Evaluating Sleep in Infants and Children

Evaluating Sleep in Infants and Children

Stephen H. Sheldon, D.O.

Diplomate, American Board of Sleep Medicine
Diplomate, American Board of Pediatrics
Director, Sleep Disorders Center
Children's Memorial Hospital, Chicago
Assistant Professor of Pediatrics
Northwestern University Medical School
Chicago, Illinois

Lippincott - Raven
P U B L I S H E R S
Philadelphia • New York

Lippincott - Raven Publishers, 227 East Washington Square, Philadelphia, Pennsylvania 19106

Made in the United States of America

Library of Congress Cataloging-in-Publication Data

Sheldon, Stephen H.
    Evaluating sleep in infants and children / Stephen H. Sheldon.
        p.   cm.
    Includes bibliographical references and index.
    ISBN 0-397-51628-2
    1. Sleep disorders in children—Diagnosis.   2. Children—Sleep.
    3. Infants—Sleep.   I. Title
    [DNLM: 1. Polysomnography—in infancy & childhood.   2. Sleep—physiology.
    3. Polysomnography—methods.   4. Child Development—physiology.
    WL 108 S544e   1996]
    RJ506.S55S538   1996
    618.92′8498—dc20
    DNLM/DLC
    for Library of Congress   95-37628
                                                                                CIP

The material in this volume was submitted as previously unpublished material, except in the instances in which credit has been given to the source from which some of the illustrative material was derived.

Great care has been taken to maintain the accuracy of the information contained in the volume. However, neither Lippincott - Raven Publishers nor the author can be held responsible for errors or for any consequences arising from the use of the information contained herein.

9   8   7   6   5   4   3   2   1

Contents

Preface

This book is an offering to health care professionals who dare to care for children during sleep.

In 1979 Anders, Emde, and Parmelee published *A Manual of Standardized Terminology, Techniques and Criteria for Scoring of States of Sleep and Wakefulness in Newborn Infants*[1] as a tool for the guidance of research into the electrophysiologic and behavioral nature of sleep in infants. It was also written, in part, as a response to the newly emerging field of sleep disorders medicine. Apparently, pediatric sleep disorders medicine had been left alone because it was too controversial, complicated, dynamic, and changing in the developing human. In short, sleep disorders medicine wanted *nothing* to do with children. There have been few centralized concerted efforts to pull together data collected over the past 23 years as a cogent and meaningful guide for the general sleep disorders medicine professional on indications, techniques, interpretation, and evaluation of sleep in infants, children, and adolescents. This book is a compilation, review, and organization of existing literature regarding sleep in the pediatric population.

Many areas of concern exist. Many data are anecdotal and speculation abounds. A majority of the literature that exists on sleep in the pediatric patient refers to neonates. Some normative data exist for adolescents, but much less exist for toddlers and youngsters during middle childhood. This may be because they are typically a healthy lot. However, adult and neonatal norms cannot be applied to these children. This segment of the population is composed of individuals with steadily changing neuroanatomic, neurophysiologic, somatic, behavioral, and social environments. Approaches in a single scientific process have been difficult and technology has not yet been available to measure those physiologic parameters required for adequate (and/or appropriate) analysis. Complicating the picture, data show that there is a wide range of variability in both internal and external organization and consistency in the developing child, making normative data quite difficult to collect and interpret. Normal developmental processes also confound attempts at standardization. How does one conduct and interpret MSLT (multiple sleep latency test) data for young children in whom diurnal sleep is still a developmentally appropriate and normal phenomenon? How can a prepubertal child of 7 or 8 years of age (Tanner stage 1) be diagnosed with narcolepsy syndrome when there is a paucity of normative MSLT data in prepubertal children and the presumed natural history of this disorder often precludes diagnosis prior to Tanner stage 5. Indeed, many youngsters, despite equivocal laboratory data, have profound performance problems in school. They may suffer sleep attacks, cataplexy for which they are labeled clumsy or epileptic, hypnogogic hallucinations for which they are misdiagnosed as having nocturnal fears, or sleep paralysis with complaints of being hard to awaken in the morning.

Many other questions exist:

- When should polysomnography be done?
- What are the indications at various developmental levels?
- Do daytime nap studies provide adequate information regarding the physiologic, developmental, and pathophysiologic answers being sought?
- If appropriate, at what age can nap studies provide comprehensive data for diag nosis and treatment?
- How long should a pediatric polysomnographic recording be conducted? Does it vary according to age?
- How many EEG channels should be monitored? How many are enough to provide adequate information regarding maturation of the central nervous system?
- What are the best methods for monitoring respiratory function?
- How should sleep states be scored and interpreted at various developmental peri ods?
- When physiologic, pathophysiologic, or pathologic sleep disorders are identified, how should they be treated?

Pediatric sleep medicine and the understanding of sleep in infants, children and adolescents have progressed significantly over the past decade. We are only beginning to understand the wide ranging implications disturbed sleep has on growth, development, maturation, and performance.

The practicing general pediatrician and academic pediatric community have felt that sleep and its disorders are purely developmental and behavioral phenomenon (except in the areas of SIDS and apnea). A comprehensive (*ecologic*) approach would include developmental and behavioral aspects of sleep, but would give equal importance to neurophysiologic, neuroanatomic, and physiologic aspects of sleep. Indeed, development and behavior have their origins in neuroanatomy, neurophysiology, and developmental biology.

Because sleep occupies a significant portion of children's lives, pathologic changes occurring during sleep, which affect central nervous system and other system development, can often result in significant morbidity. Many of these abnormalities have gone virtually unrecognized and ignored. Only a handful of general pediatricians, pediatric neurologists, pediatric pulmonologists, pediatric psychiatrists, neonatologists, and other child health care professionals have received formal training in sleep disorders medicine. Those who have received training did so in adult sleep disorders laboratories and centers. Few pediatricians have become board certified by the American Board of Sleep Medicine. Currently there are only *5 accredited pediatric sleep centers and 3 accredited pediatric sleep apnea laboratories in the United States*.[2] Comprehensive pediatric sleep medicine care is only provided in a limited number of accredited general sleep disorders centers and laboratories.

Children are not just small adults. They are remarkably different and require approaches and technologies specifically designed to meet their needs. This does not mean simply shrinking adult equipment, protocols, and technologies to smaller sizes. Children are special people. They will become our doctors, lawyers, pharmacists, bridge builders, diplomats, legislators, bus drivers, and airplane pilots. Shortly, all of us will be putting our lives and trust in their hands. It is essential that children be taken care of both day and night.

The young are the future makers and owners of the world. For their education and training and capabilities, the (physician) as the representative of medical science and art should become responsible...

Abraham Jacobi (1904)

REFERENCES

1. Anders T, Emde R, Parmelee A. *A Manual of Standardized Terminology, Techniques and Criteria for Scoring of States of Sleep and Wakefulness in Newborn Infants*. UCLA Brain Information Service, NINDS Neurological Information Network, 1971.
2. Jordan B, American Sleep Disorders Association (*personal communication*).

Acknowledgments

Many individuals unknowingly contributed to the development of this book such as the professionals who have dedicated their careers to further understanding sleep of children.

Several courageous physicians met informally one evening at the 5th annual meeting of the Association of Professional Sleep Societies, and have been carving out a niche and advocating for children within the sleep disorders medicine community since. Richard Ferber, Lee Brooks, Gerald Rosen, and Ron Dahl are acknowledged for their enthusiasm, dedication, and tireless work. Their stimulating discussions, excitement about pediatric sleep medicine, intense knowledge, and commitment to quality have been inspiring.

Encouragement from Dr. Ronald V. Marino started it all.

I also thank Jean-Paul Spire and Howard B. Levy for their constant support, trust, and unending willingness to share their vast knowledge about sleep and pediatrics.

Connie Gibbons, manager of the Lindon Seed Memorial Library, deserves particular note and thanks. Without Connie's dedication and hard work in searching the world's literature, as well as procuring articles from obscure journals at a moment's notice, compilation of materials presented in this textbook would not have occurred.

Finally, special acknowledgment is reserved for my friend, colleague, and respected developmental and behavioral pediatrician, Susan Riter. Dr. Riter critically read and reread the manuscript from its first draft to last. She has truly been bitten by the pediatric sleep disorders medicine "bug." Without her constant help and support, this book would not have been possible.

Biological Development of Sleep

...When we discover not only that there is a vast expanse of unknown, but that much which was supposed to be known is in reality a poor subterfuge of unreal facts forming structures of misleading results, which in the scientific medicine of adults would not for a second be tolerated; in fact would be laughed to scorn as relics of the dark ages of necromancy. This same misnamed medical knowledge, however, when representing the infant and child, has been accepted with but little question.

Thomas Morgan Rotch (1891)

1

Introduction

This chapter is an overview of the development of pediatric sleep medicine and provides the appropriate focus for the clinical evaluation of sleep in sleep disorders centers created and designed specifically for infants, children, and adolescents. An understanding of the evolution of sleep disorders medicine into a clinical discipline for children will place the information that follows into perspective. Parallels exist between pediatric sleep medicine and pediatrics as a specialty. A juxtaposition of these two disciplines can sensitize the reader to state of the art sleep disorder evaluations for children and, challenge those who pursue academic and clinical research into the *night life* of infants and children.

DEVELOPMENT OF PEDIATRICS AS A SPECIALTY

The most important landmark in health care for children during the 20th century was the emergence of pediatrics as an accepted medical discipline. Prior to the 1900s, specialized medical care for children and infants was virtually nonexistent. Mortality rates for infants were remarkably high and more than one third of all infants died before they reached the age of 5 years (1). Unfortunately, this high mortality rate rarely raised eyebrows and caused little excitement. Health care for children was generally left to the family. The medical community treated children much the same as adults (2), and medical care for children was considered a poor stepchild of internal medicine. Child health care practitioners were considered "baby feeders." In 1900, there probably were not more than 50 medical practitioners in the United States who took particular interest in the health care of children and less than a dozen practiced pediatrics exclusively (3) Possibly one doctor out of every 2,500 could have been classified as a pediatrician. Laboratories for clinical evaluation and hospitals for the treatment of childhood illness and disease were nonexistent (2). Great philanthropic energy was required to provide special facilities for children. Children were neither a political nor economic force and were considered the property of their parents. Disease ran rampant and the child health care practitioners' duties were based on prevention. Tea, barley water, and protein milk were common approaches to the treatment of illness during childhood. Floating hospitals and country sanatoria were occasionally utilized in the treatment of disease in children, but most treatment occurred in the home (4). Diagnosis was difficult and primarily based on clinical signs and symptoms. Bacteriologic diagnosis was not yet possible and thermometry had not yet become widely accepted. Congenital malformations were thought by some of the most respected child health care practitioners of the time to be due to "maternal impressions" (2). Treatment offered little and was completely empiric. Climatotherapy and heliotherapy were popular because it was believed that the course of many pediatric diseases "could be favorably influenced by judicious airing" (2). Appropriate climates and appropriate amounts of sunlight were accommodation for treatment of diseases such as tuberculosis, skin disorders, anemia of childhood, and particularly rickets (5). Some of these treatments were surprisingly accurate; but, most were relatively ineffective. Treatment of pneumonia in childhood often consisted of digitalis, sparteine sulfate, camphor, sodio-caffeine benzoate, strichnia, and alcohol.

The New York Babies Hospital was founded in 1887 and was the first institution in the United States dedicated exclusively to the diagnosis and treatment of children (2). At the time this hospital opened, there were less than a half-dozen *general hospitals* in the country that had wards dedicated to the care of children.

The discovery of the etiology of many of the diseases resulting in high mortality rates occurred during the first quarter of the 20th century. Pasteurization of milk and immunizations against infectious diseases placed child health care practitioners at the forefront of public health and preventive services. The discovery of antibiotics and their appropriate use in the treatment of bacterial diseases such as meningitis and pneumonia and the development of corticosteroids were also responsible for decreasing the depressingly high mortality rate that existed at the turn of the century.

During the past 30 years, progress in pediatric medicine and surgery has been staggering. Trends have turned from the treatment of infectious diseases to new, comprehensive prevention programs, developmental pediatrics, adolescent medicine, genetics, fetal and neonatal medicine, school health and community pediatrics, and many others. Different types of morbidity are being recognized. Behavioral abnormalities, family violence, child maltreatment, drug abuse, school learning problems, and developmental disabilities are beginning to attain appropriate priority. New efforts to understand and elucidate the underlying cause for many of these very significant disorders have been made and a multi-disciplinary approach to diagnosis and management has received special attention.

DEVELOPMENT OF PEDIATRIC SLEEP MEDICINE
AS A CLINICAL DISCIPLINE

At almost every juncture, pediatric sleep disorders medicine parallels pediatrics in its creation. Although a fascination with sleep has existed in literature since antiquity, sleep research can be traced back to when Berger first described spontaneous electric discharges in the brains of sleeping humans (6). Eye movements during sleep and the association of these rapid eye movements with dream mentation were suggested by Kleitman and Dement (7).

Separation of sleep into distinct states was first described by Harvey, Loomis, and Hobart in 1937 (8). But, it was not until 1953 that human rapid eye movement sleep was first described by Aserensky and Kleitman at the University of Chicago (9). In 1957, Dement and Kleitman reported the cycling of REM and NREM sleep throughout the night and proposed a system to classify NREM sleep into four distinct states (10).

These discoveries ushered in a new era in medicine and medical research. It was now not enough to evaluate and study the human patient only during waking hours. It had become clear that significant physiologic changes occurred during the one third of an individual's life spent sleeping. Physiology, pharmacology, and pathophysiology have been shown to be significantly different during sleep when compared to wakefulness (11). Sleep research progressed to a point where clinical practice could emerge. The practice of sleep medicine could then evolve in many centers during the 1970s (12).

Many clinical sleep disorders medicine services developed out of the research interests of the practitioners. Most patients were self-referrals for insomnia and a few came from physicians who were aware of such syndromes as narcolepsy and obstructive sleep apnea. Sleep disorder researchers at Stanford University Sleep Disorders Clinic demolished the notion that the majority of insomnia patients were psychiatric cases (12). European studies of sleep apnea were introduced to the United States in 1972 and the term "polysomnography" was coined in 1974 by Dr. Jerome Holland (13). By the end of the 1970s clinical sleep disorders medicine became an accepted area of practice, the American Sleep Disorders Association was formed as the American Association of Sleep Disorders Centers with five members in 1975 and the scientific journal *Sleep* was published (12). A nosology of sleep disorders was published in *Sleep* in 1979 (14) and a significant number of textbooks began to appear which focused on the science of sleep and clinical diagnosis and treatment of sleep disorders. This culminated with the publication of the landmark textbook, *Principles and Practice of Sleep Medicine,* edited by Kryger, Roth, and Dement in 1989 (15). Effective treatment for many diagnosable sleep disorders (e.g., obstructive sleep apnea with nasal CPAP) had been discovered and quickly became widespread in use. The combination of the high prevalence of obstructive sleep apnea in the United States and discovery of effective, noninvasive treatment resulted in rapid expansion of sleep medicine as a unique medical discipline. Sleep disorders medicine has become an accepted distinct specialty within the medical community.

The entire field of sleep disorders medicine is new. Many opportunities exist to evaluate and treat individuals across the entire 24-hour continuum of life. However, pediatric sleep disorders medicine had been addressed by the medical community only peripherally. In 1968, *A Manual of Standardized Terminology, Techniques, and Scoring System for Sleep Stages of Human Subjects* was published (16) in order to standardize sleep-stage scoring in adults and to eliminate serious unreliability and inconsistencies in polysomnography within and between laboratories. It soon became clear that the standards recommended by Rechtschaffen and Kales for evaluation and recording sleep stages in adult subjects were inappropriate for evaluation of sleep and its stages in newborn infants, whose physiologic sleep processes differed markedly from adults. The result of this realization was the development of an ad hoc committee to provide similar standards for newborn infants. A committee was formed and co-chaired by Drs. Anders, Emde, and Parmelee. The result of the work of this committee was the publication of *A Manual for Standardized Techniques and Criteria for Scoring of States of Sleep and Wakefulness in Newborn Infants* in 1971 (17).

However, standards for evaluating sleep in older infants, toddlers, children, and preadolescents were not addressed in this publication. Many problems existed that made standardization in the pediatric age group a formidable task. First, the nervous system as well as other physiologic processes dynamically, functionally, and anatomically change during this period of life. Attempting to define cross-sectional criteria for evaluation and comparison is quite difficult because of significant internal variability. Ranges of "normal" may be quite broad. External reliability and validity is often difficult to establish. It may be more appropriate to compare each individual child at several points in time (longitudinal evaluation or *developmental polysomnography*) to assure normal progression of maturation, rather than evaluating a single physiologic polysomnographic study at a single point. Because of these difficulties, little information has been available to provide accurate normative data, despite the evidence that sleep and its normal structure has far-reaching implications on growth, development, and learning (18,19).

Pediatric sleep disorders medicine has become an out-growth of the sleep disorders medicine movement, receiving impetus from several directions: interest in the etiology and identification of infants at risk for sudden infant death syndrome (SIDS); identification of obstructive sleep apnea syndrome and other breathing disorders occurring during sleep in infants and children; identification of the importance of sleep in the genesis of diurnal behavior disorders; the identification of behavioral impact of disordered sleep; and the effect of sleep disorders in children on day-time performance and learning.

SIDS has been discussed in the medical literature for more than 100 years (20). Despite intensive investigative efforts, the cause of SIDS is still baffling. SIDS is responsible for approximately one third of all infant deaths between the ages of 1 and 6 months and nearly half of infant mortality for children between 4 and 6 months of age (21). Because almost all of these infants die unexpectedly during sleep, especially nocturnal sleep, interest in cardiorespiratory physiology and pathophysiology during sleep in newborns and infants has thrived. Many investigators focused their research on functional variations between sleep and wakefulness as well as various sleep states (active/REM sleep and quiet/NREM sleep). Better methods for identification of sleep state have been developed. Sleep states in newborns and infants have subsequently become understood. At present, there have been more than 70 theories of the underlying cause of SIDS and still there is considerable controversy and confusion. In 1978, Marie A. Valdes-Dopena suggested that infants who die of SIDS are probably *never entirely normal* (22). She suggested that an underlying physiologic defect existed, which was at that time unknown. It was stressed that there was not one positive criterion which could be used clinically (or polysomnographically) to distinguish future victims of SIDS. Twenty years later, there has been no change. Frustration and the alarming mortality rate from SIDS focused research into cardiorespiratory control during sleep in infancy. Indeed, the electrophysiologic abnormalities are most likely quite subtle and probably consist of several complicated changes that by themselves may appear normal.

Obstructive sleep apnea syndrome and other forms of sleep disordered breathing in childhood was the second milestone in the development of pediatric sleep medicine as a discipline. In 1956, Burwell and colleagues (23) described obesity-alveolar hypoventilation syndrome and termed it a "Pickwickian syndrome" after the hypersomnolent fat boy Joe, eloquently described by Charles Dickens in the *Pickwick Papers* (24). Although sleep apnea was discovered and described simultaneously in France and Germany in 1965 (25,26), the syndrome was virtually ignored by the medical community in the United States. A series of investigations reported by Lugaresi, Tassinari, and coworkers in Italy described the sleep apnea syndrome in adults, cardiovascular effects of this form of sleep-disordered breathing, and the importance of snoring and hypersomnolence as clinical clues of the presence of sleep apnea (27).

In the early 1970s, treatment options for obstructive sleep apnea (OSA) were few. The syndrome was virtually unrecognized in the United States. Lugaresi had reported the remarkable success of tracheostomy in alleviating symptoms and sequelae of OSA (28). Similar treatment for the syndrome was strongly resisted in the United States until Guilleminault demonstrated remarkable results in managing uncontrollable hypertension in a 10-½-year-old boy with OSA by tracheostomy (27). It is fascinating that *the first successful treatment of obstructive sleep apnea syndrome in the United States was illustrated on a pediatric patient.*

Interest in obstructive sleep apnea syndrome increased dramatically, but focused mostly on the easily identifiable adult patient with OSA. Pediatricians were generally uninformed of this seemingly obscure syndrome. Even child health care practitioners who had an interest in identifying the syndrome and in diagnosing and treating other sleep disorders had virtually no place for referral since there were so few centers available to adequately evaluate sleep in infants and children.

Two important publications began to focus the pediatric health care community and emerging sleep disorders medicine professionals on the importance of sleep in childhood development and behavior. The first was publication of Dr. Richard Ferber's book for parents entitled *Solve Your Child's Sleep Problems* by Simon and Schuster (29). Based on Dr. Ferber's work done at Boston Children's Hospital, the text reviewed all aspects of sleep in childhood in a practical and informative manner. It focused on many of the developmental and behavioral aspects of sleep, the solutions of which were typically left to the parents' imagination. Pediatric textbooks and journals were virtually devoid of scientific sleep topics. For example, Nelson's *Textbook of Pediatrics*, 14th edition (30) has a total of eleven *paragraphs* devoted specifically to sleep disorders. This has been the paradigm textbook for pediatrics for the past 25—50 years and used as a reference by child health care practitioners and is studied by most students, pediatric residents, and family practice trainees.

The next important publication related to pediatric sleep medicine was edited by Christian Guilleminault and published in 1985 (31). In the Preface of his text, *Sleep and Its Disorders in Children*, Dr. Guilleminault eloquently stated:

> The text consists of a collection of papers providing seminal information on normative data. These pioneering works have become the basis for future direction in the scientific study of sleep and sleep-wake cycles during all developmental phases of infancy and childhood.

More changes in sleep-wake patterns and associated physiologic functions occur during the first 15 years of life than during the following four decades. However, we have comparatively little information regarding these developments. Likewise, information on sleep disorders in children has not been collected or presented systematically. To ascertain the prevalence and importance of sleep disorders among children requires a large data base on normal sleep/wake patterns. It must be understood how sleep develops early in infancy, how sleep and wake becomes organized over the 24-hour continuum, and how sleep/wake-day/night patterns are molded.

The many contributions presented in Dr. Guilleminault's work provided a significant base for future development of a knowledge base of understanding normal sleep in infants and children so that a clearer perception of pathologic sleep states may be developed. Care for childhood sleep disorders can then progress past the level of "camphor-strichnia-alcohol."

Clinical pediatric sleep medicine has had to rely on a nosology developed originally for adults (32). Adaptations have been attempted (33). It is apparent that simply adapting adult criteria to childhood sleep disorders has many pitfalls since the natural history of normal and abnormal physiologic states requires specific elucidation. Extensive revision of adult diagnoses and classification would be required. Dr. Guilleminault has pointed out that "before re-writing the classification for children, however, the existing classification should be applied to children's problems to test its strengths and shortcomings" (31).

The pediatrician has typically been the child health care professional to whom infants and children with sleep problems have been referred for diagnosis and management. Yet the general pediatric community has been slow to grasp the significance of the physiologic aspects of sleep and the importance of the structure of sleep to human development. A survey of major pediatric journals reveals few articles related to sleep disorders and major research meetings focus little attention to sleep related pathology or pathophysiology. (S.H. Sheldon, *unpublished data*).

Over the past 5 to 10 years pediatric pulmonologists and pediatric otolaryngologists have increasingly recognized the role of sleep and its disorders in their clinical and academic arenas, with particular focus on sleep related breathing abnormalities. During the same time period, need for comprehensive pediatric sleep medicine services has increased significantly in sleep disorders centers and laboratories. It is likely that the next 5 to 10 years will show a further increase in the need for these services within general sleep centers as well as a need for the development of specialized centers for children. Training programs, residencies and fellowships in pediatric sleep medicine require development. Comprehensive training of a cadre of clinical and academic physicians who may staff centers, consult, coordinate research, and teach is an important goal for the immediate future. Inclusion of pediatric sleep medicine in clinical curricula for undergraduate, post-graduate, and continuing medical education is a required next step.

Success of incorporating pediatric sleep medicine objectives into curricula and expansion of pediatric sleep disorders medicine services will depend much on outcome and cost-effectiveness. First, can comprehensive pediatric sleep medicine services have a significant impact on other medical illnesses such as sickle cell anemia, cystic fibrosis, neuromuscular disorders, asthma, craniofacial anomalies, congenital heart disease? Second, are higher brain functions such as learning and memory dependent on normal maturation and continuity to sleep? How might disordered sleep during early infancy and childhood affect cognitive abilities? Third, can an understanding of sleep and its disorders contribute to a better comprehension of behavioral disorders, attention span problems, and learning disabilities. Two recent articles by Wilson and McNaughton (19) and Karni and coworkers (18) have shed significant light on the importance of focusing on the sleeping brain (especially REM sleep) when assessing learning and behavior. The mystery of establishment and integrating neural networks required for learning, behavior, and performance may be locked within the sleeping brain. As was true of the development of pediatrics as a unique specialty, better appreciation of sleep, its development, and the effects of its disorders in childhood might lead to improved diagnosis, treatment, and prevention. It is clear, *the future of pediatric sleep medicine is before us.*

REFERENCES

1. Holt LE. Infant mortality ancient and modern. An historical sketch. *Arch Pediatr* 1943;30:885.
2. Cone TE Jr. *History of American Pediatrics.* Boston: Little Brown; 1979:99–130.
3. Smith RM. Medicine as a science: pediatrics. *N Engl J Med* 1951;244:176.
4. Powers GF. Developments in pediatrics in the past quarter century. *Yale J Biol Med* 1939;12:1.
5. Freeman RG. Fresh air in pediatric practice. *Trans Am Pediatr Soc* 1916;28:7.
6. Berger H. Ueber das Elektroenkephalographalogramm des Menchen. *J Psychol Neurol* 1930;40:160–179.
7. Dement WC, Kleitman N. The relation of eye movements during sleep to dream activity: an objective method for the study of dreaming. *J Exp Psychol* 1957;53:339–346.
8. Harvey EN, Loomis AL, Hobart GA. Cerebral states during sleep as studied by human brain potentials. *Science* 1937;85:443–444.
9. Aserensky E, Kleitman N. Regularly recurring periods of eye motility, and concomitant phenomena, during sleep. *Science* 1953; 118:273–274.
10. Dement WC, Kleitman N. Cyclic variations in EEG during sleep and their relation to eye movements, body motility, and dreaming. *Electroencephalogr Clin Neurophysiol* 1957;9:673–690.
11. Orem J, Barnes CD. *Physiology in Sleep.* New York: Academic Press; 1980.
12. Carskadon MA, Roth T. Normal sleep and its variations. In: Kryger M, Roth T, Dement WC, eds. *Principles and Practice of Sleep Medicine.* Philadelphia: WB Saunders; 1989:3–15.
13. Holland V, Dement W, Raynal D. Polysomnograpy: responding to a need for improved communication. *Presentation to the annual meeting of the Sleep Research Society.* Jackson Hole, Wyoming; 1974.
14. Association of Sleep Disorders Centers: Sleep Disorders Classification Committee, Roffwarg HP, chairman. Diagnostic classification of sleep and arousal disorders. *Sleep* 1979;2:1–137.

15. Kryger M, Roth T, Dement WC, eds. *Principles and Practice of Sleep Medicine*. Philadelphia: WB Saunders; 1989.

16. Rechtschaffen A, Kales A. *A Manual of Standardized Terminology, Techniques and Scoring System for Sleep Stages of Human Subjects*. Los Angeles: BIS/BRI, UCLA, 1968.

17. Anders T, Emde R, Parmelee AH, eds. *A Manual of Standardized Terminology, Techniques and Criteria for Scoring of States of Sleep and Wakefulness in Newborn Infants*. UCLA Brain Information Service, NINDS Neurological Information Network, Los Angeles, 1971.

18. Karni A, Tanne D, Rubenstein BS, Askenasy JJM, Sagi D. Dependence on REM sleep of overnight improvement of a perceptual skill. *Science* 1994;265:679–682.

19. Wilson MA, McNaughton BL. Reactivation of hippocampal ensemble memories during sleep. *Science* 1994;265:676–679.

20. Cone TE Jr. *History of American Pediatrics*. Boston: Little Brown; 1979:20.

21. Beckwith JB. *The Sudden Infant Death Syndrome*. Washington D.C.: Department of Health, Education and Welfare Publication No. (HSA)75–5137, 1975.

22. Valdes-Dapena MA. *Sudden Unexplained Infant Death, 1970 through 1975*. Department of Health, Education and Welfare Publication No. (HSA)78-5255, 1978.

23. Burwell CS, Robin ED, Wahley RD, Bickelmann AG. Extreme obesity associated with alveolar hypoventilation: a Pickwickian syndrome. *Am J Med* 1956;21:811–818.

24. Dickens C. *The Pickwick Papers*. Garden City, New York: Dodd, Mead; 1944.

25. Gastaut H, Tassinari C, Duron B. Etude polygraphique des manifestations épisodiques (hypniques et respiratoires) du syndrome de Pickwick. *Rev Neurol* 1965;112:568–579.

26. Jung R, Kuhlo W. Neurophysiological studies of abnormal sleep and the Pickwickian syndrome. *Prog Brain Res* 1965;18:140–159.

27. Dement WC. History of sleep physiology and medicine. In Kryger M, Roth T, Dement WC, eds. *Principles and Practice of Sleep Medicine*, 2nd ed. Philadelphia: WB Saunders; 1994:3–15.

28. Lugaresi E, Coccagna G, Mantovani M, Brignani F. Effects de la trachéotomie dans les hypersomnies avec respiration périodique. *Rev Neurol* 1970;123:267–268.

29. Ferber R. *Solve Your Child's Sleep Problems*. New York: Simon & Schuster; 1985.

30. Behrman RE, ed. *Nelson's Textbook of Pediatrics*, 14th ed. Philadelphia: WB Saunders; 1992.

31. Guilleminault C. *Sleep and Its Disorders in Children*. New York: Raven Press; 1987.

32. Diagnostic Classification Steering Committee, Thorpy M, chairman. *International Classification of Sleep Disorders: Diagnostic and Coding Manual*. Rochester, MN: American Sleep Disorders Association; 1990.

33. Sheldon SH, Spire JP, Levy HB. *Pediatric Sleep Medicine*. Philadelphia: WB Saunders; 1992:185–240.

2

Development of Sleep Structure

In 1963 Kleitman and Dement described the alternation of REM and NREM sleep in characteristic and reproducible cycles throughout the sleep period (1). Ultradian alternation of the basic rest–activity cycle (BRAC) was described by Kleitman (2). Observations regarding the development of rest and activity cycles as well as the structure of sleep in infants and children have been made. These cycles often appear random in their development and created, to some extent, by environmental and/or external factors.

On the one hand, development of the sleep-wake cycle and the orderly structure of sleep in the fetus, premature and term newborn, infant, and child follows a highly organized progression directly related to central nervous system (CNS) maturation and development. Structural development of sleep and sleep-wake cycles can be affected by environmental factors, genetic factors, medical factors, and biologic influences.

On the other hand, sleep architecture and the development of the structure of sleep and the sleep-wake continuum can provide quite specific and sensitive insight into the integrity of the CNS and, in certain cases, prognosis and outcome.

Despite great efforts, a clear understanding of the functions of sleep are unknown. From both human and animal experiments, there appears to be a vital nutritive function. Animals totally deprived of sleep die (3). REM sleep shows a particularly important role in learning, memory, and consolidation of memory (4,5). Continuity of sleep also appears to be quite important. When fragmented, objective and subjective symptoms of sleep deprivation occur (6).

Sleep has at least one (and most likely many) obligatory functions that cannot be accomplished during the waking state. Slow-wave sleep seems to play a critical role in accomplishing this crucial function, although the exact nature is unknown. However, this duty seems to be directly related to the brain (7). Active/REM sleep is tightly correlated with NREM sleep and plays an important role in memory and emotions (8,9), which seems to be different than the obligatory role of slow-wave sleep. Major evidence of the importance of REM sleep in facilitating recall of complex associative information has been described by Scrima (10). Recall for complex associative tasks is significantly better after REM-onset naps when compared to NREM-onset naps in narcoleptic subjects. It has also been observed that subjects learning a foreign language who made significant progress, incorporated the language into dreams earlier than the controls. In addition, significant progress was also associated with more verbal communication in their dream cognition than those who made lesser progress (11). Large quantities of active sleep during early neonatal life with its subsequent fall to adult levels throughout the first several years suggests an operative role in early human development (12). There is evidence that active sleep and quiet *alert* states correlate highly in areas of temporal maturation and this association is independent of maturational changes in the infant. Therefore, it might be assumed that active/REM sleep in early infancy performs a meaningful function by stimulating neuronal networks within the CNS during long periods of sleep. This stimulation and activation of neurons during sleep might facilitate dendritic branching and synaptic connections, development of new neuronal networks, and result in maturation of central processing and growth.

Polysomnographic recordings during the first year of life reveal clear developmental trends against a background of variability (13). The CNS functions as the executive system controlling sleep parameters, phasic activity, and body movements (see Chapter 5). REM phasic density seems to be highest in infants 36 to 38 weeks conceptional age (13).

Sustained periods of wakefulness are present in normal infants by 6 weeks of age (14). After 9 weeks of age, wakefulness is predictably distributed during late afternoon and early evening hours. The longest wake period begins to occur during the day-time hours and longest sleep period at night. REM sleep is disproportionately distributed with a higher percent of the total sleep time occurring at night. By 5 to 6 months, NREM-sleep states can be clearly demarcated and are coincident during the night with slow-wave sleep peaking during the early part of the nocturnal sleep period (14). Decreasing proportions of REM sleep during the day suggests a reciprocal relationship with wakefulness. Implications for assessment of neurophysiologic development are evident and justification for nocturnal evaluation of infants, rather than diurnal nap studies, become apparent.

State organization in terms of diurnal sleep-awake rhythm and distribution of sleep states in preterm infants with good neurologic outcome seems to be accelerated over those infants with a poorer prognosis (15). Viable infants born after the shortest gestations tend to have longer time awake at conceptional term than viable preterm infants born closer to conceptional term. Curzi-Dascalova and coworkers in studying sleep states in normal premature infants characterized the development of state between 30 and 41 weeks conceptional age (16). All infants studied fell asleep in active sleep. The first active sleep episode after sleep onset was significantly shorter than the next active sleep episode. Mean sleep cycle duration increased from approximately 46 minutes at 31–34 weeks to 70 minutes at 35–36 weeks conceptional age. Stable-active and quiet-sleep periods were observed. These stable states lasted continuously, without interruption for 5 minutes or longer. Indeterminate sleep constituted about 30% of the sleep period time at 31–34 weeks and decreased to about 12% of the sleep cycle by 35–36 weeks. Both duration and percentage of active and quiet sleep increased at 35–36 weeks and remained stable up to 39–41 weeks of conceptional age. However, quiet-sleep percentage was reduced when defined by traditional criteria as well as by respiratory rate, tonic chin EMG activity, and movements. The contrast, starting from 31–34 weeks conceptional age, between active sleep and quiet sleep as defined by EEG and REM criteria could account for state differences in the control of many physiologic variables in the premature infants.

Most observations regarding the development of sleeping and waking states, however, have been done in the prematurely born infant. Specific bias regarding state development may then exist. State formation of the fetus in utero has been studied by Shinozuka and colleagues (17). Fetal rapid eye movements, breathing movements, and trunk movements were observed through the use of three ultrasonic real-time scanners. Each movement was recorded with an event marker and quantitatively analyzed in relation to the development of the sleep-wakefulness cycle by a computer-assisted system. The number of rapid eye movements increased with gestational age. REM/NREM cycle rhythm was distinguishable after 32 weeks. The relationship between REM sleep eye movements and body movements increased with gestational age. The time of occurrence of each phasic movement of the trunk had no correlation to that of rapid eye movements when analyzed in short-term epochs. But, the incidence of phasic body movements was high during active sleep.

In general, ontogeny of the sleep-wake state is comparable in premature and full-term infants (18). Development of sleep-wake states in the premature group, however, is more variable across the first year of life, even though both the premature and term infant demonstrate individual stability of some sleep-wake variables over the first year. Anders and coworkers described sleep-wake state organization, neonatal assessment, and development in premature newborns during the first year of life (19). Infants were evaluated in their homes at seven different ages during the first year of life to determine whether sleep-wake state organization was related to either neonatal assessment or short-term developmental outcome measures. Sleep-wake state variables and neonatal assessment items were related to each other, and both predicted developmental outcome at 6 months and 1 year of age. Concordance was present primarily in the domain of motor activities. Waking motor development and maturation of motor activity in sleep seem to independently reflect an infant's level of developmental organization.

Individual sleep-wake state variables are influenced by both biologic and environmental factors. Ontogeny of quiet sleep is predominantly biologically determined, as evidenced by its relationship to the infant's gestational age or birth weight; the infant's behavior that results in being taken from the crib during the night, and the course of his/her sleep that occurs between midnight and morning are dependent on both biologic factors, and post-birth experiences. Apparently, the course of active sleep and wakefulness are dependent solely on environmental influences, and not on maturity at birth.

EEG sleep measures have been compared in healthy full-term and preterm infants at matched conceptional age (20). Major differences in each sleep organization for the preterm infants included:

1. a longer ultradian sleep cycle (70 minutes versus 53 minutes);
2. more abundant tracé alternant pattern (34% versus 28%); and,
3. less abundant low-voltage irregular active sleep (13% versus 17%).

Although no differences were observed for sleep-onset latency and sleep efficiency, the preterm infants had fewer number and shorter duration of arousals, fewer body movements, and rapid eye movements, particularly during quiet sleep. It has been concluded that extrauterine experience or the earlier birth of the preterm infant may influence specific sleep structure and continuity measures when compared with the sleep of full-term infants who experienced a complete intrauterine gestation.

Other factors also influence the development of basic rhythms in the newborn and infant. Feeding patterns seem to induce development of ultradian cycles during the early newborn period and these patterns are based both on metabolic demands and external, parental influences. The effects of feeding on sleep and wakefulness were examined by Matsuoka and coworkers (21). Analysis of the frequency of sleep epochs after feeding in 4-hour periods across the 24-hour day revealed specific patterns during each week of post-natal life. By 2 weeks of age, sleep epochs appeared most frequently in time periods between midnight and 0400 and 0400 and 0800. These periods also had high rates of sleep after feeding. After 6 weeks of age, both the number of sleep epochs and the frequency of episodes of sleep after feeding in time periods from 0800 to 2000 tended to decrease. These results suggested that the development of the circadian oscillation of the sleep-wake cycles begin with sleep epochs occurring first during the time period from midnight to 0800. In addition, feeding seemed to have no role as a time cue in the first 4 months of life, but influenced the ultradian cycle during later infancy.

Circadian rhythm of wakefulness and sleep is clearly established as early as 4 months of age and consolidated mostly during nocturnal hours between 6 and 7 months (22). Some ages (6 to 7 months; 10 to 12 months; and 13 to 15 months) are characterized by significant changes in the daily distribution and duration of sleep periods. These latter observations suggest the existence of several ultradian rhythms that successively prevail from one age to the next throughout child development. Longitudinal evaluation of sleep and wake states of the young child allows better assessment of the influence of factors related to developmental disorders and dysfunction.

Sleep behavior of preterm infants at 3 years of age can vary considerably. Sleep disturbances are frequently noted in prematures at 3 years of age. By 5 years of age, however, the number of reported sleep problems decreases. Children with remaining sleep problems at 5 years of age tend to be different children than those who had sleep problems at 3 years (23). Surprisingly, the children with the greatest sleep onset and settling difficulties at 3 years of age were children with the fewer neonatal medical problems, higher scores on the Bayley scales, and more positive social interactions with their caregivers during the first two years. These data suggest that environmental influences may contribute to the development of sleep difficulties, especially settling problems, after a critical time of CNS bio-physiologic development.

Three months of post-term conceptional age appears to be a critical time period for neurophysiologic development. Early bioelectric maturation may reflect the development of neural mechanisms that are also the substrate for later cognitive and behavioral functioning.

Sleep-state organization at 3 months post-term can often be utilized as a benchmark for CNS development (24). At this age, more mature adult-like sleep stages begin to emerge. The presence of NREM organization, characteristics, and stage sequencing suggest that sleep-regulatory mechanisms are approaching a level of functional maturity in the human infant at about 10 to 12 weeks of post-conceptional term. There appears to be a relationship between sleep staging at 3 months post-term and mental and motor performance at 12 months post-term. Sleep organization and state development are as directly related to CNS development as other traditional measurements. Physiologic sleep measurements may provide a more sensitive and objective indicator of maturational level than traditional appraisals. Many explanations for current findings of limited group differences between premature and term infants at comparable conceptional ages can be identified, but remain buried in the data as currently presented (25).

Environmental influences on the development of state organization and sleep-related behaviors can be influenced in some areas by extrauterine environment. When preemies and term newborn are compared according to respiratory variables and behavioral state observations, the premature infant appears to be more mature by measures of some variables than the term newborn and less mature by others. These observations suggest the presence of global differences in state organization, although neither the cause nor the consequences of these differences are currently known (26).

At times, state differences in polysomnographic parameters between term and premature newborns at conceptional term can be affected by laboratory conditions. Without habituation to the laboratory environment, physiologic sleep and sleep-waking behaviors in older infants, children, and adults occur making normative data difficult to collect in any systematic way. Simple videotaping conditions, as well as complex polygraphic recording of 2- and 8-week-old infants in the laboratory, have been shown to affect state organization (27). Under either conditions and at both ages increased crying and fussiness and decreased alertness have been shown to occur during the first 4 hours in the laboratory.

Decreased fussiness and increased alertness can be demonstrated in the following sleep-wake periods, indicating adaptation to the laboratory conditions.

Because of this "laboratory effect," efforts have been made by home health care companies to provide in-home evaluations. Home studies have a theoretical advantage of performing the procedure in a familiar environment. It is also said to be more cost effective since the costs incurred in the laboratory and by having the study continuously attended by a technologist are not required. Unfortunately, these contentions have not been validated in the pediatric population. The studies are unattended and littered with technical difficulties. Behavioral observations of the patient are vital during pediatric polysomnography and are impossible during an unattended study. Home studies are also typically limited in scope (routine sleep-state scoring utilizing EEG, EOG, and EMG are not performed). Cost effectiveness is also controversial since most home studies are nearly as expensive as in-laboratory investigations. Home studies frequently require laboratory confirmation by comprehensive polysomnography when results are equivocal.

Sleep-onset latency seems to be shorter and drowsiness increased under laboratory polygraphic recording. At 8 weeks of age, quiet sleep appears to be increased and active sleep decreased. Observational and polygraphic studies seem to be stressful even for young infants and time for adaptation is needed. Short nap studies without a period of adaptation, therefore, may be affected by reaction to laboratory conditions, even during early infancy. Cross-sectional studies may fail to reveal deviation from state development and progression characteristic of the infant's chronologic age. When studies are conducted longitudinally, however, there is a "within-individual" consistency in the development of CNS control of behavioral states across the sleep-wakefulness cycle despite the diverse activities of the environment (28). These factors can be accommodated in the laboratory assessment of the development of state in infants and children.

In addition to laboratory effect, sleep posture also appears to affect behavioral states in newborns. Newborn infants in the United States tend to sleep more in the prone position than supine. Recently, the American Academy of Pediatrics has made changes in recommendations for sleeping positions in newborn infants (29). The prone sleeping position has been show to be epidemiologically associated with SIDS (30,31). The supine position has resulted in a significant decrease in the incidence of SIDS. Although this recommendation is still controversial the AAP has recommended the supine or lateral decubitus position for sleep in newborns and infants (29).

In the prone position, quiet sleep occupies a greater portion of the sleep period than in the supine (32). Gross movements, jerky movements, and twitches occur less frequently in the prone than in the supine position. There appear to be no differences in localized movement or tremor-like movement in the two positions. Respiration is more regular in the prone position, which may be state dependent on quiet sleep. Sleep apnea (greater than or equal to 6 seconds) is less in the prone position. The pulse rate during quiet sleep was also higher in the prone position than supine (32).

Term infants between 1 week and 6 months of age reveal a consistent emergence of temporal distribution of quiet sleep, active sleep, motility, and circadian influences on heart rate during sleep (33). With increasing age, an increased percentage of active sleep begins to cluster toward the end of the night and an increased percentage of quiet sleep toward the beginning of the sleep period. When the 24-hour period is split into two distinct episodes (day-time/night-time) it can be seen that quiet sleep increases only during the night-time while active sleep and indeterminate sleep decrease during the day-time (34). Quiet sleep in older subjects becomes mainly located at the beginning of the night-time period, when particularly long phases take place. However, prior to one year of age, slow-wave sleep appears to be distributed evenly across the nocturnal sleep period. Although slow-wave sleep decreases across the night for adults and children, it does not decrease across the sleep period for infants (35). The distribution during the night-time of active sleep (in terms of the percentage and mean duration) does not change notably with age. A circadian influence upon heart rate can be observed in active sleep and indeterminate sleep prior to existence in quiet sleep. At 2 months and 3 months of age, motility in quiet sleep and active sleep increases linearly during the night (33).

Temporally patterned stimulation can have a significant effect on development. When appropriately instituted, premature infants can manifest a decreased rate of activity while in the hospital, fewer abnormal reflexes, and better orienting responses (36). At 2 years of age, premature infants who had experienced patterned auditory and kinesthetic stimulation scored higher on the Mental Development Index of the Bayley Scales (36). Both temporal patterning and contingent responsiveness in the preterm infant's early waking state contribute positively to some aspects of the development of such infants.

Arousal thresholds appear to be greater in children than adults. In one study Busby and Pivik showed no behavioral responses or sustained awakenings for any child studied during the first cycle of sleep to stimuli at intensities up to 123 dB sound pressure, intensities more than 90 dB above waking threshold values (37). Half of the arousals to stimulation during stage 2 and one quarter during stage 4 elicited only a partial physiologic arousal manifested by brief EEG desynchronization and/or change in skin potential response or respiratory activity rates. These arousals were short-lived, with the subjects returning to sleep event with continued increased stimulus intensity. Therefore, both intrinsic and extrinsic stimuli are required to result in an arousal response.

It is clear that sleep occupies a major portion of newborns', infants', and children's lives. A term newborn spends more than 70% of every 24 hours sleeping. Because sleep occupies such a large portion of the newborns' day, major developmental work most likely occurs during this state.

Spontaneous fetal movements can be identified at approximately 10 weeks of gestation, and rhythmic cycling of activity can be recorded in utero by 20 weeks conceptional age (38). At 28 to 30 weeks of age, brief quiet periods begin to appear, although their periodicity is not yet stable (39). By 32 weeks conceptional age, body movements are absent in 53% of 20-second epochs during 2- to 3-hour sleep recordings (40). The number of epochs containing no recordable movements increase to 60% at conceptional term.

State development in the prematurely born infant may be influenced by physical and biologic conditions that require continuous medical or surgical interventions. The neonatal intensive care unit affords a quite different environmental milieu than the normal intrauterine environment. Preterm infants born after the shortest gestation typically suffer from significant medical and/or surgical abnormalities. Extrauterine development of the infant occurs either in a 24-hour lighted environment or, more recently, under cycled lights rather than within a 24-hour dark environment. The effect of light and frequent medical interventions on development of the CNS and sleep cycling has not yet been elucidated.

As previously stated, during the first 3 months of life, striking changes occur in many physiologic activities. Ten to 12 weeks of age appears to be a critical period of CNS reorganization. Infantile patterns of sleep behavior and physiology shifts to a more mature form. Sleep-wake patterns and organization change. In the newborn infant, total sleep time is about 16 to 17 hours (40). Total sleep time gradually decreases, reaching 14 to 15 hours by 16 weeks of age and 13 to 14 hours by 6 to 8 months of age.

Maturation of attentive-waking behaviors in infancy seems to occur concomitantly with the development of quiet-sleep and sustained-sleep patterns. These maturational changes seem to suggest continued development of inhibitory and controlling feedback mechanisms secondary to the increasing complexity of neural networks and neurochemical maturation (40). By 10 to 12 weeks of age, development of these systems produces a relatively stable diurnal distribution of sleep and wake. There is also a remarkably regular alternation of active and quiet sleep across the normal nocturnal sleep period (41). Prior to 12 weeks of age, concordance of physiologic variables is remarkably high (42). This may be due to lack of maturation of essential feedback control. A lack of variability is occasionally seen in cardiovascular dysfunction, resulting in little variability and minimal beat-to-beat variation. Periodic breathing common during REM sleep becomes rare after 7 weeks of age (43).

Major consolidation of sleep at night occurs between 3 and 6 months of life. Changes occur in the duration of single-sleep periods and their placement during the 24-hour continuum. Coons has shown that at 3 weeks of age, the mean length of the longest sleep period was 211.7 minutes, or 23.2% of the total 24-hour sleep time. In comparison, by 6 months of age, the longest sleep period was 358 minutes, or 48% of the total sleep time. Between 3 and 6 weeks of age, the longest sleep periods lengthened considerably, but were randomly distributed throughout the 24-hour day. By 6 weeks of age, the longest sleep period was no longer randomly distributed through the 24-hour period, but more consistently occurred during the nocturnal period. Similarly, the longest wake period occurred during day-time hours. A nocturnal pattern of sleep and diurnal pattern of wake is relatively well established by 12 to 16 weeks of age (40). By 6 months of age, the longest sleep period follows the longest wake period (44). By 12 weeks of age, diurnal wake period continues to develop and day-time sleep consolidates into discrete naps (45).

Brief awakenings from nocturnal sleep are more frequent from quiet sleep during the first 8 weeks than at older ages (41). Younger infants are more likely to awaken from active sleep.

Sleep onset occurs through REM sleep in the newborn infant. During the first 12 weeks of life, these sleep-onset REM periods gradually begin to change to sleep onset through NREM. At 3 weeks of age, an infant is likely to have two-thirds of sleep periods beginning with REM sleep (44). Younger infants manifest REM latencies shorter than 8 minutes (46). Older infants produce a mixed distribution of short and long REM latencies. By 6 months of age, the percentage of sleep-onset REM has decreased to 18% (44). Between 4 and 13 months of age, the total distribution of REM latencies appears to be bimodal, with latencies either shorter than 8 minutes or longer than 16 minutes (46). In this age range, the temporal distribution of latencies constitutes a diurnal rhythm, with the longest latencies appearing between noon and 1600 and a tendency for shorter latencies to occur between 0400 and 0800. REM latencies also appear to be dependent upon the *length* of the prior period of wakefulness. Long REM latencies are more often preceded by long episodes of wakefulness than short REM latencies. By 6 months of age, the longest sleep period is only 20% more likely to have REM-sleep onset (44). The ratio of active sleep to quiet sleep is sometimes considered an indicator of maturation (41). Active-sleep time exceeds quiet-sleep time during the first months of life. A reversal of this relationship is noted in 60% of infants at 3 months of age and 90% of infants at 6 months of age.

Changes in the percentage of REM sleep during the sleep period also occur. REM sleep occupies about 50% of the total sleep time at conceptional term. During the first 6 months of life, this volume decreases dramatically. This decrease seemingly represents a redistribution of sleep stages, since only a relatively small decrease in the total sleep time occurs during this time. This change is also considered an important indicator of CNS maturation (47). Interestingly, the reduction in REM sleep is balanced by an increased proportion of the 24-hour day spent in wakefulness.

Between 2 and 5 years of age, growth and development continue in a very steady manner. Sleep becomes consolidated into a long nocturnal period of approximately 10 hours (48–51). Diurnal naps continue. Early during this age period, the first diurnal nap occurs about mid-morning and the second early in the afternoon. The morning nap is gradually abandoned first, and by 3–5 years of age all naps are given up and sleep consolidated into a single nocturnal sleep period.

Between 9 and 12 months, REM sleep averages about 30% to 35% of the total sleep time. Small and large body movements associated with REM sleep during infancy become less frequent. REM periods are of approximately uniform length, despite day-time naps. As the CNS matures, the first REM period shortens and becomes quite brief. Successive REM periods become longer and more intense. Overall cycle length also seems to increase slightly (52). At 2 to 3 years of age, cycle length remains about 60 minutes (the first REM period occurs about 60 minutes after sleep onset). By 5 years of age the cycle length has increased gradually from 60 to 90 minutes. However, on the first recording night in the laboratory, the first REM period is often missed.

Between 2 and 5 years of age, REM volume gradually decreases to the adult level of about 20% to 25%. Changes in the percentage of REM sleep appear to be correlated to the augmented periods of wakefulness during the day. Diminution of REM volume progresses until day-time napping is abandoned. By this age, distinct differences between REM episodes, sleep cycles, and occurrence of slow-wave sleep during early and late portions of the sleep period have emerged (52)

Children in this age group will cycle approximately 7 times during a single nocturnal sleep period (51). Sleep-onset latency is generally about 15 minutes and lengthens to about 15 to 30 minutes. Slow-wave sleep predominates during the first third to first half of the sleep period and as much as 2–3 hours may be spent in slow-wave sleep. EEG amplitude is remarkably high. Stage 2 first appears about 3–4 minutes after sleep onset and slow-wave sleep appears about 7 to 10 minutes later (50). Indeed, children during this age period descend rapidly into deep sleep during the early portion of the sleep period.

Unique characteristics of the physiology of sleep occurring during this developmental period may signify stabilization of maturation of the sleep state (49,50,53):

1. A relatively small number of state changes occur per hour of sleep (about 3.5 shifts per hour, which is significantly different from young adults);
2. EEG amplitude is consistently higher in all states;
3. Slow-wave sleep is considerably longer;
4. There is a relatively smooth progression of stages across the sleep period, whether moving deeper or lighter; and,
5. Transition between stages is relatively regular and consistent, in comparison to adults who often move abruptly across several stages at a time.

After 5 years of age, growth and development remain relatively constant and progressive. This time, however, is not a period of quiescence, but characterized by activation and change, searching and exploring, learning, memory, and increasingly sophisticated decision making. It is a period of consolidation of prior experiences, preparation, and trial (54). The structure of sleep has nearly reached adult characteristics, although there is considerable variability. There appears to be a relative stability of patterns, and the percentage of time spent in each sleep stage and the number of sleep stages remain remarkably constant from night to night (50). Total sleep time during middle childhood is about 2.5 hours longer than in healthy young adults. This time is equally distributed throughout all sleep stages.

Body movements are seen more often in this age group than in adolescents and young adults (13). Slow-wave sleep volume decreases from about 2 hours in the preschool child to 75 to 80 minutes during the latter portion of middle childhood (52). Naps during this period of development are very rare. Consistent day-time napping during this developmental period often represents a pathologic process. Prepubertal children are generally exquisitely alert throughout the entire day (55,56)

REFERENCES

1. Dement WC, Kleitman N. Cyclic variations in EEG during sleep, their relation to eye movements, body motility, dreaming. *Electroencephalogr Clin Neurophysiol* 1957;9:673–690.
2. Kleitman N. *Sleep, Wakefulness.* Chicago: University of Chicago Press; 1963:131–194.
3. Rechtschaffen A, Gilliland MA, Bergmann BM, Winter JB. Physiological correlates of prolonged sleep deprivation in rats. *Science* 1983;221:182.
4. Karni A, Tanne D, Rubenstein BS, Askenasy JJM, Sagi D. Dependence on REM sleep of overnight improvement of a perceptual skill. *Science* 1994;265:679–682.
5. Wilson MA, McNaughton BL. Reactivation of hippocampal ensemble memories during sleep. *Science* 1994;265:676–679.
6. Roehrst T, Merlotti L, Petrucelli N, Stepanski E, Roth T. Experimental sleep fragmentation. *Sleep* 1994; 17:438–443.
7. Cai ZJ. The function of sleep: further analysis. *Physiol Behav* 1991;50:53–60.
8. Jenkins J, Kallenbach K. Oblivescence during sleep, waking. *Am J Psychol* 1924;35:605.
9. Van Ormer EG. Retention after intervals of sleep, waking. *Arch Psychol* 1932;137:5.
10. Scrima L. Isolated REM sleep facilitates recall of complex associative information. *Psychophysiology* 1982;19:252.
11. DeKoninck J, Christ G, Hebert G, Rinfret N. Language learning efficiency, dreams, REM sleep. *Psychiatr J Univ Ottawa* 1990;15:91–92.
12. Denenbert VH, Thoman EB. Evidence for a functional role for active (REM) sleep in infancy. *Sleep* 1981;4:185–191.
13. Hoppenbrouwers T. Polysomnography in newborns, young infants: sleep architecture. *J Clin Neurophysiol* 1992;9:32–47.
14. Coons S, Guilleminault C. Development of sleep-wake patterns, non-rapid eye movement sleep during the first six months of life in normal infants. *Pediatrics* 1982;69:793–798.
15. Yokochi K, Shiroiwa Y, Inukai K, Kito H, Ogawa J. Behavioral state distribution throughout 24-hour video recordings in preterm infants at term with good prognosis. *Early Human Dev* 1989;19:183–190.
16. Curzi-Dascalova L, Peirano P, Morel-Kahn F. Development of sleep states in normal premature, full-term newborns. *Dev Psychobiol* 1988;21:431–444.
17. Shinozuka N, Okai T, Kuwabara Y, Mizuno M. The development of sleep-wakefulness cycle, its correlation to other behavior in the human fetus. *Asia Oceania J Obstet Gynaecol* 1989;15:395–402.
18. Anders TF, Keener M. Developmental course of night time sleep-wake patterns in full-term and premature infants during the first year of life. I.*Sleep* 1985;8:173–192.
19. Anders TF, Keener MA, Kraemer H. Sleep-wake organization, neonatal assessment, development in premature infants during the first year of life. II. *Sleep* 1985;8:193–206.
20. Scher MS, Steppe DA, Dahl RE, Asthana S, Guthrie RD. Comparison of EEG sleep measures in healthy full-term, preterm infants at matched conceptional ages. *Sleep* 1992;15:442–448.
21. Matsuoka M, Segawa M, Higurashi M. The development of sleep, wakefulness cycles in early infancy, its relationship to feeding habit. *Tohoku J Exp Med* 1991;165:147–154.
22. deRoquefeuil G, Djakovic M, Montagner H. New data on the ontogeny of the child's sleep-wake rhythm. *Chronobiol Int* 1993;10:43–53.
23. Ungerer JA, Sigman M, Beckwith L, Cohen SE, Parmelee AH. Sleep behavior of preterm children at three years of age. *Dev Med Child Neurol* 1983;25:297–304.
24. Crowell DH, Kapuniai LE, Boychuk RB, Light MJ, Hodgman JE. Day-time sleep stage organization in three month old infants. *Electroencephalogr Clin Neurophysiol* 1982; 53:36–47.
25. Parmelee AH. Neurophysiological, behavioral organization of premature infants in the first months of life. *Biol Psychiatry* 1975;10:501–512.

26. Booth CL, Leonard HL, Thoman EB. Sleep states, behavior patterns in preterm, full-term infants. *Neuropediatrics* 1980;11:354–364.
27. Sostek AM, Anders TF. Effects of varying laboratory conditions on behavioral-state organization in two, eight week old infants. *Child Dev* 1975;46:871–878.
28. Becker PT, Thoman EB. Organization of sleeping, waking states in infants: consistency across contexts. *Physiol Behav* 1983;31:405–410.
29. AAP Task Force on Infant Positioning, SIDS. Positioning, SIDS. *Pediatrics* 1992;89:1120–1126.
30. Engelberts AC, deJonge GA. Choice of sleeping position for infants: possible association with cot death. *Arch Dis Child* 1990;65:462–467.
31. Taylor BJ. A review of epidemiological studies of sudden infant death syndrome in southern New Zealand. *J Pediatr Child Health* 1991;27:344–348.
32. Hashimoto T Hiura K, Endo S, Fukuda K, Mori A, Tayama M, Miyao M. Postural effects on behavioral states of newborn infants—a sleep polygraphic study. *Brain Dev* 1983:5:286–291.
33. Hoppenbrouwers T, Hodgman JE, Harper RM, Sterman MB. Temporal distribution of sleep states, somatic activity, autonomic activity during the first half year of life. *Sleep* 1982;5:131–144.
34. Fagioli I, Salzarulo P. Sleep state development in the first year of life assessed through 24-hour recordings. *Early Hum Dev* 1982;6:215–228.
35. Bes F, Schulz H, Navelet Y, Salzarulo P. The distribution of slow-wave sleep across the night: a comparison for infants, children, adults. *Sleep* 1991;14:5–12.
36. Barnard KE, Bee HL. The impact of temporally patterned stimulation on the development of preterm infants. *Child Dev* 1983;54:1156–1167.
37. Busby K, Pivik RT. Failure of high intensity auditory stimuli to affect behavioral arousal in children during the first sleep cycle. *Pediatr Res* 1983;17:802–805.
38. Sterman MB. The basic rest-activity cycle, sleep: developmental considerations in man, cats. In: Clemente CD, Purpura DP, Mayer FE, eds.*Sleep, the Maturing Nervous System.* New York: Academic Press; 1972.
39. Dryfus-Brisac C. Ontogénese du sommeil chez le premature humain: étude polygraphique. In: Minokowski A, ed. *Regional Development of the Brain in Early Life.* Oxford, England: Blackwell; 1967.
40. Parmelee AH, Stern E. Development of states in infants. In: Clemente CD, Purpura DP, Mayer FE, eds. *Sleep, the Maturing Nervous System.* New York: Academic Press; 1972.
41. Hoppenbrouwers T. Sleep in infants. In: Guilleminault C, ed. *Sleep, Its Disorders in Children.* New York: Raven Press; 1987.
42. Harper RM, Leake B, Miyahara L, Hoppenbrouwers T, Sterman MB, Hodgman J. Development of ultradian periodicity, coalescence at 1 cycle per hour in electroencephalographic activity. *Exp Neurol* 1981;73:127.
43. Metcalf D. The ontogenesis of sleep-awake states from birth to 3 months. *Electroencephalogr Clin Neurophysiol* 1979;28:421.
44. Coons S. Development of sleep, wakefulness during the first 6 months of life. In: Guilleminault C, ed.*Sleep, Its Disorders in Children.* New York: Raven Press; 1987.
45. Parmelee A, Wenner WH, Schulz HR. Infant sleep patterns from birth to 16 weeks of age. *J Pediatr* 1964;65:576.
46. Schultz H, Salzarulo P, Fagiolo I, Massetani R. REM latency: development in the first year of life. *Electroencephalogr Clin Neurophysiol* 1983;56:316.
47. Stern E, Parmelee AH, Akiyama Y, Schulz MA, Wenner WH. Sleep cycle characteristics in infants. *Pediatrics* 1969;43:65.
48. Mattison RE, Handford HA, Vela-Bueno A. Sleep disorders in children. *Psychiatr Med* 1987;4:149.
49. Kohler WC, Coddington D, Agnew HW. Sleep patterns in 2-year old children. *J Pediatr* 1968;72:228.
50. Ross JJ, Agnew HW Jr, Willimas RL, Webb WB. Sleep patterns in pre-adolescent children: an EEG-EOG study. *Pediatrics* 1968;42:324.
51. Williams RL, Karacan I, Hursch CJ. *Electroencephalography (EEG) of Human Sleep: Clinical Applications.* New York: Wiley; 1975.
52. Roffwarg HP, Dement WC, Fisher C. Preliminary observations of the sleep-dream pattern in neonates, infants, children, adults. In: Harms E, ed. *Problems of Sleep, Dreams in Children.* New York: MacMillan; 1964.
53. Sheldon SH, Spire JP, Levy HB. *Pediatric Sleep Medicine.* Philadephia: WB Saunders; 1992.
54. Levine ME. Middle childhood. In: Levine ME, ed. *Developmental—Behavioral Pediatrics.* Philadelphia: WB Saunders; 1983.
55. Carskadon MA, Keenan S, Dement WC. Night time sleep, day time sleep tendency in preadolescents. In: Guilleminault C, ed. *Sleep, Its Disorders in Children.* New York: Raven Press; 1987.
56. Carskadon MA, et al. Pubertal changes in day-time sleepiness. *Sleep* 1980;2:453.

3

Development of Sleep-Related Respiratory Function

A large segment of pediatric sleep medicine literature and research has centered on the respiratory system and the effects of sleep and its various states on breathing. Much of this research has been driven by the presumption that sudden infant death syndrome (SIDS) was primarily an abnormality in the central control of breathing, ventilation, and/or cardiorespiratory function. Therefore, a considerable amount of literature exists regarding respiratory function during sleep in infants and children.

Chapter 3 addresses issues related to the ontogeny of respiratory function during sleep, assessment of monitoring respiratory effort, hemoglobin oxygen saturation, respiratory airflow, identification and classification of breathing abnormalities, and home monitoring of respiratory function and ambulatory diagnosis.

ONTOGENY OF BREATHING

Intricacies in the control of respiration in infants and small children differs greatly from the adult. Regulation of breathing is affected significantly by the processes of maturation from gestation throughout post-natal life and early childhood development. The most dramatic changes occur at the time of birth when respiratory activity switches from behavioral breathing movements to sustained respiratory activity essential for ventilation.

Sleep states significantly influence both mechanical relationships of respiratory muscles and the control of ventilation (1). Neurophysiologic immaturity and mechanical characteristics of chest wall compliance that may compromise respiration and ventilation present special challenges for the infant and small child.

Fetal Breathing Movements

Although suggested almost 100 years ago, fetal respiratory movements were first described in some detail by Dawes and coworkers in 1972 (2). Cyclic breathing movements were studied in fetal lambs and confirmed in humans by Boddy and Robinson (3). It has become apparent that fetal respiratory activity is essential for normal pulmonary development during gestation (4,5). Indeed, fetal breathing activity has been demonstrated in every mammalian species investigated and is clearly a required part of normal fetal development.

Control of fetal breathing movements in utero differs from mechanisms of control after birth (6). Inhibitory influences are prominent in utero where conservation of energy may be advantageous during fetal development. Control of breathing movements also seems to be in part under chemical control. Kitterman and colleagues have shown administration of inhibitors of prostaglandin synthesis causes marked stimulation of fetal breathing movements in lambs (7). Four parameters changed after administration of sodium mechlofenamate and/or indomethacin. Incidence of fetal breathing movements almost doubled. Average amplitude and maximal amplitude of change in tracheal pressure during fetal breathing movements increased substantially. Finally, the duration of the longest continuous episode of breathing movements increased from 37 minutes to 229 minutes. Infusion of prostaglandin E2 after blockade results in a dose-dependent increase in fetal breathing and restoration of physiologic cycling with electrophysiologic state (8).

Fetal breathing movements also appear to vary according to state, and control of respiratory activity in the fetus seems to be state dependent. Breath-to-breath intervals show respiratory differences during active and quiet fetal-time periods (9). Irregular fetal respiratory movement patterns are noted during fetal-active periods. Regular fetal respiratory movements correlate with quiet periods in the term fetus. This behavior suggests that a quiet-sleep state may exist in utero in the near term fetus. This can be corroborated by the presence of quiet-sleep state in the prematurely born infant near term.

In the fetal lamb, breathing movements generally occur during low-voltage, high-frequency electrocortical activity. However, during infusions of prostaglandin inhibitors, breathing movements also occur during high-voltage, low-frequency electrocortical activity (7). Therefore, there appears to be both central (mediated at the level of the upper pons) and chemical (mediated by prostaglandins) inhibitory influences on fetal breathing movements.

Newborn

Action of respiratory muscles are state dependent. Skeletal muscle tone and monosynaptic reflexes are actively inhibited during REM sleep (10,11). Motor inhibition involves active hyperpolarization of 1-α spindle afferent fibers by descending inhibitory fibers originating in the pons. Superimposed upon this active hyperpolarization of alpha and gamma efferents, unorganized phasic motor activity occurs resulting in muscle twitches and saccadic extra-ocular eye muscle activity. This behavioral activity associated with desynchronization of EEG collectively comprises active sleep. During quiet sleep, tonic skeletal muscle activity persists, but may be somewhat lower than in the waking state.

These changes, which occur in the skeletal musculature and central nervous system, exert a significant influence on respiration. Increased chest wall compliance in the newborn also has an effect on breathing. Maintenance of inspiratory muscle tone in the preservation of functional residual capacity (FRC) is crucial in the newborn. In a study conducted by Lopes and coworkers (12) a decrease in diaphragmatic and intercostal muscle tone was associated with a decrease in the anteroposterior diameter of both rib cage and abdomen, indicating a fall in the FRC. These changes in diameter of chest and abdomen were more marked during quiet sleep than in active sleep, indicating that inspiratory muscle tone is a major determinant of FRC in the newborn. In the premature newborn, however, Moriette and coworkers found no differences in FRC between active and quiet sleep (13).

A significant relationship was identified between active sleep and paradoxic breathing and between active sleep and irregular breathing. As the diaphragm shortens during active sleep in the newborn, the chest moves inward and abdominal displacement increases, leading to paradoxic breathing, which appears to be normal during active sleep (1). As the infant matures, distortion of the chest wall decreases, improving the mechanical stability of the chest during ventilatory efforts (14). During quiet sleep, tonic activity of the intercostal muscles (as well as other accessory muscles of respiration) helps to stabilize the chest wall (15,16). Quiet sleep in the term newborn is remarkably stable and respiratory rate is regular and monotonous. As maturation continues, chest wall contribution to tidal volume increases (17).

It has been postulated that during periods of paradoxic breathing in active sleep, increased chest wall compliance resulting in collapse could also lead to deflation of the lungs, reduced oxygen stores, and the rapid development of hypoxemia. Henderson, Smart, and Read have demonstrated that thoracic gas volume (TGV) measured by occlusion plethysmography was significantly reduced during active sleep and was associated with rib cage collapse and increased abdominal-diaphragmatic excursions (i.e., paradoxic breathing) (18). The average reduction in TGV was almost one third of that measured during quiet sleep. This reduced lung volume during active sleep could have implications for the regulation of breathing in that state. A reduction of oxygen stores during active sleep suggests an ontogenetic vulnerability of the premature newborn, term newborn, and young infant to hypoxemia (18). However, FRC does not appear to differ between sleep states. Beardsmore and colleagues (19) reported no significant changes in FRC between states using a specially constructed, closed-circuit, helium dilution technique. Similarly, Stokes and coworkers (20) showed that FRC variations during sleep-state changes were smaller than those seen within a defined sleep state, and they concluded that changes in sleep state were not associated with variations in FRC.

Regional Airway Contribution to Respiration

Upper-airway musculature plays an important role in contributing to total pulmonary resistance, even very early in life. Airway diameter and muscle activity in the larynx, pharynx, and nose contribute to dynamic changes in the resistance to airflow during breathing both during wakefulness and sleep (1). The larynx is the most important variable resistor to respiratory airflow (21). Five intrinsic muscles of the larynx modulate laryngeal resistance during breathing through their action on the movement of the vocal cords. These muscles include the cricothyroids, lateral cricoarytenoids, transverse aryntenoids, thyroarytenoids, and posterior cricoarytenoid (22).

High Upper-Airway Resistance

The upper-airway serves a variety of functions including ventilation, protection of the lower airway, and phonation. Significant literature exists regarding the role of the upper airway in these and other functions, as well as activity of upper-airway musculature in the pathogenesis of obstructive sleep apnea (23).

The frequency and prevalence of sleep-disordered breathing during childhood is unknown. It has been estimated to range from 1.6% to 3.4% (24). Clinical presentation of children with obstructive sleep apnea syndrome (OSAS) differs significantly from symptoms occurring in adults. Obesity is much less common in childhood obstructive sleep apnea and failure-to-thrive occurs in one third to one half of infants with OSAS (24). Upper-airway obstruction from hypertrophied tonsils and adenoids is reportedly the most common etiology. Approximately one third of patients with OSAS of childhood have some degree of facial dysmorphism.

Diagnosis of occlusive upper-airway disease is best made through use of polysomnography. Two groups of children with clinically diagnosed occlusive upper-airway diseases can be identified: (i) those with clearly identifiable obstructive events on a polysomnogram, and (ii) those where clear occlusive events are not manifest when typical instrumentation is used. Indeed, *labored breathing may be the only finding of high upper-airway resistance* (25).

Physiologic Expiratory Apnea

There is considerably less known regarding the function of the upper airway and larynx in breathing during sleep in neonates, and only a paucity of studies regarding normal and abnormal pharyngeal and laryngeal respiratory function in prepubertal children. Peculiar (but seemingly common) respiratory events have been described that manifest an expiratory occlusive pattern characterized by sleep-related post-inspiratory upper-airway obstruction similar to post-inspiratory expiratory braking described in animals and children undergoing anesthesia induction with ketamine (26,27). Ketamine is an N-methyl-D-aspartate (NMDA) antagonist and blockade of NMDA receptors results in an increase in inspiratory time (T_i), without increasing expiratory time (T_e), causing an apneustic (prolonged inspiratory activity) breathing pattern (28).

In 18 children studied by Schulman and colleagues (27), T_i was twice as long when compared to pre-induction resulting in a significant increase in T_i/T_e. There was a more rapid increase in lung volume in early inspiration and a slower decrease in volume early in expiration. In addition, occasional early expiratory breath-holding (lasting up to 3 seconds) was identified. Apneustic inspiratory pattern and expiratory braking resulted in an increase in mean lung volume.

During the normal respiratory cycle, the laryngeal airway is widely patent during inspiration and narrow during expiration (29). Phasic changes in glottic aperture principally result from activity (contraction and relaxation) of the posterior cricoarytenoid muscles (PCA) and the pharyngeal constrictor (PC) muscles (30). PCA functions to widen the glottis and is the principal abductor of the vocal cords (31). Along with the PC muscles, the lateral cricoarytenoid, oblique and transverse arytenoid, and thyroarytenoid (TA) muscles function to close the glottis by adduction of the vocal cords. Controlled decline in PCA activity acts in concert with a decrease in activity of thoracic inspiratory muscles to cause expiratory *braking*. Expiratory braking, reflexively controls regulation of expiratory airflow and end-expiratory volume (32). This type of breathing has been shown to occur in the normal newborn puppy (33).

In studying the differential organization of medullary post-inspiratory neuronal activity, Richter, Ballantyne, and Remmers demonstrated that activation of laryngeal and high-threshold pulmonary receptor afferents excited bulbar post-inspiratory neurons (34). Hering and Breuer described an active respiratory response to the magnitude of rapid lung inflation which results in inhibition of the next inspiratory effort when the vagi were intact (35). There is a popular view that the Hering-Breuer reflex may be present only for the first few days of life. With vagal blockade, however, prolonged breath holding to a degree where frank cyanosis occurs can be induced (36).

Importance of the upper airway in regulating the respiratory cycle is critical (36). There is increasing evidence to suggest that the upper airway has to dilate before the diaphragm initiates inspiration. During quiet sleep in lambs several weeks of age, endogenous expiratory pressures of 5 to 7 cm of water pressure develop (37). Opening a tracheal window results in immediate slowing and irregularity of respiration. Expiration becomes prolonged and during expiration, redundant glottic constriction occurs. During apneustic breathing, neurons active only during portions of inspiration or expiration and those neurons whose activity spanned both phases of respiration change markedly; some reveal tonic changes and others exhibit complete cessation of activity (38). Such marked changes can be observed in all laryngeal expiratory neurons. This change in activity may be partly responsible for prolonged respiratory pauses following augmented breaths (signs).

In 1985, Southall and coworkers described 10 children between the ages of 2 and 87 months who demonstrated prolonged expiratory apnea (39). In one infant, glottic closure was demonstrated during sleep-related cyanotic spell by microlaryngoscopy. In addition, similar glottic (vocal cord) adduction has been demonstrated in children who had suffered an ALTE (40).

Reflex glottic closure can result from superior laryngeal nerve stimulation (41). Closure may be facilitated by decreased $PaCO_2$, increased PaO_2, negative intrathoracic pressure, and the expiratory phase of breathing. Arterial chemoreceptors provide a powerful excitatory input to inspiratory hypoglossal motoneurons, both during inspiration and expiration (42). In obstructive sleep apnea, the longest time of post-inspiratory activity of diaphragmatic EMG is associated with the highest inspiratory volumes in the same breath (43), suggesting increased expiratory effort against a closed or partially closed upper airway.

Thyroarytenoid (TA) muscle and post-inspiratory diaphragmatic activity is consistently high during quiet wakefulness and quiet sleep (44). Expiratory TA activity decreases dramatically and post-inspiratory diaphragmatic activity becomes highly variable during REM sleep. Breath-holding (physiologic expiratory apnea) seemed to take place only during non-REM sleep. No sleep-related breath-holding (SRBH) events have been identified during REM-sleep periods.

Polysomnographic characteristics of SRBH are very similar to post-sigh central apneas (PSCA) and graphic appearance often depends upon polygraph amplifier filter settings and sensitivities. However, SRBH appears to differ from PSCA in several important (*but subtle*) aspects. A sigh with a PSCA begins with a deep inspiration and is followed by a complete expiration. Respiratory pause occurs at or near the functional residual capacity. On the one hand, the first post-pause breath appears to be inspiratory; it is not associated with audible expiratory breaking or glottic noise and no significant EKG variability occurs. On the other hand, SRBH similarly begins with a deep inspiration, but is followed by post-inspiratory braking and an incomplete expiration. The post-inspiratory respiratory pause arises at a higher lung volume than the pre-inspiratory functional residual capacity. The first post-pause breath is typically *expiratory*. The recorded pause may be associated with an audible expiratory break or expiratory glottic stridor.

The clinical significance of SRBH is unknown. In Southall's group of 10 patients with expiratory apnea (39), 8 were severely neurologically impaired and it was difficult to determine causality of their respiratory manifestations. The remaining two patients had stormy prenatal and natal courses. In addition, one infant was the twin of a sibling who had died of SIDS. Stephenson subsequently described a prolonged expiratory apnea (breath-holding spell) which resulted in fatality (45). The patient's underlying etiology was secondary to neurologic malformation of the brainstem and cerebellum.

Although there had been risk factors associated with gestation in all six patients with physiologic expiratory apnea, none exhibited significant neurologic abnormalities at the time of presentation. All had been prescribed continuous home cardiorespiratory monitoring and had exhibited frequent alarms due to both apnea and bradycardia. Comprehensive endoscopic evaluations conducted on two patients revealed their upper airways to be widely patent, without apparent anatomic causes for expiratory obstruction, although one patient exhibited a loud voice and small vocal cord nodules. These same two patients had been evaluated comprehensively by different pediatric cardiologists because of bradycardia occurring during sleep. Both had normal cardiovascular examinations, but had exhibited brief episodes of what was considered "benign bradycardia" on continuous 24-hour ambulatory EKG monitoring. None exhibited evidence of significant classical OSAS or desaturations during polysomnography. Each exhibited a tachy-bradydysrhythmia with each SRBH event, similar to those seen during the Valsalva maneuver. Frequent monitor alarms resulted in significant familial stress and parental/sibling/patient sleep disruption.

Subsequent to the initial sleep laboratory studies, one patient continues to have SRBH events resulting in monitor alarms. Observed events have been described by the patient's parents as "apneas" associated with "bright reddening and swelling of his face, like he was blowing up a balloon." Of particular interest, the child's father made "expiratory creaking noises as a child" (which resolved during adolescence). A second child had very frequent episodes of expiratory stridor ("glottic creaking") at 2 years of age, but it had resolved by 4 years.

Many questions remain. Is the glottic closure a pathologic process or is it an exaggeration of normal laryngeal function? Does the length of the event determine the clinical presentation of cyanotic spells during sleep? Do symptomatic children have other concomitant neurologic or neuromuscular dysfunction (e.g., laryngeal dystonia)? These questions await elucidation. It is evident that:

1. SRBH (post-inspiratory upper-airway obstruction) occurs in pre-pubertal children;
2. This respiratory pattern may result in EKG irregularities secondary to mechanical, chemical, and/or autonomic factors; and
3. This pattern of breathing may result in prolonged utilization of apnea/cardiorespiratory monitors.

Further exploration of SRBH and its clinical significance is needed.

Nasal Occlusion and Airway Resistance

The nose has an effect on breathing during sleep (46). Both chemical factors and mechanic stimulation appear to be involved. Muscle activity of the alae nasi decreases resistance to airflow (47). Sleep-state differences were obscured when breathing was stimulated by CO_2. Increased nasal dilation may be a compensatory response to overall increased total pulmonary resistance during REM sleep. End-tidal CO_2 during nose-obstructed breathing is lower than that during sleep with the nose unobstructed. Furthermore, apnea during nasal occlusion has been shown to occur, most frequently after transition to a deeper sleep state (48). This suggests that diminished PCO_2 stimulus combined with behavioral activity play an important role for disordered breathing in nose-obstructed sleep.

Mechanic effects are also significant. Increases in minute ventilation and mean-inspiratory flow rate have been shown to occur during stage 2 NREM sleep with delivery of 4 liters of added nasal airflow via nasal prongs (49), although ventilatory frequency did not change. Laryngeal and pharyngeal dilatation occurs during inspiration (50) that suggests an active muscular process. Negative airway pressure would, therefore, promote collapse of the pharynx unless the negative pressure created by diaphragmatic contraction was opposed. Muscular inhibition that occurs during sleep affects pharyngeal musculature similarly to other skeletal muscles. This loss of tone during REM sleep affects pharyngeal dilation and contraction and may contribute to airway collapse (51). However, upper-airway reflexes that promote upper-airway patency by dilating the pharyngeal lumen continue to operate during sleep in the normal infant (1). Some infants reveal increased frequency of airway obstruction during active sleep because of increased negative pressure generated during inspiratory effort against an added pharyngeal compliance (52).

Respiratory Frequency

Ontogenetic changes occur in respiratory frequency. Respiratory rates are normally higher at all ages when term newborns and infants 18 weeks of age are compared (53). During transitions from one well-defined sleep state to another, respiratory rate showed an intermediate level. Transition from active to quiet sleep showed a progressive slowing of respiratory frequency. Although, transition from quiet sleep to active sleep occurs relatively abruptly, with sudden acceleration in respiratory rate, considerable variability in respiratory rate and pattern occurs during active sleep. In contrast to this variability, there is no difference between the beginning, middle, and end of quiet-sleep episodes (53).

Respiratory frequency appears to be higher in 2- to 10-week-old age groups when compared to newborns and 11- to 18-week-old infants. Measurement of respiratory rate by observation, however, is less reliable than by stethoscope (54) or airflow measurement. During the first 3 years of life, there is a decrease in respiratory frequency during both wakefulness and sleep. It is also faster in the first few months of life in both states and there is also a greater dispersion of rates (54). Rusconi and coworkers have developed reference percentile values for children in the first 3 years of life (Tables 3-1 and 3-2, Figs. 3-1 and 3-2).

Brief respiratory pauses are common in normal term neonates but occur more frequently in premature infants. These physiologic apneas are more prevalent during active sleep in both preterm and term infants (55). Waite and Thoman have shown that brief apneas of 2–5 seconds and apneas of longer duration (6–16 seconds) positively correlate with state in terms of rate per hour, average length, and longest episode in both quiet

TABLE 3-1. *Reference values for respiratory variables during wakefulness: the first 3 years of life (awake)*

Age (months)	Awake				
	−2SD	−1SD	Mean	+1SD	+2SD
0–2	29.8	38.9	48.0	57.1	66.2
2–6	24.3	34.2	44.1	54.0	63.9
6–12	22.1	30.6	39.1	47.6	56.1
12–18	22.9	28.7	34.5	40.3	46.1
18–24	22.4	27.2	32.0	36.8	41.6
24–30	17.6	23.8	30.0	36.2	42.4
30–36	18.9	23.0	27.1	31.2	35.3

Modified from: Rusconi F, Castagneto M, Gagliardi L, et al. Reference values for respiratory rate in the first 3 years of life. *Pediatrics* 1994;94:350–355, with permission.

TABLE 3-2. *Reference values for respiratory variables during sleep: the first 3 years of life (asleep)*

Age (months)	Asleep				
	−2SD	−1SD	Mean	+1SD	+2SD
0–2	31.1	39.8	48.5	57.2	65.9
2–6	19.4	26.4	33.4	40.4	47.4
6–12	15.6	22.6	29.6	36.6	43.6
12–18	16.0	21.6	27.2	32.8	38.4
18–24	16.1	20.7	25.3	29.9	34.5
24–30	13.9	18.5	23.1	27.7	32.3
30–36	14.1	17.8	21.5	25.2	28.9

Modified from: Rusconi F, Castagneto M, Gagliardi L, et al. Reference values for respiratory rate in the first 3 years of life. *Pediatrics* 1994;94:350–355, with permission.

sleep and active sleep. The magnitude of correlation decreased slightly with age in active sleep, whereas in quiet sleep the association showed a positive increase.

Brief respiratory pauses of 3 seconds or longer followed by normal breathing for 20 seconds or less is termed periodic breathing. Periodic breathing is common in active sleep and constitutes a significant percentage of active-sleep time in the premature. This decreases in percentage as term is reached. By 3 months of age, periodic breathing during active sleep is generally less than 3% of the total active sleep time (Fig. 3-3) (56).

Rate (breaths/minute)

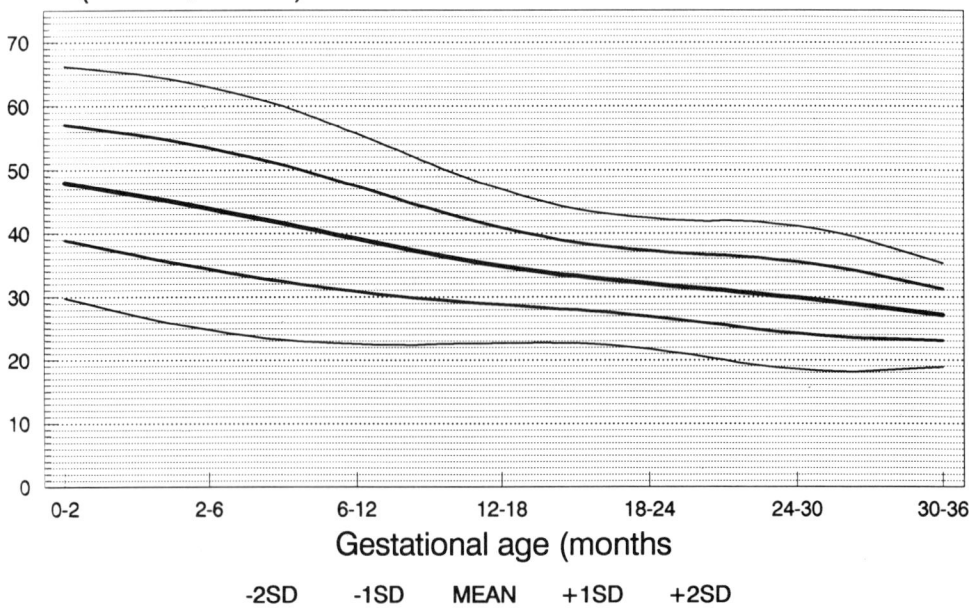

FIG. 3-1. Reference values for respiratory variables during wakefulness: the first 3 years of life (AWAKE)—nomogram. (Modified from: Rusconi F, Castagneto M, Gagliardi L, et al. Reference values for respiratory rate in the first 3 years of life. *Pediatrics* 1994;94:350–355, with permission.)

Rate (breaths/minute)

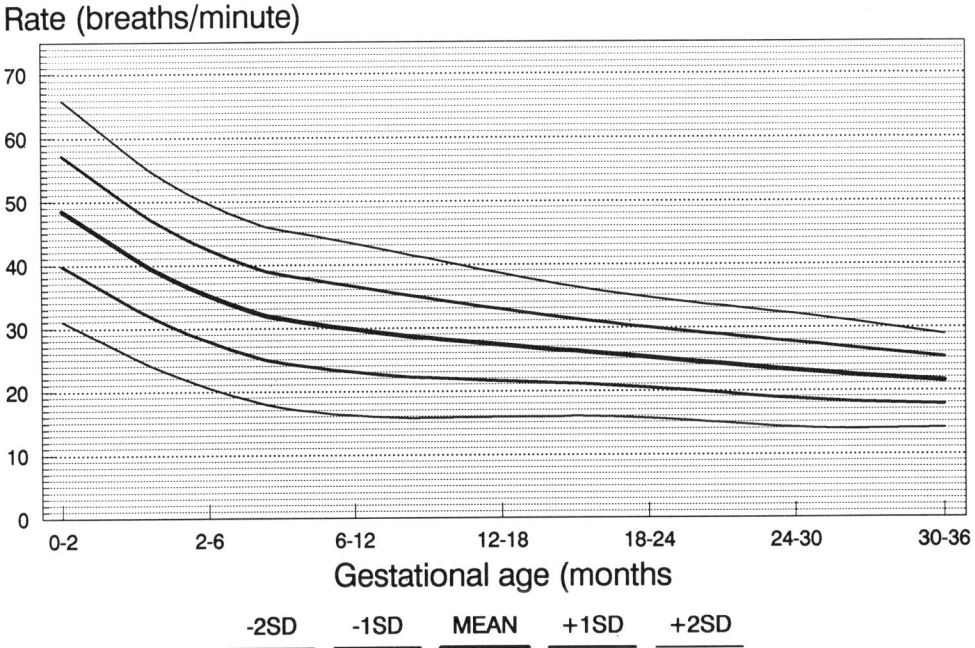

FIG. 3-2. Reference values for respiratory variables during wakefulness: the first 3 years of life (ASLEEP)—nomogram. (Modified from: Rusconi F, Castagneto M, Gagliardi L, et al. Reference values for respiratory rate in the first 3 years of life. *Pediatrics* 1994;94:350–355, with permission.)

Periodic breathing can arise as a result of unstable behavior of the respiratory control system. Longobardo, Cherniack, and Gothe utilized a mathematic model of the respiratory control system to investigate the effect of severity of disturbance to respiration and certain system parameters on periodic breathing during sleep (57). Effects of hypoxia and hypercapnia on upper-airway musculature were excluded. This model revealed that as circulation time increased, the number of central apneas associated with periodic breathing increased. As sensitivity of peripheral controller responsiveness to CO_2 increased, the frequency of apneas also increased, although periodic breathing occurred with lower controller sensitivity as circulation time increased. There were more apneas with hypoxia. Apneas increased in frequency with sleep-associated reduction in metabolic rate. The quicker the rise in resting PCO_2 at sleep onset, the greater the likelihood of recurrent apneas.

Sleep-Disordered Breathing: High Upper-Airway Resistance

A great deal of research has been conducted to identify etiologies of sleep-disordered breathing in adults. A paucity of information has been available regarding causes of sleep-related upper-airway obstruction in children. Most data on sleep-disordered breathing during childhood have been either extrapolated from adult data or gathered from preliminary observations, studies conducted with very small sample sizes, and data from investigations into infant sleep apnea and SIDS. Many of these data are observational and anecdotal. Despite limitations, information suggests that *sleep-disordered breathing in children is clearly a different disorder than sleep-disordered breathing in adults.*

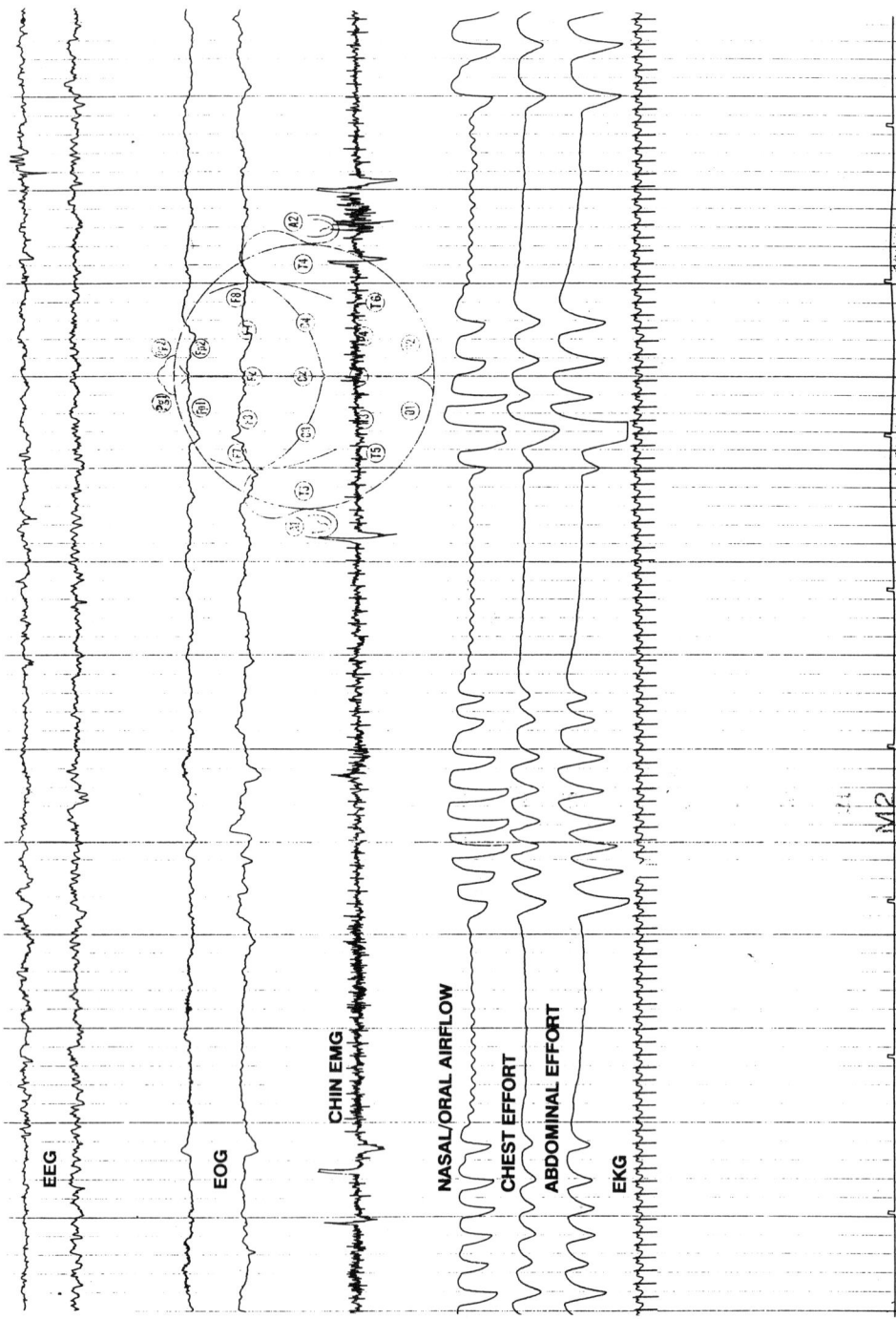

EEG

EOG

CHIN EMG

NASAL/ORAL AIRFLOW

CHEST EFFORT

ABDOMINAL EFFORT

EKG

Definitions of pathologic respiratory events and thresholds for abnormality vary considerably. For example, during childhood the duration of abnormal occlusive respiratory events seems to be less important than in adults. In infants and small children, complete occlusion of the airway with absence of measurable nasal and oral airflow in the presence of at least two respiratory efforts can be considered an abnormal event regardless of the length. Abnormal respiratory events are typically associated with arousal, decreased heart rate, and/or decrease in oxygen saturation (58). Profound cardiac and hemodynamic abnormalities may occur even with very brief events. Significant occlusive respiratory events may occur *without changes in airflow* and are characterized only by increased upper-airway resistance. During NREM sleep, increased resistance to airflow results in intensified respiratory efforts and recruitment of accessory respiratory muscles. Although resistance has increased, this augmentation of effort results in maintenance of airflow.

During infancy, central apneas of 20 seconds or longer are considered pathologic (55). Central apneas less than 20 seconds in length which are associated with bradycardia and/or hemoglobin oxygen desaturation are also considered abnormal. However, criteria seem to be different when considering toddlers and older children.

Resistance to flow can be increased at any point of the airway, including (but not limited to) the anterior nasal valve; nasopharynx (adenoids); oropharynx (tonsils and tongue); hypopharynx (peripharyngeal soft tissue, musculature and pharyngeal constrictor muscles); larynx (vocal cords and laryngeal musculature); and lower-airway smooth muscles. All pathologic changes in airway function have not been elucidated and a complete understanding of the pathophysiology of abnormal increases in airway resistance is still controversial. A multifactorial etiology is most likely. In addition, it is unknown whether various types of occlusive airway phenomena during childhood are separate entities with different etiologies or a single disorder with various manifestations on a continuum of severity.

Anatomic abnormalities (hypertrophic tonsils and adenoids) are the most common cause for upper-airway obstruction during sleep in children (59). This may not be true for all youngsters. Clearly, other anatomic abnormalities of the face, head, and neck as well as many neuromuscular disorders are associated with airway obstruction and increased upper-airway resistance. Etiologies of upper-airway obstruction and increased airway resistance during infancy may be as different from older children as the childhood disorder is from adult obstructive sleep apnea syndrome. Systematic research and collaborative efforts are required in order to better describe and understand underlying pathophysiology.

Other types of normal and abnormal occlusive respiratory events have been described. Significance of these respiratory pauses is controversial. Exact cause of these events is poorly understood. For example, a sigh is considered to be a normal respiratory phenomenon. Often a sigh is followed by a central respiratory pause (60). The event begins with an augmented breath which is characterized by a deep inspiratory effort followed by an exhalation, generally to the functional residual capacity (FRC) of the lungs. During sleep, the "central" respiratory pause may last a few seconds or may continue for a relatively prolonged period. The direction of the first post-pause respiratory effort is typically inspiratory. Sighs are commonly seen in infants and children during NREM stage 2 and slow-wave sleep. At times the respiratory pause following the sigh is associated with

FIG. 3-3. A–B: Active sleep–periodic breathing. Note the respiratory pauses for 3 seconds or greater followed by less than 20 seconds of normal breathing.

mild EKG changes and minimal oxygen desaturation. Clinical significance of isolated sighs and post-sigh pauses during sleep is unclear and these respiratory events have been considered to be normal physiologic phenomena.

Isolated NREM-sleep expiratory apneas have also been identified (26). These unusual respiratory events appear polysomnographically similar to a sigh. However, they can be differentiated by several criteria. Compared to a sigh, the expiratory phase stops short of the FRC. Direction of airflow immediately after the respiratory pause is expiratory. In addition, there is a greater degree of change in heart rate between sighs and these expiratory-obstructive apneas. In many patients, the site of airway occlusion seems to be at the level of the glottis. Some of these peculiar respiratory pauses are associated with only partial occlusion during expiration. Glottic "noise" or prolonged expiratory stridor can be heard during the event, indicating continued expiratory effort and airflow against partially closed vocal cords during the *central* portion of the respiratory pause.

METHODS OF MONITORING RESPIRATION DURING SLEEP

Over the past 25 years, methods of measuring respiration during sleep have varied considerably from impedance pneumography to measurement of end-tidal CO_2. Each of these methods involve different technology and have their own strengths and weaknesses. The first method of measurement of respiration during sleep involved direct observation. This was clearly inadequate due to the inability to both monitor and record airflow.

Impedance pneumography involves placement of electrodes on either side of the chest and measurement/recording of impedance changes. Changes in distance between the two electrodes results in fluctuation in impedance, thereby providing a source for recording chest and/or abdominal wall movement. Unfortunately, sensitivities and specificities for measuring respiratory efforts by impedance is poor (56). False-negatives (absence of effort when effort is actually present), false-positives (recording of respiratory activity when it is actually absent), frequent movement artifact, and lack of ability to measure airflow using impedance pneumography makes its usefulness quite doubtful.

Polysomnography utilizing a variety of newer methods for measurement of respiration and breathing is recognized as the most reliable and accepted method. A variety of instrumentation has been developed over the past 10 years that provides accurate and reproducible results, as well as yielding good internal and external validity.

Measurement of Respiratory Effort

Strain Gauges

Mercury-filled strain gauges have been a fairly reliable method of measuring respiratory effort. These sensors involved encircling the chest and abdomen with a belt and adjusting the belt tightly enough around the chest or abdomen so that outward movement of the rib cage or abdomen stretched a mercury-filled, flexible column. An electric current was passed through the mercury and resistance measured. With elongation of the mercury column, the resistance varied and resulted in an analog output through a differential amplifier. Many advantages existed over impedance pneumography. Specificity was considerably improved since the measurement of effort involved movement of the chest and/or abdomen and fewer endogenous artifacts occurred. Sensitivity was still somewhat poor. Mercury strain gauges were also quite fragile and were easily damaged, requiring frequent replacement.

Plethysmography

Plethysmography has many advantages over other forms of measurement of respiratory effort. Plethysmography measures changes in volume and, therefore, chest and abdominal circumference changes reflecting volumetric variations during the respiratory cycle can be easily recorded. However, plethysmographic recording can be difficult on small infants, neonates, and premature newborns. Belts and halters must be appropriately sized and recordings may be affected by body movements and improper position. Plethysmography also uses summation potentials (adding chest and abdominal movements). Paradoxic efforts generally are considered to depict absence of airflow and upper-airway obstruction. However, because of the increased chest wall compliance of small infants and newborns, paradoxic respirations are common, even in the absence of an obstructed upper airway. Therefore, certain methodologic difficulties potentially exist when dependent upon plethysmography *alone* for monitoring respiratory effort.

Intercostal and Diaphragmatic EMG

Measurement of respiratory activity using surface EMG has many advantages over other forms of effort recording. Set up is relatively easy and displacement of electrodes from body movements is uncommon and minimal. In adults, intercostal EMG is often highly effective in identifying obstructive respiratory events since recruitment of accessory muscles of respiration with increasing obstruction can easily be recorded. In addition, the intercostal space is large enough to permit accurate placement of electrodes in order to obtain accurate and reproducible output. On smaller infants, however, the size of even the smallest recording electrodes may be too large to utilize in the intercostal space. The size of the electrode may be great enough to cover two ribs (and/or intercostal spaces) with minimal contact on accessory respiratory musculature. Inhibition of skeletal muscle tone during active sleep might also result in misleading graphic output and "central" events may be recorded even in the presence of respiratory muscle activity. Diaphragmatic EMG is exquisitely difficult to obtain from surface recording electrodes and may be significantly affected by interference by abdominal accessory muscle recruitment.

Pneumatic Transduction

Pneumatic transduction involves utilization of belts containing air-filled bladders similar to a blood pressure cuff. One chest and one abdominal belt are utilized. With inspiratory and expiratory efforts, movement of air within the bladder results in movement of a small diaphragm within the transducer, which is then converted into an electric current producing an analog output on a polygraph. Advantages include ease of application of the belts and limited expense. Disadvantages are many. Air leakage from the bladder is common. Sensitivity is limited. Belts are frequently displaced and limited sizes are available. Even the smallest belts often will not fit smaller premature infants. In addition, because of the presence of an air-filled bladder, re-inflation is required prior to each use. Deflation of the bladder often occurs during the course of a study and artifact is frequent if the patient moves and lays on the bladder.

Peizo Crystal Belts

Peizo electric crystal belts are generally smaller, readily adjustable for infants and children of all sizes. Soft Velcro is used. Some manufacturers provide belts that may be cut to size in order to fit even the smallest premature infant. The crystal emits an electric current when tension is placed on the belt and the amplified signal may be recorded on either an analog or digital output device. Sensitivity is excellent. Specificity is also good. Cardiogenic pulse artifact may be noted. Since the belts are quite thin (when compared to other methods of measurement of respiratory effort), proper positioning is rather simple. However, if the belts are not positioned appropriately or if displacement occurs, a poor signal can result.

Proper Placement of Respiratory Effort Belts

In obtaining an accurate effort recording, effort belt sensors must be properly placed in order to obtain the best signal. Belt tension must be to a degree that slippage or displacement is minimized, but not so tight that respiratory effort is impeded. Proper positioning of the chest belt should assure that the rib cage is surrounded at the level of the nipple line. It should fit comfortably under the axillae. Protrusions and connection fittings should be appropriately placed off the midline and away from the sternum and other bony prominences so that with movements, the sensors are minimally intrusive or disruptive to the continuity of sleep. The abdominal belt should be positioned at the level of the umbilicus, or at the point of maximal expansion of the abdomen with respiratory movements. Observations of direction of movement of the chest and abdomen during inspiration and expiration should be recorded on the tracing and polarity adjusted so that when chest and abdominal movements are in the same direction during the respiratory cycle, graphic output will be in-phase on both recording channels. Documentation of concordance of chest and abdominal motion during calibration will assist in identifying respiratory efforts which are paradoxic (i.e., chest and abdominal movements are 180° out of phase). Although paradoxic breathing is normal during active/REM sleep, continuous and periodic alteration in the phase angle of abdominal and chest effort during the respiratory cycle might suggest the presence of high airway resistance, respiratory distress, or periodic upper-airway obstruction.

Measurement of Nasal and Oral Airflow

Several methods of measuring airflow at the nose and mouth are available. Each is fairly reliable and have certain advantages and disadvantages. Airflow measurement is generally accomplished by interposing a sensing device within the airstream from the nose and mouth. Newborn infants are generally obligate nasal breathers (61), however oral breathing has been shown to occur and accurate assessment of airflow also requires measurement at both locations. Unfortunately, the majority of techniques for measuring airflow have significant drawbacks. Utilization of masks which cover both the nose and mouth to accurately measure end-tidal CO_2 require a tight seal. Significant pressure is placed on the face, especially in the region of the mandibular and maxillary division of the fifth cranial nerve. Afferent impulses from this region caused by airflow has been shown to induce apnea in the newborn (62,63). It is unclear whether respiration during sleep may be affected by a tight fitting mask. In addition, sensory afferents from the pressure of the mask has the potential to disrupt the continuity of sleep and the sleep-wake cycle, again limiting the effectiveness of this technique. All other methods involve interposing small sensors into the airstream from the nose and mouth. These methods appear to be significantly less intrusive than the face mask and involve measuring temperature changes at the nose and mouth or assessing expired carbon dioxide (capnography). However, most sensors have been designed to measure airflow in the adult patient and sensors for children have been merely smaller versions of the adult design. This often creates placement difficulties. Infants, neonates, and children have different anatomic relationships from the adult and require sensing devices created and designed specifically for their anatomy.

Thermocouples

Measurement of the airflow at the nose and mouth may be accomplished using a thermocouple. This involves pairing of wires of different metallic composition that conduct heat at different rates. When the thermocouple is interposed into the airstream from the nose and/or the mouth, the temperature difference between inspired and expired air results in a change in conductance. This change is amplified and recorded on an oscillograph. The major advantage of using a thermocouple is that the technique is relatively inexpensive. However, sensitivity is not very high and responsiveness is relatively slow. Even with minor displacement of the thermocouple, artifact and poor signal occur.

Thermistry

Thermistry measures airflow at the nose and mouth in a manner similar to a thermocouple. However, it differs in that actual temperature change is measured by the sensor and transformed into an electric signal that may be recorded on an oscillograph or by digital equipment. Generally, thermistors require a cable containing a battery. Therefore, thermistry is somewhat more expensive because of the need for occasional cable replacement (more frequent than thermocouple cable). Thermistry, however, appears to be more sensitive. Specificity appears to be similar. Disadvantages are similar. Thermistors are easily displaced from the airstream. They have also been designed for adults. Neonatal and pediatric probes are merely smaller versions of the adult sensors, often making accurate placement difficult. Because of the different anatomic structure of the mid-face of an infant and child compared to an adult, the adult probe may not fit appropriately and provides a poor quality signal. Several disposable thermistors are commercially available and may be "cut-to-fit." These thermistors have the advantage of better placement of the probe in the airstream, but cutting the firm plastic has the potential to leave sharp edges, increasing the risk of irritation to the youngster's face. In addition, signal quality seems poorer and validation of signal sensitivity and specificity studies have not been conducted in children.

Capnography

Capnography measures changes in carbon dioxide at the nose and mouth. It is a very close estimate of the end-tidal CO_2, however, it is not a completely true measurement since there is some mixing of expired CO_2 with room air because a tight fitting mask is not used. The probe is similar to some thermistor probes, however it consists of prong-like tubes placed into the anterior nares. A third tube extends from the nasal tubing and is interposed into the oral airstream. The capnograph is calibrated using known concentrations of CO_2 prior to the study. Sensitivity and specificity are excellent for measurement of expired CO_2. Additional advantages include the ability to obtain quantifiable values for expired carbon dioxide. This may assist in identifying increasing levels of expired CO_2 associated with upper-airway obstruction during sleep, especially when there is limited or minimal changes in nasal/oral airflow. Several disadvantages do exist. CO_2 probes, like other devices, are smaller versions of those designed for adults. Nasal prong width is fixed and may not fit smaller infants or those with mid-face malformations. In addition, easy displacement of the prongs often results from body and head movements causing poor signal quality and/or artifact. In addition, tubing frequently becomes clogged, limiting signal quality and requiring a significant amount of technician time for maintenance during the course of nocturnal polysomnography. Finally, capnography measures CO_2 concentration, not flow. It estimates flow indirectly. Therefore, significant mixing with room air can result in poor signal quality.

Most laboratories utilize one technique for measurement of airflow. Nasal and oral flow may be coupled and linked on a single channel. This provides an opportunity to easily visualize total decrease in airflow due to decreased effort or airway obstruction. However, in order to accurately determine airflow changes due to obstruction requires very careful calibration at the beginning of the study, and compulsive maintenance of probe patency. If sensor position at the mouth results in an airflow signal that appears reduced compared to flow through the nose, false-positive respiratory occlusive events might be recorded. The degree and severity of sleep-disordered breathing may be considerably over-estimated. Therefore, in younger children, children who will not (or cannot) understand patient calibration instructions, infants, and neonates, linking of nasal and oral airflow to a single channel can be done. This must be done very carefully or the signals should be split onto two separate recording channels.

Two channel recording of airflow (one nasal and one oral) has the major advantage of being able to determine whether flow is mainly through the nose and/or mouth. If nasal occlusion occurs and mouth breathing results, this can be easily identified by two-channel recording. Unfortunately, similar problems exist with calibration and hypopnea may be quite difficult to assess if the oral signal is low, despite adequate oral airflow.

Because of the technical disadvantages of thermistry and capnography, some laboratories utilize both techniques for assessment and monitoring of airflow. Measurement by both techniques increases the sensitivity of the procedure. On the one hand, cost is greater and more polygraph channels are required. On the other hand, one technique may provide backup for the other if technical difficulties are encountered. However, it is not uncommon to have technical problems with both airflow/capnography channels simultaneously requiring technician intervention to maintain interpretable signals.

Measurement of Oxygen Saturation

The most common and widely accepted method for measuring changes in oxygenation during sleep is *pulse oximetry*. This noninvasive technique involves spectrographic analysis of light transmitted through a digit or ear lobe (foot or hand in the case of small premature infants). Oxygenated hemoglobin absorbs light within a relatively narrow spectral range. When deoxygenated hemoglobin absorbs more/less of the transmitted light, this change in absorption can be converted into an analog or digital output signal. Advantages of pulse oximetry are many. Ease of application of the probe, lack of invasiveness of the procedure, relative high sensitivity and specificity, and low cost make it a desirable method of continuously measuring oxygen saturation.

Oximetry is a widely used, clinically accepted, noninvasive technique for assessing oxygen saturation despite limited normative data in the newborn and young child. Limited data are available regarding reliability of pulse oximetry in the newborn and less is known regarding the affect of altitude on normal oxygen saturation values. At 5,280 feet above sea level, mean oxygen saturation at 24 to 48 hours of age remains relatively stable at about 92% to 93%. This is affected little by the infant's activity. With increasing postconceptional age there is a tendency for oxygen saturation during awake states to increase from 93% to 94%, while oxygen saturation during sleep stays the same or even decreases slightly (64). The lower end of the reference range (2 standard deviations below the mean) can be as low as 85% during feeding at 24 to 48 hours and 86% during quiet sleep at 1 and 3 months of age, with 88% to 89% being the lower limit in other activities at all ages.

However, the degree of desaturation during sleep varies significantly and can depend upon the percent of hemoglobin F, hemoglobin A1, and other hemoglobin types (which are the principal determinants of P50), pH, temperature, as well as the type of oximeter utilized (65,66).

Measurement of oxygen saturation by pulse oximetry is distorted by movement artifact (65). Movement artifacts are common regardless of the instrument utilized and can be more significant with some pulse oximeters than others. In addition, different manufacturers' instruments will yield different values for the same infant (65,66). This is due to different algorithms used to calculate oxygen saturation. Visual display and the ability to record pulse signal simultaneously with the oximetry output will assist in identifying artifact associated with movement.

Location of probe placement should be easily accessible, permit adequate light transmission and be minimally intrusive to the study. Prematures and newborns typically require utilization of the foot and/or hand. Fingers and/or earlobes are too small. Older children and adolescents are best monitored by utilization of a finger probe or placement of the probe on a toe.

Transmission artifacts can be caused by hyperpigmented skin resulting in poor light transmission and a variety of chromophobic and chromophilic circulating compounds. Also, the degree of oxygen desaturation associated with changes in PaO_2 varies significantly with the position of the P50 (partial pressure of oxygen where 50% of hemoglobin is saturated). The position of the P50 is determined by the type of hemoglobin present, the level of 2,3-DPG, pH, and temperature.

Although a relatively benign procedure, pulse oximetry is not without potential complications. Broken probes and probes manufactured for different oximeters and interchanged can result in significant burn injuries. Serious burns have been reported when probes have been interchanged between equipment (67,68).

Degree of oxygenation can also be monitored in the sleep laboratory by other noninvasive techniques. Monitoring of *transcutaneous PO_2* (TcPO$_2$) was quite popular during the 1980s. This technique provided continuous monitoring of oxygen concentration (not saturation) in high risk neonates, infants, and young children requiring ventilator therapy. This methodology obviated the need for frequent, continuous blood drawing in order to assess the adequacy of ventilation. Premature neonates' blood volume is not great and often transfusion was required to replace blood that was required for blood gas analysis.

$TcPO_2$ monitoring provided the ability to continuously monitor oxygenation in these high risk infants without risking complications from blood withdrawal and transfusion. Unfortunately, in order to obtain a signal, the probe was required to significantly heat the underlying skin and subsequent burns limited $TcPO_2$ usefulness, especially when other noninvasive techniques could be utilized that did not carry the same burn risk. Because pulse oximetry does not required heating of the skin, complications are much less frequent and it has virtually replaced routine $TcPO_2$ monitoring. However, nocturnal (sleep-related) blood gas determination, blood gas determination upon waking, and diurnal blood gas assessments may be quite helpful in determining the presence of alveolar hypoventilation.

Measurement of *transcutaneous PCO_2* ($TcPCO_2$) to assess ventilation has been associated with fewer complications than measurement of $TcPO_2$ and can be utilized in management of ventilator-dependent youngsters. Utilization in the sleep laboratory has been limited since $EtCO_2$ by capnography provides breath-to-breath assessment of exhaled CO_2 yielding more information regarding upper-airway obstruction and airflow, and can provide some information regarding adequacy of ventilation. It is also less affected by circulation time. Assessment of congenital central hypoventilation syndrome, however, and assessment of sleep-related disorders on chronic ventilator patients may provide for greater utilization of this technique.

Monitoring intrathoracic pressure typically requires insertion of an indwelling esophageal catheter connected to a manometer. This technique is rather invasive, however, it provides a number of significant advantages in assessing ventilatory function during the respiratory cycle in children. Often, significant airway obstruction is present without significant changes in airflow. Increased respiratory effort results in increased negative intrathoracic pressure and arousal prior to a point where frank apnea occurs. This has been termed the upper-airway resistance syndrome (UARS) (69). UARS may be more prevalent than overt obstructive sleep apnea syndrome in children. The only clear mechanism to make an accurate diagnosis is by utilization of this indwelling esophageal balloon. Intrathoracic pressure changes can be accurately measured and recorded. Several major limitations exist. Esophageal manometry requires a moderately invasive procedure. Although polysomnography carries almost no risk, esophageal manometry is a relatively simple and safe procedure, it adds considerably to potential risks and complications. Often, parents are hesitant to permit invasive procedures to be performed. Children may be hesitant to permit placement of the catheter. Finally, and perhaps equally important to parent and patient discomfort, placement of a catheter into the esophagus results in the artificial creation of a pharyngeal foreign body. Pharyngeal visceral afferent activity might result and cause artificial active and or passive splinting of the airway. False-positive and/or false-negative studies might result rendering data questionable. Other noninvasive techniques have been developed to preclude the use of an indwelling esophageal catheter. When increased negative intrathoracic pressure occurs during the respiratory cycle, the suprasternal notch retracts. Noninvasive sensors have been developed to detect and record this retraction and provide qualitative data which approximates quantitative intrathoracic pressure measurements. Further validation study is necessary, but preliminary data are quite encouraging.

Audio and video monitoring are quite helpful in assessing respiratory variables during sleep (as well as movement and seizure disorders). Documenting snoring, increased respiratory effort, movement arousals, environmental influences (e.g., parents snoring), and expiratory glottic stridor can greatly assist in interpretation of the polysomnogram.

REFERENCES

1. Eichenwald EC, Stark AR. Respiratory motor output: effect of state and maturation in early life. In: Haddad GG, Farber JP, eds. *Developmental Neurobiology of Breathing.* New York: Marcel Dekker; 1991: 551–587.
2. Dawes GS, Fox HE, Ledue BM, Liggins GC, Richards RT. Respiratory movements and rapid eye movement sleep in the foetal lamb. *J Physiol* 1972;220:119–143.
3. Boddy K, Robinson JS. External method for detection of fetal breathing in utero. *Lancet* 1971;2:1123–1233.
4. Alcorn D, Adamson TM, Malone JE, Robinson PM. Morphologic effects of chronic bilateral phrenectomy or vagotomy in fetal lamb lung. *J Anat* 1980;130:683–695.
5. Goldstein JD, Reid LM. pulmonary hypoplasia resulting from phrenic nerve agenesis and diaphragmatic amyoplasia. *J Pediatr* 1980;97:282–287.
6. Jansen AH, Chernick V. Fetal breathing and development of control of breathing. *J Appl Physiol* 1991; 70:1431–1436.
7. Kitterman JA, Liggins GC, Clements JA, Tooley WH. Stimulation of breathing movements in fetal sheep by inhibitors of prostaglandin synthesis. *J Dev Physiol* 1979;1:453–466.
8. Wallen LD, Murai DT, Clyman RI, Lee CH, Mauray FE, Kitterman JA. Regularion of breathing movements in fetal sleep by prostaglandin E2. *J Appl Physiol* 1986;60:526–531.
9. Timor-Tritsch IE, Dierker LJ Jr, Hertz RH, Chik L, Rosen MG. Regular and irregular human fetal respiratory movement. *Early Hum Dev* 1980;4:315–324.
10. Jouvet M. Neurophysiology of the states of sleep. *Physiol Rev* 1967;47:117–177.
11. Kubota K, Iwamura Y, Niimi Y. Monosynaptic reflex and natural sleep in the cat. *J Neurophysiol* 1965; 28:125–138.
12. Lopes J, Muller NL, Bryan MH, Bryan AC. Importance of inspiratory muscle tone in maintenance of FRC in the newborn. *J Appl Physiol* 1981;51:830–834.
13. Moriette G, Chaussain M, Radvanyi-Bouvet MF, Walti H, Pajot N, Relier JP. Functional residual capacity and sleep states in the premature newborn. *Biol Neonate* 1983;43:125–133.
14. Heldt GP. Development of stability of the respiratory system in preterm infants. *J Appl Physiol* 1988;65: 441–444.
15. Prechtl HFR, Van Eykern LA, O'Brien MJ. Respiratory muscle EMG in newborns: a non-intrusive method. *Early Hum Dev* 1977;1:265–283.
16. Thach BT, Abroms IF, Frantz ID III, Sotrel A, Bruce EN, Goldman MD. Intercostal muscle reflexes and sleep breathing patterns in the human infant. *J Appl Physiol* 1980;48:139–146.
17. Hershenson MB, Colin AA, Wohl MEB, Stark AR. Changes in the contribution of the rib cage to tidal breathing during infancy. *Am Rev Respir Dis* 1990;141:922–925.
18. Henderson-Smart DJ, Read JD. Reduced lung volume during behavioral active sleep in the newborn. *J Appl Physiol* 1979;46:1081–1085.
19. Beardsmore CS, MacFadyen UM, Moosavi SS, Wimpress SP, Thompson J, Simpson H. Measurement of lung volumes during active and quiet sleep in infants. *Pediatr Pulmonol* 1989;7:71–77.
20. Stokes GM, Milner AD, Newball EA, Smith NJ, Dunn C, Wilson AJ. Do lung volumes change with sleep state in the neonate? *Eur J Pediatr* 1989;148:360–364.
21. Bartlett D, Remmers JE, Gautier H. Laryngeal regulation of respiratory airflow. *Respir Physiol* 1973;18: 194–204.
22. Quiring DP, Warfel JH. *The Head, Neck, and Trunk: Muscles and Motor Points.* Philadelphia: Lea & Febiger; 1967.
23. Mortola JP, Fisher JT. Upper airway reflexes in newborns. In: Mathew OP, Ambrogio GS, eds. *Respiratory Function of the Upper Airway.* New York: Marcel Dekker; 1988:303–357.
24. Gaultier CL. Clinical and therapeutic aspects of obstructive sleep apnea syndrome in infants and children. *Sleep* 1992;15:s36–s38.
25. Sheldon SH. Diagnosis and management of upper-airway resistance syndrome in children. *RT* 1994;7: 59–64.
26. Sheldon SH, Önal E, Lilie J, Spire JP. Sleep-related post-inspiratory upper-airway obstruction in children. *Sleep Res* 1993;22:270.
27. Schulman D, Bar-Yishay E, Godfrey S. Drive and timing components of respiration in young children following induction of anaesthesia with halothane and ketamine. *Can J Anaesth* 1988;35:368–374.
28. Foutz AS, Champagna J, Denavit-Saubie M. N-methyl-D-aspartate (NMDA) receptors control respiratory off-switch in cat. *Neurosci Lett* 1988;87:221–226.
29. Mathew OP, Remmers JE. Respiratory function of the upper airway. In: Saunders NA, Sullivan CE, eds. *Sleep and Breathing.* New York: Marcel Dekker; 1984:163–200.
30. Bartlett D Jr. Effects of hypercapnia and hypoxia on laryngeal resistance to airflow. *Respir Physiol* 1979; 37:293–302.
31. Quiring DP, Warfel JH. *The Head, Neck, and Trunk: Muscles and Motor Points.* Philadelphia: Lea & Febiger; 1967:128.

32. Remmers JE, Bartlett D Jr. Reflex control of expiratory airflow and duration. *J Appl Physiol* 1977;42: 80–87.
33. Griffiths GB, Noworaj A, Mortola JP. End-expiratory level and breathing pattern in the newborn. *J Appl Physiol* 1983;55:243–249.
34. Richter DW, Ballantyne D, Remmers JE. The differential organization of medullary post inspiratory activities. *Pflugers Arch* 1987;410:420–427.
35. Phillipson AE. Regulation of breathing during sleep. *Am Rev Respir Dis* 1977;115(Suppl):217.
36. Johnson P. Prolonged expiratory apnoea and implications for control of breathing. *Lancet* 1985;2: 877–880.
37. Johnson P. Comparative aspects on the control of breathing during development. In: von Euler C, Lagerkrantz H, eds. *Central Nervous Control Mechanisms in Regular, Periodic, and Irregular Breathing.* Oxford: Pergamon Press; 1979:337–350.
38. St. John WM, Bianchi AL. Comparison of activities of medullary respiratory neurons in eupnea and apneusis. *Respir Physiol* 1983;51:361–377.
39. Southall DP, Talbert DG, Johnson P, Morley CJ, Salmons S, Miller J, Helms PJ. Prolonged expiratory apnoea: a disorder resulting in episodes of severe arterial hypoxaemia in infants and young children. *Lancet* 1985;2:571–577.
40. Ruggins NR, Milner AD. Site of upper airway obstruction in infants following an acute life-threatening event. *Pediatrics* 1993;91:595–601.
41. Ikari T, Sasaki CT. Glottic closure reflex: control mechanisms. *Ann Otol Rhinol Laryngol* 1980;89: 220–224.
42. Mifflin SW. Arterial chemoreceptor input to respiratory hypoglossal motoneurons. *J Appl Physiol* 1990; 69:700–709.
43. Cibella F, Marrone O, Sanci S, Bellia V, Bonsignore G. Expiratory timing in obstructive sleep apneas. *Eur Respir J* 1990;3:293–298.
44. England SJ, Kent G, Stogryn HA. Laryngeal muscle and diaphragmatic activities in conscious dog pups. *Respir Physiol* 1985;60:95–108.
45. Stephenson JBP. Prolonged expiratory apnea in children [Letter]. *Lancet* 1985;2:953.
46. Orr WC, Cohen DE. *The Nose at Night.* Chanhassen, MN: CNS; 1993.
47. Carlo WA, Martin RJ, Bruce EN, Strohol KP, Fanaroff AA. Alae nasi activation (nasal flaring) decreases nasal resistance in preterm infants. *Pediatrics* 1983;72:338–343.
48. Tanaka Y, Honda Y. Nasal obstruction as a cause of reduced PCO_2 and disordered breathing during sleep. *J Appl Physiol* 1989;67:970–972.
49. NcNicholas WT, Coffey M, Boyle T. Effects of nasal airflow on breathing during sleep in normal humans. *Am Rev Respir Dis* 1993;147:620–623.
50. Bosma J, Lind J. Upper respiratory mechanisms of newborn infants. A clinical essay.*Acta Paediatr Suppl* 1962;135:32–44.
51. Hudgel DW, Hendricks C. Palate and hypopharynx: sites of inspiratory narrowing of the upper airway during sleep. *Am Rev Respir Dis* 1988;138.1542–1547.
52. Knill R, Andrews W, Bryan AC, Bryan MH. Respiratory load compensation in infants. *J Appl Physiol* 1976;40:357–361.
53. Curzi-Dascalova L, Gaudebout C, Dreyfus-Brisac C. Respiratory frequencies of sleeping infants during the first months of life: correlations between values in different sleep states. *Early Hum Dev* 1981;5: 39–54.
54. Rusconi F, Castagneto M, Gagliardi L, et al. Reference values for respiratory rate in the first 3 years of life. *Pediatrics* 1994;94:350–355.
55. Sheldon SH, Spire JP, Levy HB. *Pediatric Sleep Medicine.* Philadelphia: WB Saunders; 1992.
56. National Institutes of Health Consensus Development Conference: Infantile apnea and home monitoring. Bethesda, MD: US Department of Health and Human Services, Oct 1, 1987, NIH Pub. No. 87-2905.
57. Longobardo GS, Cherniack NS, Gothe B. Factors affecting respiratory system stability. *Ann Biomed Eng* 1989;17:377–396.
58. Guilleminault C. *Sleep and Its Disorders in Children.* New York: Raven Press; 1987:195–211.
59. Brouillette RT, Ferbach SK, Hunt CE. Obstructive sleep apnea in infants and children. *J Pediatr* 1982; 100:31–40.
60. Miller MJ, Martin RJ, Carlo WA. Diagnostic methods and clinical disorders in children. In: Edelman NH, Santiago TV, eds. *Breathing Disorders During Sleep.* New York: Churchill Livingstone; 1986: 157–180.
61. Nelson WE, Vaughn VC, McKay RJ, eds. *Textbook of Pediatrics.* Philadelphia: WB Saunders; 1987:868.
62. Abu-Osba YK, Mathew OP, Thach BT. An animal model for airway sensory deprivation producing obstructive apnea with postmortem findings of sudden infant death syndrome. *Pediatrics* 1981;68: 796–801.
63. Haddad GG. Control of breathing in children. In: Edelman NH, Santiago TV, eds. *Breathing Disorders During Sleep.* New York: Churchill Livingstone; 1986:57–80.
64. Thilo EH, Park-Moore B, Herman ER, Carson BS. Oxygen saturation by pulse oximetry in healthy infants at an altitude of 1610 m (5280 ft). What is normal? *Am J Dis Child* 1991;145:1137–1140.

65. Poets CF, Southall DP. Noninvasive monitoring of oxygenation in infants and children: practical considerations and areas of concern. *Pediatrics* 1994;93:737–746.
66. Levene S, Lear GH, McKenzie SA. Comparison of pulse oximeters in healthy sleeping infants. *Respir Med* 1989;83:233–235.
67. Murphy KG, Secunda JA, Rockoff MA. Severe burns from a pulse oximeter. *Anesthesiology* 1990;73: 350–352.
68. Sobel DB. Burning of a neonate due to a pulse oximeter: arterial saturation monitoring. *Pediatrics* 1992; 89:154–155.
69. Guilleminault C, Winkle R, Korobkin R, Simmons B. Children and nocturnal snoring: evaluation of the effects of sleep related respiratory resistive load and day-time functioning. *Eur J Pediatr* 1982;139: 165–171.

4

Polysomnographic Development
of the EKG

This chapter focuses on the development of cardiac function and specific changes that occur during fetal and neonatal development. Focus is principally on cardiac function and dynamics during ontogenetic development of sleep and the effect of sleep and state on cardiac function. Generation of the EKG and identification and significance of typical arrhythmias/dysrhythmia seen during polysomnography will be covered. Continuous cardiac monitoring, home monitoring of cardiac function, and polysomnographic evaluation of continuous cardiac function during sleep will be presented.

EMBRYOLOGIC CONSIDERATIONS

Little is known of the physiologic development of the heart in humans. Direct observational and experimental data have been almost impossible to collect. Therefore most of what is known about the development and ontogeny of the heart beat and electric activity of the developing heart has been extrapolated from experimental data on chick embryos (1). Studies suggest that the human heart begins to beat at about 22 weeks gestation (2,3). At this point in development, the heart is a tubular organ and consists of only a conus and part of the unpaired ventricles. The caudal-most differentiated tissue in the tubular heart is in the middle of the future ventricular region. As the tube elongates by addition of pre-cardiac mesoderm at the caudal end, it undergoes its characteristic curvature and the pacemaker zone moves progressively to the caudal-most portion. Pacemaker activity begins at a primitive stage in cardiac development, before atrial or nodal sinoatrial tissue differentiates (1). The heart increases more than 1,000-fold in size during fetal development while the time required for propagation of excitation remains relatively constant. Spread of impulses matches the increasing size of the early heart because the conduction velocity increases pace in the ventricle.

During fetal development the cardiac rate-setting mechanism is complex. Intrinsic rate of any part of the heart at any fetal age depends upon the surface density and activities of a variety of ion channels and pumps, each of which is synthesized and inserted into the heart cell membrane over a period of hours or days during development. Throughout embryo/fetogenesis, the various parts of the heart show a gradient of intrinsic beat rate, with rostral tissue (conus) beating slowly and more posterior regions each having a progressively faster rate. At all stages of development, the caudal-most tissue acts as pacemaker for the rest of the heart.

When the heart starts to beat, the action potential for cardiac tissue is different than it is in the adult. It undergoes significant changes in size, shape, and pharmacology as the heart differentiates. Changes suggest progressive alteration in underlying action currents (4). Many of the conditions and properties of the embryonic action potential resemble those seen in the ischemic adult heart (1).

DEVELOPMENT OF CARDIAC FUNCTION

The anatomy and function of the fetal cardiovascular system differ profoundly from that of extrauterine life. Although right and left heart function is parallel during fetal life, immediately after birth the right side and left side are required to function in series. Significant anatomic and physiologic changes in the respiratory and cardiac systems occur immediately at the time of birth. Alveolar fluid within the lung is expressed and absorbed, being replaced immediately with air. Pressure changes and oxygenation result in closure of the ductus arteriosus and ventricular and atrial septal communicating channels, isolating the pulmonary and systemic circulation.

Heart rate generally decreases during natural sleep. In general, heart rate is about 4 to 8 beats per minute slower when heart rate during quiet wake (QW) is compared to quiet sleep (QS) (5). During tonic periods of REM sleep, a decrease in rate of approximately 8% less than QW has been reported. Reduction in heart rate during sleep appears to parallel sleep-related alterations in blood pressure (6). In addition, heart rate variability is clearly greater in REM sleep than in slow-wave sleep (7). Although there is a significant decrease in heart rate during tonic periods of REM sleep, heart rate is also significantly influenced by phasic activity during REM sleep (8). During phasic activity of REM sleep, there are clear episodes of short-lasting tachycardia, followed occasionally by a rebound brief bradycardia before return to baseline levels. Variations in heart rate differ significantly according to sleep state. Before 37 weeks of gestational age, the sequential curves of heart rate show periodic variations present in both active and quiet sleep (9). After 37 weeks, slow periodic variations are still present in active sleep, but superimposed by fast variations synchronous to respiratory cycles. Fast variations prevail in quiet sleep. In newborns suffering from pathologic conditions (medical or surgical), smaller variability associated with respiration is seen with prematurity, young age at recording, and hypercapnia. But, this diminished respiratory-related heart rate variation can be very transient. Pronounced variations similar to those in babies without abnormalities are observed in two thirds of the patients with or without ventilatory assistance (9). Baust and Gagel described the development of periodicity of heart rate and respiration during sleep in newborn babies (10). The period durations obtained by power spectral analysis showed two maxima. In many cases cycles of respiration and heart rate were not identical. Their experiments showed that newborns have two separate cycles with different period durations. Most probably the shorter cycle originates from fetal life, the longer one represents the development of a more mature periodicity. In studying respiration and heart rate variation in normal infants during quiet sleep over the first year of life, Litscher and colleagues showed that the respiratory rate during quiet sleep decreases and the respiratory variability decreases with age (Table 1) (11). A comparison of the cardiorespiratory data from the first and last quiet-sleep period showed no significant differences within any of the age groups studied.

Heart rate in siblings of SIDS victims was higher than in normal infants during quiet sleep over the first 6 months of life and was higher than normal in the waking state at 3

TABLE 4-1. *Cardiorespiratory variations in infants during the first year of life*

	RR[a]	CV[b]	HR[c]	HRv[d]
6 weeks	37.2 ± 5.4	2.3 ± 0.7	127.4 ± 11.5	3.8 ± 1.5
6 months	30.1 ± 4.9	3.2 ± 1.1	119.4 ± 17.3	4.2 ± 1.7
1 year	24.1 ± 1.8	3.4 ± 1.0	110.3 ± 21.5	5.8 ± 2.3
Adult	14.8 ± 1.8	4.5 ± 1.0	59.2 ± 8.5	4.3 ± 2.2

[a] Respiratory rate (breaths per minute).
[b] Coefficient of respiratory rate variation (increasing coefficient indicates decreasing variation).
[c] Heart rate (beats per minute).
[d] Heart rate variation expressed at percent (%).
Modified from: Litscher G, Pfurtscheller G, Bes F, Poiseau E. Respiration and heart rate variation in normal infants during quiet sleep in the first year of life. *Klin Padiatr* 1993;205:170–175.

months of age (12). The siblings of SIDS victims also have lower variability in heart rate at one week of age during quiet sleep.

Van Geijn and colleagues studied heart rate as an indicator of states in newborn infants (13). During quiet sleep, the R-R interval length was longer, the long-term irregularity index lower, and the interval difference index higher than in the immediately preceding or following active sleep. For non-consecutive quiet and active sleep states, a maximum separation was obtained and with discriminant function analysis correctly classified in 93% of quiet- and active-sleep epochs. These data have specific implications for identification of state in the fetus without the need for antepartum invasive monitoring.

Heart rate and its variability, however, can be affected by certain medications. In one study by Gabriel and Albani, it was demonstrated that the amount of active sleep, as well as the incidence of apnea and/or cardiac slowing occurring predominantly during active sleep, were decreased at therapeutic levels of phenobarbital (14). With declining serum drug levels, active sleep showed a rebound effect; at the same time, apnea and/or cardiac slowing relapsed. These findings tend to confirm that neonatal apnea is facilitated by active sleep-inhibitory brain mechanisms and these mechanisms have significant effects not only on the respiratory system, but on the cardiovascular system as well.

Beat-to-beat variability of heart rate has been used as an index of integrity of the autonomic nervous system in early infancy (15). Mazza and coworkers have shown that the beat-to-beat heart rate variability during active sleep and quiet sleep correlated very well with the instantaneous heart rate (R-R interval). The correlation coefficient range was 0.49 to 0.92 in quiet sleep and 0.50 to 0.03 in active sleep. Regression analysis supported a linear approximation of the beat-to-beat heart rate variability to the instantaneous heart rate over the instantaneous heart rate range investigated. The slopes of these linear functions were similar in both active sleep and quiet sleep in infants from birth to 4 months of age (15).

Assessment of vagal tone may be a significant method of assessing the periodic variation of heart rate associated with respiration (respiratory sinus arrhythmia). Arendt and colleagues, studied vagal tone in 20 full-term infants and found that heart period and heart period variability were highly correlated with vagal tone (16). Variation in vagal tone between states was also detected. Repeated assessments revealed that average vagal tone values collected in the same state were not significantly correlated across successive days. This short-term variability both between and within individuals does not support the notion that a single assessment of vagal tone can, by itself, be used to identify infants at risk for sudden unexpected death during sleep or predict neuro-developmental outcome. Successive assessments, however, might provide a greater degree of information.

In older infants and children, heart rate reveals significant respiratory modulation. This is termed a normal sinus arrhythmia (Fig. 1). In newborn infants, however, respiratory modulation of heart rate is variable. Hathorn, using spectral analysis on ventilation and instantaneous heart rate has shown that during quiet sleep, the relative magnitudes of the high-frequency and lower-frequency peaks for heart rate depend on the respiratory rate and the variability of the T_{tot} (Fig. 1) (17).

During active sleep, most of the power in the heart rate spectrum was concentrated in the low-frequency range. Weighted coherence between ventilation and heart rate was higher during quiet sleep than active sleep, but in the high-frequency and low-frequency spectra. Low-frequency power was higher during active than quiet sleep in both ventilation and heart rate. The results suggest that the pattern of breathing has a marked effect on the shape of the heart rate spectrum. In most infants, however, there is no fixed phase relationship between oscillations in ventilation and the heart rate, at high or low frequencies. These oscillations are affected by sleep state and hence, by implication, by central nervous system rhythm generators.

Particular types of heart rate variation are enhanced during periods of slow heart rate and diminished when heart rate is high. Shechtman and Harper have shown that the maturational patterns of heart rate by heart rate variation correlation were strongly influenced by sleep-waking state and were dissimilar to those previously reported for correlations between cardiac and respiratory measures (18). Their findings suggested dissimilar developmental patterns for autonomic and somatic motor systems, and include a discontinuity in autonomic development at approximately 1 month of age. They speculated that these trends reflected a change in the nature of sleep states as forebrain connections develop.

State-dependent variations also occur over the first year of life. Litscher and colleagues performed spectral analysis of breathing and heart rate patterns during the first and last episode of quiet sleep recorded over an 8-hour all-night period on 19 infants at 6 weeks, 6 months, and 1 year of age. A total of 43 recordings were analyzed. Their results demonstrated that the respiratory rate decreased during quiet sleep and the respiratory variability decreases with age. Calculations of heart rate in beats-per-minute and heart rate variability (%) revealed a slowing of the heart rate and an increase in the variability (Table 1). A comparison of the cardiorespiratory data from the first and last quiet-sleep period showed no significant differences within either age group.

When Haddad and coworkers studied the state dependence of the QT interval in normal infants at 2 weeks, 1 month, 2 months, 3 months, and 4 months of life, they found that the QT index (defined as QT interval/square root of the RR interval) was significantly greater during quiet sleep than during REM sleep. This significant difference was present at all age groups studied (19).

Cardiac output is also coupled to heart rate during wakefulness. During sleep, however, cardiac output is only slightly decreased during slow-wave sleep (5,20). Decrease in cardiac output is more significantly pronounced during the tonic REM state, its average being about 9% less than during QW. Changes in cardiac output are not accompanied by changes in stroke volume, which tends to remain constant during QW, slow-wave sleep, and REM sleep.

Blood pressure also varies significantly between QW and sleep. There is a relatively modest decrease in blood pressure during NREM sleep (approximately 14 mmHg) (7). It decreases to an even greater extent during tonic REM sleep. Blood pressure variation during REM sleep is complex and notable. Periods of relative hypotension are interrupt-

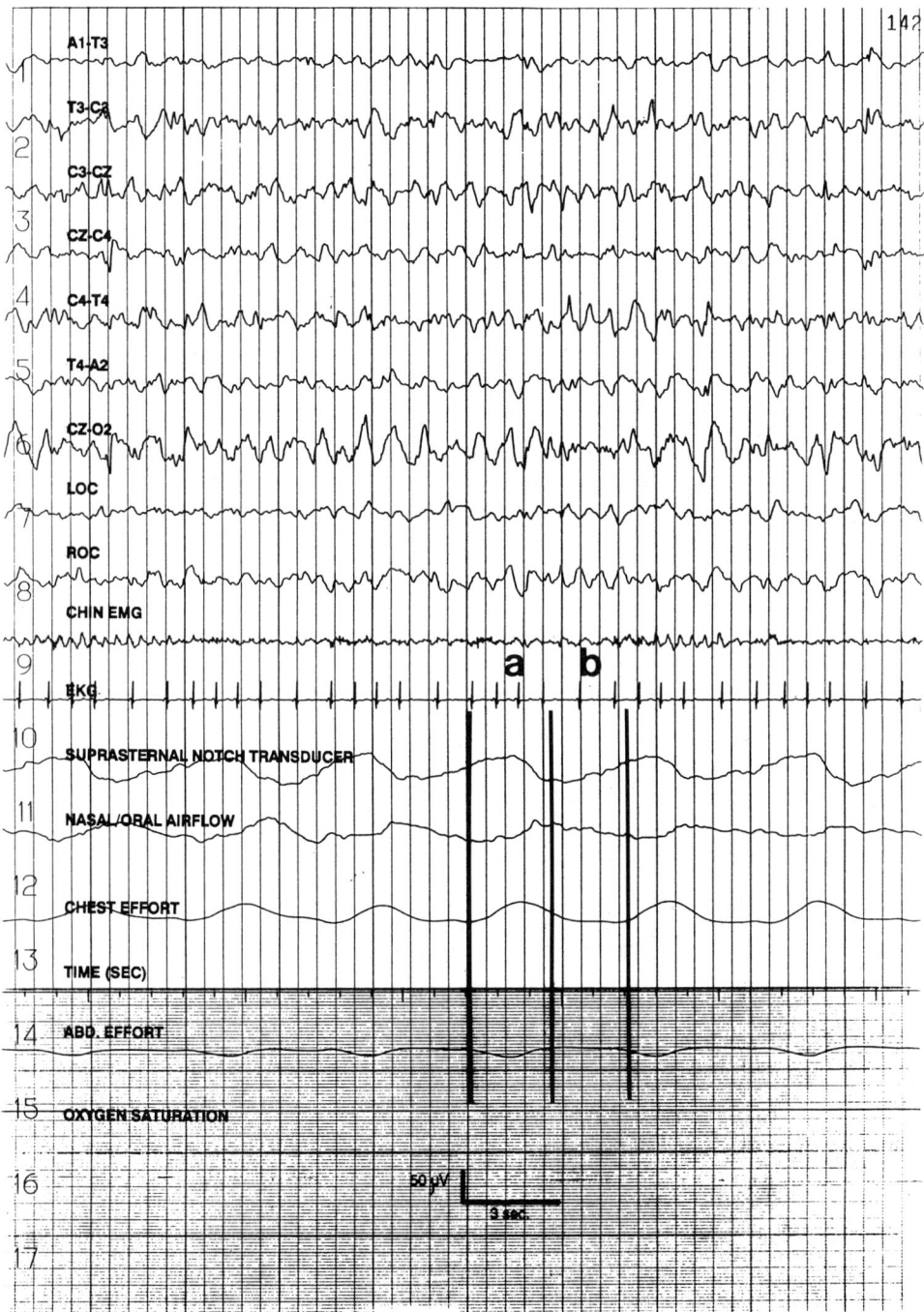

FIG. 4-1. Sinus arrhythmia. Note variation in R-R intervals of the EKG tracing. **a:** R-R interval is decreased with inspiration (instantaneous heart rate increases); **b:** R-R interval is increased with expiration (instantaneous heart rate decreases).

ed by brief sharp increases in mean arterial pressure (8). Oscillations in blood pressure appear to be related to phasic phenomena of REM sleep. Blood pressure increases appear to occur shortly before or shortly after the onset of bursts of phasic activity (eye movements or phasic muscle twitches) (8).

Abnormalities and intercurrent medical conditions can affect the variability and state dependence of heart rate, and contribute to arrhythmias. Fagioli and colleagues have shown that there is a high frequency of sinus pauses in malnourished infants (21). This arrhythmia was mainly identified during quiet sleep. After nutritional rehabilitation of the infants studied, there was a dramatic reduction in the frequency of these sinus pauses. They concluded that the large number of sinus pauses seen in infants suffering from severe malnutrition may reflect a disturbance of neuro-vegetative regulation that is intensified by sleep-related physiologic changes.

Cardiac and other cardiovascular variations during sleep in newborns, infants, and children are complex and appear to hold particular and consequential clinical relevance. Phasic excitation of the heart and vascular changes in the coronary, systemic, and cerebral circulations may profoundly influence the course of other medical conditions in the fragile child.

REFERENCES

1. DeHaan RL. The embryonic origin of the heartbeat. In: Hurst JW, Schlant RC, eds. *The Heart.* New York: McGraw-Hill; 1990:72–77.
2. Davis CL. Development of the human heart from its first appearance to the stage found in embryos of 20 paired somites. *Carnegie Inst Contr Embryol* 1927;19:245.
3. DeHaan RL, O'Rahilly RO. Embryology of the heart. In: Hurst JW, et al., eds. *The Heart*, 4th ed. New York: McGraw-Hill; 1978:6.
4. DeHaan RL. Differentiation of excitable membranes. *Curr Topics Dev Biol* 1980;16:117.
5. Mancia G, Baccelli G, Adams DB, Zanchetti A.. Vasomotor regulation during sleep in the cat. *Am J Physiol* 1971;220:1086–1093.
6. Sheldon SH, Spire JP, Levy HB. *Pediatric Sleep Medicine.* Philadelphia: WB Saunders; 1992:46–57.
7. Guazzi M, Zanchetti A. Blood pressure and heart rate during natural sleep of the cat and their regulation by carotid sinus and aortic reflexes. *Arch Ital Biol* 1965;103:789–817.
8. Gassel MM, Ghelarducci B, Marchiafava PL, et al. Phasic changes in blood pressure and heart rate during rapid eye movement episodes of desynchronized sleep in unrestrained cats. *Arch Ital Biol* 1964;102: 530–544.
9. Radvanyi MF, Morel-Kahn F. Sleep and heart rate variations in premature and full term babies. *Neuropadiatrie* 1976;7:302–312.
10. Baust W, Gagel J. The development of periodicity of heart rate and respiration in newborn babies. *Neuropadiatrie* 1977;8:387–396.
11. Litscher G, Pfurtscheller G, Bes F, Poiseau E. Respiration and heart rate variation in normal infants during quiet sleep in the first year of life. *Klin Padiatrie* 193;205:170–175.
12. Harper RM, Leake B, Hodgman JE, Hoppenbrouwers T. Developmental patterns of heart rate and heart rate variability during sleep and waking in normal infants and infants at risk for sudden infant death syndrome. *Sleep* 1982;5:28–38.
13. Van Geijn HP, Jongsma HW, deHaan J, Eskes TK, Prechtl HF. Heart rate as an indicator of the behavioral state. Studies in the newborn infant and prospects for fetal heart rate monitors.*Am J Obstet Gynecol* 1980;136:1061–1066.
14. Gabriel M, Albani M. Rapid eye movement sleep, apnea, and cardiac slowing influenced by phenobarbital administration in the neonate. *Pediatrics* 1977;60:426–430.
15. Mazza NM, Epstein MA, Haddad GG, Law HS, Mellins RB, Epstein RA. Relation of beat-to-beat variability to heart rate in normal sleeping infants. *Pediatr Res* 1980;14:232–235.
16. Arendt RE, Halpern LF, MacLean WE Jr, Youngquist GA. The properties of V in newborns across repeated measures. *Dev Psychobiol* 1991;24:91–101.
17. Hathorn MK. Respiratory modulation of heart rate in newborn infants. *Early Hum Dev* 1989;20:81–99.
18. Schechtman VL, Harper RH. Minute-by-minute association of heart rate variation with basal heart rate in developing infants. *Sleep* 1993;16:23–30.
19. Haddad GG, Krongrad E, Epstein RA, et al. Effect of sleep state on the QT interval in normal infants. *Pediatr Res* 1979;13:139–141.

20. Kumazawa T, Baccelli G, Guazzi M, et al. Haemodynamic patterns during desynchronized sleep in intact cats and cats with sinoatrial deafferentiation. *Circ Res* 1969;24:923–937.
21. Fagioli I, Salzarulo P, Salomon F, Ricour C. Sinus pauses in early human malnutrition during waking and sleeping. *Neuropediatrics* 1983;14:43–46.

Development of the EOG, EMG, and Movement Behaviors During Sleep

THE ELECTRO-OCULOGRAM

Recording of eye movements during sleep provides important information regarding identification of state. Although dysconjugate eye movements can occur during wakefulness in premature and term neonates, fixation of the eyes follows a clear developmental course. Visual fixation to a single patterned stimulus has been recorded in premature newborns as early as 30 weeks conceptional age (1). Evaluating visual fixation by corneal reflection technique has permitted determination of the presence of discriminable waking states (crying wake by behavioral observations, quiet wake, and drowsiness). Younger infants seem to spend more time in drowsiness whereas older infants spend more time in quiet wake as determined by fixation. Fixation time during quiet wakefulness increases with increasing gestational age and fixation occurs more frequently in quiet wake when compared to drowsiness.

Measuring eye movements to determine state of wakefulness has been over-shadowed by the usefulness of the electro-oculogram (EOG) in determining sleep state and sleep/ wake transitions. Evaluation of eye movements during sleep is clearly required in determination of the REM-sleep state.

The eye is a functional dipole with the cornea being between 7 to 100 microvolts positive when compared to the retina (2). Using electro-oculographic techniques (in contrast to measuring eye movements by visual fixation), conjugate and non-conjugate eye movements can be recorded with the eyelids closed. Recording electrodes are conventionally placed at the outer canthus of each eye and offset from the horizontal by approximately 0.5 to 1.0 cm. These distances may be modified depending upon the size of the infant. Offsetting the electrodes from the horizontal plane (one above the horizontal and one below the horizontal) is crucial in identification of vertical and oblique eye movements.

Conjugate eye movements occur in saccades during wakefulness and in saccadic bursts during active (REM) sleep. Slow rolling eye movements and dysconjugate eye movements can occur during quiet wakefulness, drowsiness, sleep/wake transitions, and in certain medical/surgical abnormalities present (e.g., extraocular muscle paralysis, brainstem anatomic abnormalities, disorders that affect the cranial nerves). Because of the mechanism of retinal development in premature infants, with migration of vasculature from the region surrounding the optic disc toward the periphery (as well as the development of central control of eye movements), the EOG may reveal both saccadic eye movements and dysconjugate movements in younger prematures. Since EMG characteristics may not be as reliable as the EEG and EOG, identification of REM sleep requires a characteristic EEG pattern and the presence of at least *some* rapid conjugate eye movements.

Human infants can fixate and focus accurately for considerable periods before they are able to perceive all the details obtained in a visual image projected onto the retina. During the first year of life accurate fixation and focusing occurs in about 13% of 3-month-old infants (3). This increases almost fivefold over the next 3 months and is present in more than three-quarters of 1-year-old children.

Development of clear conjugate eye movements during wakefulness depends to a great extent upon the stage of retinal development and the maturational level of fixation. However, the saccadic eye movements during sleep do not require retinal development or conscious fixation. Control may be mediated through a number of different, but interrelated, central neurologic mechanisms including (but not limited to) cerebral and cerebellar cortical and subcortical development, oculomotor/trochlear/abducens nuclei development, and maturation of central vestibular nuclei. Development of the vestibular system is important for fixation during wakefulness and ocular saccades during active sleep (4).

Ocular movements have been identified by traditional visual inspection of saccades beneath the closed eyelid. This technique may have specific limitations especially in the sleep laboratory. Electro-oculography is considerably more reliable, cost-effective, and eye movements can be identified by post-hoc inspection of the polysomnographic tracing. Unfortunately, specific limitations of electro-oculography are present in smaller infants. Smaller premature neonates' eyes present weaker dipoles and there may be considerable difficulty with subjective analysis of the EOG when dysconjugate movements are present. In an attempt to resolve these obstacles, automated methods of analysis of rapid eye movements during active sleep in infants has been described (5). Computer analysis of slope and amplitude threshold criteria have been performed. Digital filtering is used to improve effectiveness and identification and quantification of ocular movements. The method has been shown to be highly reliable and useful in differentiating between tonic and phasic states during active sleep. This differentiation of REM sleep into two distinct states by the presence or absence of phasic muscle and extraocular muscle activity may hold specific significance in evaluation of studies of sleep-related cardiorespiratory physiology during infancy. In healthy adults, different physiologic characteristics of tonic and phasic REM can be clearly identified (6). This may also be true of infants.

Eye movement density and bursts of saccades may hold special significance in evaluating and predicting mental development of the child. If this is proven to be true, evaluation of the EOG may provide additional information regarding prognosis, long-term outcome of neonatal illness, morbidity, and development in young infants and children.

Dream-related and non-dream-related ocular movements occur in both humans and animals (7). It appears that only high-amplitude rapid eye movements and eye movements occurring in bursts have any possibility of corresponding to visual images. Intense rapid eye movements during sleep have been investigated as possible indications of delay in neural development of infants (8). Becker and Thoman evaluated the occurrence of "REM storms" in first-born infants during the second through fifth post-natal week and again at 3, 6, and 12 months of age. The amount of REM within each 10-second interval of active sleep was rated on a scale based on frequency and intensity of eye movements. Bayley scales of mental development were administered to the cohort of infants at 12 months of age. A significant negative correlation was found between the frequency of REM storms and Bayley scores. By 6 months of age, REM storms seemed to express dysfunction or delay in the development of central inhibitory feedback control for sleep organization and phasic sleep-related activities.

Although few studies exist in infants and children, eye movement density has been shown to be significantly decreased during the second and third REM period of the night after a night of complete and partial sleep deprivation (9). Slow-wave sleep rebound is generally confined to the first NREM-sleep period and 0.05 to 3 Hz activity amplitude increases.

Peizo-electric strain gauge transducers have also been used to evaluate eye movements during sleep (10). These sensors have been shown to be highly sensitive to fine micro-tremor activity during wakefulness. This micro-nystagmoid activity diminishes during NREM sleep and increases during REM sleep. It is intriguing to note that micro-tremor ocular activity also increases after presentation of an auditory stimulus to subjects during NREM sleep. Similar increased micro-tremor activity also occurs *with the appearance of K-complexes* in the EEG.

EMG AND MOVEMENT ACTIVITY DURING SLEEP

Body movements are characteristic of sleep-state changes especially at the termination of a slow-wave-sleep period with lightening (ascent) of state and the termination of the sleep cycle with a REM episode. The REM period generally ends with a major body movement or abrupt increase in chin muscle EMG activity. The next sleep cycle then begins.

Intermittent body movements occur frequently during sleep without significant change in state or beginning of a new sleep cycle. These movements without state change involve both brief phasic activity lasting less than 6 seconds and gross slower body movements (squirming) lasting longer than 6 seconds. Development and maturation of this skeletal muscle activity also follows a regular and predictable maturational pattern. During wakefulness, development of gross motor and fine motor activity form the basis of half of the tests of developmental screening. Maturation of gross motor, fine motor, and phasic muscle movements during sleep may also be sensitive markers of neurologic development.

During quiet wakefulness, random muscle activity usually does not occur. However, a wide range of elementary and complex motor activities are known to occur during sleep. Random minute electric activity constitutes the basic physiologic condition of the skeletal muscles during sleep (11). During NREM sleep, random minute motor activity decreases considerably when compared to the quiet-waking state. During REM sleep, there is a sudden increase in isolated motor unit action potentials. Particular structural features of the anterior tibialis muscle makes it seemingly the most active muscle during sleep (11) and monitoring of the anterior tibialis EMG activity during sleep is recommended during nocturnal polysomnography in *all* neonates, infants, children, adolescents, and adults.

Although a significant decrease in the number of body position shifts occurs during sleep across the life cycle (12), during middle childhood there does not appear to be a difference in the number and frequency of major body movements and position shifts in normal youngsters. During early childhood, there appears to be an increase in the duration of maintenance of body position and in the number of periods of more than 30 minutes of positional immobility. In middle childhood prone, supine, and lateral decubitus positions occupy an equal proportion of the sleep period time. Sleeping in the prone position is characteristically abandoned as maturation continues.

Characteristic body and muscle movements in premature newborns and term neonates during quiet sleep appear similar to startle (Moro-like) reflexes, generalized phasic movements (13), or tonic increase in submental muscle activity. In contrast to the total simultaneous pattern of motor activity seen during quiet sleep, active sleep is characterized by a more uncoordinated and localized pattern of movements such as generalized phasic movements, local tonic activity, localized phasic activity, and brief clonic muscle activity. With increasing conceptional age, there is a decrease in the occurrence of the startle reflex, generalized phasic movements, and localized phasic movements. Localized tonic activity tends to remain constant with increasing conceptional age. The differences in decreasing tendencies among these movements may indicate the differences of maturational changes in different parts of the central nervous system (13).

Degree of phasic activity during sleep may reflect the maturity of the developing brainstem. Dissociation of sleep-related phasic motor phenomena may hold special clinical significance in some infants. In assessing possible causes for ALTE and SIDS, Kohyama and coworkers postulated brainstem immaturity as a possible cause. They calculated and utilized a "dissociation index" between body movements and density extraocular eye movements in a group of infants who exhibited cyanosis during feeding (14). When motor activity was evaluated, with respect to extraocular muscle activity, there was no difference in eye movement density and body movements greater than 2 seconds in infants with cyanosis during feeding who ultimately suffered an apparent life-threatening event or who subsequently died of SIDS, when compared to infants with cyanosis during feeding who did not suffer either of these catastrophic events. However, infants with cyanosis during feeding in the ALTE/SIDS group exhibited a significantly higher decrease in dissociation of extraocular movements and body movements when compared with the control group.

On the one hand, they concluded that cyanosis during feeding may be a mild expression of brainstem immaturity and rapid conjugate eye movements and body movements can be useful indicators of the maturation of the CNS in infants with nonspecific cyanosis during feeding. On the other hand, types of skeletal muscle movement show specific developmental relationships with respect to conceptional age. Fukumoto and colleagues (15) described the ontogenetic evolution of three types of movements: (i) gross movements, (ii) localized movements, and (iii) phasic movements (twitches lasting less than 0.5 seconds). All body movement parameters decreased in frequency with maturation. Interestingly, each type of movement behavior showed a fairly specific and individual time course. Earliest decrease between 30 weeks conceptional age and 18 months chronologic age occurs in phasic activity. This takes place relatively early in development of the infant. Second, localized movements decreased in frequency next and gross movement continued unchanged until a basal level is reached at approximately 9 to 13 months of post-natal age. The number of epochs without body movements increases steadily until about 8 months of age.

Gross movements, localized movements, and phasic movements are controlled by the central nervous system at different organizational levels. Phasic activity is more ontogenetically simple and decreases early during maturation. Gross movements are quite complex and require a greater degree of central nervous system integration. Therefore, these types of movements are correlated to maturational processes of the CNS and provide an additional window and indicator of normal and abnormal development. Evaluation of these types of movements during polysomnography can provide an additional assessment, when coupled with traditional developmental appraisals.

Evolution of movements and specific spontaneous behaviors during sleep in neonates have been reported by Meyers (16). Frequency distribution of time intervals between spontaneous behaviors showed that movements were typically spaced closely in time. However, none of these spontaneous motor activities occur with a set interval between successive behaviors. Spontaneous muscle activity in the sleeping neonate conform to a single pattern of temporal organization regardless of the specific movement displayed or the state of sleep. The pattern approximates a systematic alternation of periods of increasing and decreasing time intervals between successive behaviors.

When clear NREM states can be identified, body movements reveal a clear state-dependent relationship (17). A continuum of movements can be demonstrated with decreasing frequency, respectively, between wakefulness, stage 1 (transitional sleep), REM sleep, stage 2 NREM , and slow-wave sleep. The relative frequency of body movements, therefore, seems to be regulated by state-dependent mechanisms and body movements may be a reliable measure of the development and organizational maturation of sleep-state differentiation particularly if the time base is long enough. When the maturational progression of these states does not follow the expected developmental pattern, support of the diagnosis of delay in maturation of the central nervous system may be considered. Prolonged uninterrupted sleep states without body movements or position change might indicate abnormal development of the arousal response and constitute a subtle indication of underlying central nervous system control abnormality.

Body position may have a significant effect on state organization and might suggest that the central vestibular system contributes to the development and organization of state. Hashimoto and colleagues studied the contribution of the prone and supine body position to both physiologic and behavioral correlates during sleep in neonates (18). Quiet sleep occupied a greater percentage of the total sleep time when the newborn was in the prone position when compared to supine. Gross movements, and phasic muscle activity were also less frequently observed in the prone position, although there was no difference in localized movements between the two body positions. Expectedly, since there was an increase in quiet sleep, respiration was more regular in the prone position. Interestingly, the pulse rate during quiet sleep was higher in this position.

Type and frequency of body movement activity during sleep may provide significantly useful information regarding the integrity of the central nervous system in term newborns. Hakamada and coworkers (19) studied body movements in term newborns with significant illnesses or malformations such as perinatal asphyxia, purulent meningitis, meconium aspiration syndrome, gastrointestinal bleeding, porencephaly, and hydranencephaly. Newborns who had recovered from transient vomiting were also evaluated and used as a comparison group. Generalized body movements, localized tonic movements, and generalized phasic movements were evaluated. On the one hand, patients with minimally depressed background EEG activity showed an increase in generalized movements and localized tonic movements during quiet sleep. On the other hand, hydrancephalic infants showed an increase in generalized phasic movements in active and quiet sleep and a profound decrease in generalized movements during sleep when EEG abnormalities were markedly severe. Although the absence of, or a significant decrease in generalized body movements, or an increase in generalized phasic muscle activity might indicate a very poor prognosis for particular infants, the presence of localized tonic movements (even in small amounts) suggest the preservation of cortical function.

Spontaneous body movements and behaviors appear to be controlled by an interaction of endogenous rhythms that do not appear to run independently (20). Instead, a system of interaction between endogenous oscillations exists. By 2 weeks of age, an ultradian 3- to 4-hour cycle can easily be identified. This cycle is typically related to feeding patterns and may be controlled by hypothalamic mechanisms and metabolic requirements. A 50-minute basic rest—activity cycle (the BRAC cycle) originally described by Kleitman (21) can be identified and a circadian cycle is present at about 8 to 12 weeks of age.

The BRAC described by Kleitman (21) appears to trigger sensory and motor mechanisms characterizing both the phases of enhanced stereotypic motor activity during the day and night in children with developmental disabilities with stereotypic behaviors during wakefulness and sleep (20). Peak frequency of stereotypic behaviors seem to follow the same mean REM-to-REM interval on consecutive nights.

New methods of digital statistical analysis of EEG, EMG, and EOG activity has the potential to describe the structural and temporal characteristics of tonic electrophysiologic activity during sleep (22). Three components can be identified: slow-fast component, hemispheric shift, and ocular movement activation. Cycles of tonic electrophysiologic activity that are both slower and faster than the typical 90 minute ultradian rhythm of sleep states can be identified by utilization of these components in older children and adults.

Activity monitoring accelerometry can also provide significant information regarding disturbed sleep in infants and children. First, state monitoring by actigraphy is generally consistent with polysomnography when assessing certain parameters of sleep and the sleep-wake cycle in children (23). Sadeh and coworkers have described actigraphic sleep/wake scoring in sleep-disturbed children compared to a control group of healthy children (23). Movements measured actigraphically characteristic of wakefulness lasting longer than 5 minutes were significantly greater in the sleep-disturbed group of children clearly showing poorer sleep quality in these children (12 to 18 months of age). Sleep measures showed significant night-to-night stability in both groups. The stability of specific measures and their age trends were different between the groups. These data clearly showed that measurement of body movements during sleep at home could discriminate between sleep-disturbed and healthy children with a highly correct assignment rate.

Other motor disorders of childhood have significant sleep-related correlates and motor behaviors which can be monitored and assessed polysomnographically. Gadoth and coworkers studied sleep-related body movements and periodic limb movements in unrelated patients with L-dopa-responsive hereditary progressive dystonia. Also studied were their unaffected family members (24). All patients with dystonia had an increase in major body movements during REM sleep. Most unaffected parents and siblings had either similar REM-related body movements, periodic limb movements, or both. Therefore, a common mechanism for the dystonia, body movements, and periodic limb movements may exist and a causative relationship between these two motor phenomena during sleep seems to be implied.

REFERENCES

1. Hack M, Muszynski SY, Miranda SB. State of awakeness during visual fixation in preterm infants. *Pediatrics* 1981;68:87–92.
2. Sheldon SH, Spire JP, Levy HB. *Pediatric Sleep Medicine.* Philadelphia: WB Saunders; 1992.
3. Molteno AC, Hodgkinson IJ, Hewitt CJ, Sanderson GE. The development of fixing and focusing behaviour in normal human infants as observed with the Otago photoscreener. *Aust NZ J Ophthalmol* 1992;20: 197–205.
4. Tomko DL, Paige GD. Linear vestibuloocular reflex during motion along axes between nasooccipital and interaural. *Ann NY Acad Sci* 1992;656:233–241.
5. Gopal IS, Haddad GG. Automatic detection of eye movements in REM sleep using the electrooculogram. *Am J Physiol* 1981;241:R217–R221.
6. Orem J, Barnes CD. *Physiology in Sleep.* New York: Academic Press; 1980.
7. Soh K, Morita Y, Sei H. Relationship between eye movements and oneiric behavior in cats. *Physiol Behav* 1992;52:553–558.
8. Becker PT, Thoman EB. Rapid eye movement storms in infants: rate of occurrence at 6 months predicts mental development at 1 year. *Science* 1981;212:1415–1416.

9. Feinberg I, Baker T, Leder R, March JD. Response of delta (0–3 Hz) EEG and eye movement density to a night with 100 minutes of sleep. *Sleep* 1988;11:473–487.
10. Coakley D, Williams R, Morris J. Minute eye movement during sleep. *Electroencephalogr Clin Neurophysiol* 1979;47:126–131.
11. Askenasy JJ, Yahr MD. Different laws govern motor activity in sleep than in wakefulness. *J Neural Transm Gen Sect* 1990;79:103–111.
12. DeKoninck J, Lorrain D, Gagnon P. Sleep positions and position shifts in five age groups: an ontogenetic picture. *Sleep* 1992;15:143–149.
13. Hakamada S, Watanabe K, Hara K, Miyazaki S. Development of the motor behavior during sleep in newborn infants. *Brain Dev* 1981;3:345–350.
14. Kohyama J, Watanabe S, Iwakawa Y. Phasic sleep components in infants with cyanosis during feeding. *Pediatr Neurol* 1991;7:200–204.
15. Fukumoto M, Mochizuki N, Takeishi M, Nomura Y, Segawa M. Studies of body movements during night sleep in infancy. *Brain Dev* 1981;3:37–43.
16. Myers A. Organization of spontaneous behaviors of sleeping neonates. *Percept Motor Skills* 1977;45:791–794.
17. Wilde-Frenz J, Schlz H. Rate and distribution of body movements during sleep in humans. *Percept Motor Skills* 1983;56:275–283.
18. Hashimoto T, Hiura K, Endo S, et al. Postural effects on behavioral states of newborn infants—a sleep polygraphic study. *Brain Dev* 1983;5:286–291.
19. Hakamada S, Watanabe K, Hara K, Miyazaki S, Kumagai T. Body movements during sleep in full-term newborn infants. *Brain Dev* 1982;4:51–55.
20. Meier-Koll A, Fels T, Kofler B, Schulz-Weber U, Thiessen M. Basic rest activity cycle and stereotyped behavior of a mentally defective child. *Neuropadiatrie* 1977;8:172–180.
21. Kleitman N. *Sleep and Wakefulness.* Chicago: University of Chicago Press; 1963:131–194.
22. Sussman P, Moffitt A, Hoffmann R, Wells R, Shearer J. The description of structural and temporal characteristics of tonic electrophysiological activity during sleep. *Waking-Sleeping* 1979;3:279–290.
23. Sadeh A, Lavie P, Scher A, Tirosh E, Epstein R. Actigraphic home-monitoring sleep-disturbed and control infants and young children: a new method for pediatric assessment of sleep-wake patterns. *Pediatrics* 1991;87:494–499.
24. Gadoth N, Costeff H, Harel S, Lavie P. Motor abnormalities during sleep in patients with childhood hereditary progressive dystonia, and their unaffected family members. *Sleep* 1989;12:233–238.

6

Evaluation of the History and Physical Examination

Clinical evaluation of the neonate, infant, and child is clearly the most important approach in the process of assessment and management of sleep and its disorders in the pediatric population. The clinical history is the mainstay of the clinical problem-solving process and most important means of diagnosis and management.

THE PROCESS OF SOLVING CLINICAL PROBLEMS

Clinical problem solving in pediatric sleep medicine begins in an identical manner to solving any clinical problem. The experienced clinician begins with three steps: (i) perception of the patient situation, (ii) perception of particular cues, and (iii) hypotheses generation (1). These initial tasks in arriving at a diagnosis are internalized, occur instantaneously during the earliest part of the clinical encounter, and are generally unconscious. Most clinical hypotheses regarding potential diagnosis (either general or specific) are generated before any historic or physical investigations occur. Hypotheses form the basis of inquiry into a patient's presenting problem(s). By testing each hypothesis in parallel with questions to identify certain patterns and performing a physical examination to further test remaining hypotheses, the hypothesis set is reorganized into a differential diagnosis. Laboratory testing and polysomnography is needed only when the various components of the hypothesis set cannot be differentiated based on clinical grounds. It may also be required to confirm or refute significant diagnoses that may result in morbidity and/or mortality, or to characterize two or more diagnoses requiring different treatments.

EVALUATION OF THE CLINICAL HISTORY

Establishing an initial hypothesis set and subsequent testing by clinical inquiry requires a knowledge base of patterns of symptoms that are related to primary or secondary sleep disorders. An understanding of pathophysiology, natural history, clinical manifestations, and *diurnal* symptoms are essential for accurate diagnosis and subsequent treatment. Sleep disorders are common and must assume a proper place in the clinical evaluation. The National Commission on Sleep Disorders Research has reported the prevalence of sleep disorders being much more extensive than previously believed (2).

Parents will often seek medical attention early for the sleepless child. Clearly, the sleepless child *disturbs parents* during the middle of the night and the awakening causes symptoms of sleep deprivation *in the parents*. Seeking help from the primary care practitioner early is common for these disorders. Unfortunately, a comprehensive knowledge of pediatric sleep disorders has not been included in medical curricula at the undergraduate or graduate medical education level. Therefore, the approach to diagnosis and management is often inappropriate and based on limited scientific and/or clinical information. Consequently, the sleepy child reaches appropriate professional care very late in the course of his/her disorder and often suffers significant morbidity well before professional attention is obtained. Profoundly sleepy children may reach the sleep professional early, if they tend to fall to sleep at inappropriate times (e.g., during meals, talking on the phone, while opening presents at a birthday party). However, the youngster with intermediate sleepiness as an infant may be considered a "wonderful child" who never bothers anyone. Parents have their own personal time, time together when the youngster is sleeping and does not require parental attention. Unfortunately, these "wonderful children" may have significantly greater medical and/or developmental difficulties than the sleepless child. When a youngster has an intermediate degree of sleepiness and/or develops a state of hypo-arousal, symptoms are considerably different. Intermediate degrees of sleepiness and hypo-arousal states are most often manifested by diurnal hyperactivity and attention span problems. Youngsters are easily distracted, have rapid mood swings, learning problems in school, and become easily frustrated. These symptoms are typically addressed in a behavioral manner and limited searching of the sleep history is the rule rather than the exception. Screening the medical sleep history generally takes a short period of time, and provides the practitioner insight into the well being of his/her patient during a very large portion of their lives.

It has been shown in one study of 202 children consecutively presenting to a developmental and behavioral pediatric practice, that parents and other primary caretakers infrequently report that their child has a sleep problem, even when symptoms suggesting a sleep disorder are present (3). In fact, parents rarely report the presence of disordered sleep, even when they recognize their child is having difficulties sleeping at night. Simply asking the parent whether or not the child has a sleep problem is inadequate to establish a hypothesis set or to test hypotheses regarding pathologic sleep.

Clearly, many sleep-related problems during the early neonatal period and/or infancy are identified early by the health care professional and parents/caretakers. Apnea of prematurity is typically diagnosed prior to discharge from the neonatal nursery. Apparent life-threatening events (ALTEs) are alarming to parents and result in early medical evaluation and intervention. In other situations, early medical attention does not occur and clinical evaluation is rather difficult.

A sleep history obtained from a frustrated, sleepy parent is commonly not very genuine or specific. Parents will often relate the child's sleep pattern that has been the worst *for them* over the preceding months or will often present only the sleep pattern of the youngster from the night before. A history of habitual sleep patterns is often very difficult to obtain. Frequently information offered is not reproducible since it changes from night to night. A more accurate depiction of the sleep patterns across time requires the informant to maintain a diary, log, or chart. Prior to the first visit, the parent can be asked to maintain a sleep log or diary for a period of 2 to 4 weeks. This log then becomes very helpful in identifying habitual sleep-wake cycle patterns and provides documentation of abnormalities occurring from night-to-night (4). Maintaining a sleep log seems to improve observational skills of the child's caretaker, increases validity of observational data, and *is commonly therapeutic*. Parents can often identify patterns without assistance and can distinguish methods of intervention to assist their child resolve the problem(s).

When the sleep disorders professional reviews the diary, it also becomes the focus of assessment. The sleep log provides a focus for intervention, can mirror success of management, and documents longitudinal improvement of symptoms (or lack thereof).

It is important, however, for parents to receive explicit instruction on proper maintenance of the diary and an amount of time must be spent with the caretaker regarding methods for appropriately recording data. Functional status of the caretaker and the ecologic milieu must be assessed at the first visit. When caretaker/child dysfunction is present, it may be the root of the problem. Requesting maintenance of a sleep log may add to family dysfunction, especially if the caretaker does not know exactly how to properly maintain the diary. For example, the caretaker who has inappropriate expectations regarding the sleep-wake cycle of his/her child, may find maintenance of the diary difficult because of a feeling that a loss of sleep must occur nightly as they document sleep-wake processes. At other times, the requirement of maintenance of the log may provide focus for the caretaker and identify exactly where the inappropriate expectations exist, thus assisting with resolution of the problem. Therefore, a sleep log or diary used judiciously is a vital first step in clinical assessment of the youngster with disordered sleep.

The clinical history is the most important aspect of assessment of disordered sleep in children (as well as in adults). Obtaining appropriate information by searching the history is based on knowledge of patterns of symptoms and grounded on the wide variety of hypotheses generated from the initial patient contact, patient situation, and cue perception. Information regarding the presentation and natural history of most sleep disorders is rarely presented at *any* level of medical education. It is important, therefore, to begin with a screening process which may provide insight or cues to the practitioner that a problem may be present requiring further investigation, referral, or testing. As previously pointed out, simply asking the question whether the youngster has a sleep problem is insufficient to identify those children in need of further evaluation. A structured approach to screening the history has been tested and validated (3). An important first step is obtaining information regarding the typical/habitual sleep patterns and difficulties.

HISTORIC DETAILS

Bedtime, Sleep Latency, and Normal Time of Sleep Offset

The history can begin with obtaining three important time parameters and intervals. First, what time is the youngster's habitual bedtime? Although there is no "right time" for children to go to bed, knowledge of parental perception of appropriate bedtime can provide insight into their perceptions of normal sleep in childhood and also provides a focal point for assessment of other very important parameters in the sleep/wake continuum. For example, a 9-year-old child whose bedtime is 1930 most likely will be in bed at a time when his/her circadian rhythmicity will not permit easy settling. Information regarding this early bedtime may provide information regarding other aspects of the caretakers' lives and perceptions which will aid in intervention into the youngster's sleep problem. Similarly, a 2-year-old child whose bedtime is 0100 because the mother or father works at night and wants to spend time with the child before the parent goes to bed will most likely develop either a sleep-phase delay that will present problems later in life when social responsibilities (e.g., school) emerge, or develop an insufficient sleep syndrome that can result in profound diurnal problems (e.g., behavior problems, attention span difficulties, school failure).

The *length of time it takes for the youngster to fall to sleep* can provide information regarding the ease of settling at night. This information combined with the habitual bedtime can help in determination of the presence of behavioral sleep-onset difficulties, parental limit setting problems, circadian rhythm abnormalities, anxiety-related sleep disorders, sleep-onset association problems, as well as biologic/physiologic abnormalities resulting in sleep-onset delays during childhood. Behavioral abnormalities resulting in sleep-onset difficulties are much more common than biologic, medical, and/or physiologic abnormalities in children. When a medical or physiologic problem is present, it typically presents with the youngster having *difficulty falling to sleep anywhere and under any circumstances.* Therefore, obtaining a history that the youngster can fall to sleep easily and without difficulty when at her grandparents' house, or in the parents' bed, or on the sofa in front of the television strongly suggests a behavioral etiology rather than a biologic cause for the sleeplessness. Prolongation of the sleep latency must be assessed in conjunction with bedtime in order for accurate interpretation. For example, a 4-hour sleep-onset latency has different meaning when the bedtime is 1900 when compared with a bedtime of 2200 in a 9-year-old child. At the present time there are no normative data nor accurate suggestions for parents regarding a "normal bedtime" and a "normal" sleep-onset latency. Each is relative and each individual child is different. Times and latencies may vary according to age, according to biologic susceptibility, according to social responsibilities, according to maturity, and will vary over time. Each of these bits of information must be assessed in conjunction with all other information obtained and only provides an initial insight into the sleep-wake cycle of the child.

Normal time of morning sleep offset should also be obtained in the general sleep history and systems review. Habitual time of morning sleep offset provides the basis for determination of total nocturnal sleep time. It should also be determined whether sleep offset is spontaneous or prompted by parents, clocks, or other environmental stimulus. Morning sleep offset is also the most powerful point of circadian rhythm entrainment and inconsistent times of sleep offset might suggest a sleep-wake schedule abnormality.

In addition to the habitual time of morning sleep offset on weekdays (school days), it is equally important to determine these times on weekends and holidays. Late sleep offset on weekends and holidays might suggest a sleep-phase delay syndrome. A non-24 hour sleep-wake schedule, might be suspected in a youngster with neurologic/neurophysiologic abnormalities. Children presenting with very early sleep-offset time will come to the attention of the professional early, because the youngster will wake early in the morning and disrupt the parents' sleep. Inability of the parents to sleep as long as they require and the youngster who is ready to begin the day "before the sun comes up" might suggest the presence of a sleep-phase advance syndrome, although this is much less common than a phase delay. It also might suggest an environmental sleep disorder or congenital short-sleep period. Sleep-maintenance insomnia is fairly common in adult patients with affective disorders. Similar sleep-related symptoms of affective disorders do not seem to be reproducible in children.

Continuity of Sleep

Children as well as adults not only have sleep-onset difficulties, but sleep-continuity problems occur as well. Determination of nocturnal wakings will provide information regarding behavioral aspects of the sleep-wake cycle and assist in determining the presence of a physiologic basis for the youngster's sleep disorder. Sleep-onset difficulties accompanied by sleep-continuity problems in the absence of physiologic abnormalities suggest the presence of behavioral etiologies and these should be pursued historically. Often, limit setting and insufficient parental tolerance are easy to detect since similar difficulties exist during the day and discipline/day-time limit-setting abnormalities are also present. When sleep-maintenance problems exist, it is important to determine the timing, frequency, and duration of the wakings. Answers to these questions will also assist in differentiating sleep-onset association disorders from behavioral problems and excessive nocturnal fluids. Again, physiologic, biologic, and medical abnormalities resulting in sleep-maintenance problems are typically present all the time and the youngster will sleep neither continuously nor well in any environmental or behavioral situation.

Excessive Day-Time Sleepiness

Determination of day-time sleepiness is vitally important in assessing the child with sleep complaints. It is extremely difficult to determine excessive sleepiness in young infants, toddlers, and young children. Infants' sleep time occupies most of their day. Total sleep time ranges from about 16–18 hours in the newborn to about 8–9 hours by late childhood. There is a progressive decline in total sleep time as maturation occurs. After about 12 weeks of age, circadian rhythmicity of the sleep-wake cycle begins to emerge and the longest sleep period tends to occur at night while the longest wake period occurs during the day. At this time, day-time sleep typically occurs in about three sleep episodes. Naps then begin to consolidate during the first year of life into two briefer sleep periods. During the second year, these day-time sleep episodes consolidate into one early afternoon sleep period until naps are completely given up (between 3 and 5 years of age). There also appears to be a wide variation of normal, but youngsters napping after 6–7 years of age, may be exhibiting symptoms of day-time sleepiness.

It is difficult to determine significant day-time sleepiness in infants and younger children. The basis for these difficulties rests with the absence of reliable norms in these age groups. How can one accurately determine excessive sleepiness in a youngster who is supposed to habitually nap during day-time hours? Therefore, only the most severe forms of excessive sleepiness will come to the attention of the practitioner early in the course of the disorder. In addition, the sleepier infant and child is too often considered a "good baby." They are no bother to the parents, sleep most of the time, and rarely disturb their parents' nocturnal sleep.

Children are different in diurnal manifestations of intermediate degrees of sleepiness. Whereas an adult will manifest classical behavioral characteristics of sleepiness (yawning, lethargy, droopy eye lids, listlessness, and frequently manifest sleep), intermediate degrees of sleepiness in young children rarely present in this manner. There may be indirect evidence of sleepiness, for example day dreaming and occasionally falling to sleep during soporific conditions (e.g., in the school classroom or while riding in an automobile). Often, however, these youngsters will manifest sleepiness by presenting with *hyperactivity*. Hyperactivity often alternates with other symptoms of sleepiness including (but not limited to) day dreaming, withdrawal, aggressiveness with other children, learning difficulties, behavior problems, attention span problems, excessive fidgetiness and motor activity, rapid mood swings, and/or easy distractibility.

One clue the practitioner may use in determining the presence of excessive sleepiness is determining whether the youngster *habitually naps*. Diurnal naps are typically abandoned by 5 years of age. A school-age youngster who habitually naps may be manifesting symptoms of excessive sleepiness. The practitioner should then pursue this possibility by further questioning the parents and child regarding possible biologic, physiologic, and/or behavioral causes for the sleepiness. It must also be remembered that the ability to tolerate and perform during intermediate degrees of sleepiness varies between individuals making the assessment of disorders of excessive somnolence difficult to diagnose early in childhood. Longitudinal evaluation and continuity of care is essential to follow the natural history of the development excessive sleepiness in children.

Parasomnias

Parasomnias should also be searched for during the history. A wide variety of REM and NREM parasomnias exist, but simple questions can provide information regarding the presence or absence of these disorders. Identification of the presence of these symptoms, however, does not indicate the presence of a *disorder*, nor does it require intervention in most cases. Parasomnic symptoms are fairly common during the toddler period and during early childhood. Symptoms decrease in frequency or resolve as the child develops. Indications for further evaluation, including polysomnography, depend upon the age of the child, the frequency of symptoms, the severity of symptoms, and the presence of concomitant symptomatology. Further diagnosis and treatment is generally based on the probability of injury from the disorder or the presence of other precipitating phenomena. It is important to determine whether the youngster rocks or bangs her head before or during sleep. Symptoms typically surround the sleep-wake transition period. Symptoms that occur only during wakefulness and are not associated with sleep-wake transitions most likely reflect behavioral or psychologic pathology and should be further evaluated in those contexts.

Does the youngster *grind her teeth*? Does this occur only during sleep or does it also occur during wakefulness? Bruxism can result in wearing away of the crowns of the teeth causing morbidity and requiring dental intervention. It also may result in temporomandibular joint dysfunction, morning headaches, as well as symptoms of day-time sleepiness. Dental evaluations and mouth guards are often required when symptoms are clinically significant. The sound created when the youngster is bruxing is very characteristic, often quite loud, and can result in disruption of sleep in other members of the family.

Does the child *walk or run during sleep*? NREM disorders such as somnambulism, agitated sleep walking, paroxysmal nocturnal wanderings, sleep-related eating/drinking syndrome can result in injury, and can be potentially fatal due to injury during the episode. Similarly, REM-sleep motor disorder has been described during childhood (5) and is also potentially fatal due to injury.

Does the youngster have *nightmares*? This simple question and its resultant answer can be very complicated in interpretation. It is often difficult for a parent to differentiate the variety of occurrences during sleep that may appear similar to nightmares. Caretakers will often report "nightmares" for sleep-related symptoms associated with the youngster waking and crying or screaming. Unfortunately for diagnostic purposes, *all that screams during the night is not nightmares*. It is important to determine whether the child was sleeping at the time. This may also be difficult. Nightmares typically occur later in the sleep-period time, during early morning hours (although they may occur at any time during the sleep period). They occur during REM sleep and are considered anxiety dreams, similar to adults. There may be an abrupt awakening from the dream, crying, and/or screaming that is associated with a waking state. Autonomic discharge is generally mild and the waking is often associated with difficulty returning to sleep. In addition, the dream recall, if present, is often vivid and there is a clear story quality to the dream report. Other anxiety-related symptoms may be present during diurnal hours.

In contrast, *sleep terrors and other paroxysmal disorders* associated with screaming at night are amnestic. Children rarely recall the occurrences, but may exhibit anxiety secondary to the presentation without recall. Autonomic discharges during sleep terrors is much more extreme. Sleep terrors generally are heralded by a "blood curdling" scream, excessive panic, and profound autonomic discharge including pupillary dilation, diaphoresis, tremor, tachycardia, tachypnea, and other sympathetic manifestations. They tend to occur during the early portion of the sleep period, during slow-wave sleep. The youngster may appear to speak and report dream mentation during the episode, however, it is often garbled, confused, and unintelligible. There may or may not be displacement from the bed. If there is displacement from bed, the likelihood of injury is significant and potentially fatal. Story-like quality is most frequently absent. The arousal is brief, lasting only several minutes (although at times may be prolonged and last hours). The youngster rapidly returns to sleep and there is amnesia for the event the next morning.

It may be difficult to differentiate other paroxysmal disorders from sleep terrors. Sleep-related temporal lobe seizures may appear remarkably similar to sleep terrors. They occur at random, appear stereotypic, and are often associated with abnormal EEG findings (if a relatively complete montage is recorded during sleep). There may be displacement from the bed, and injury may occur. Differentiation is important since treatment programs would vary considerably.

It is important to determine whether the youngster sleeps soundly or is *restless during sleep*. Restlessness during sleep is subjectively assessed by the caretaker(s). It may be observed intermittently during the night. It may be assessed by dishevelment of the bed in the morning, or may be directly observed during co-sleeping episodes. In any case, if the subjective assessment is accurate, restless sleep can have diagnostic import and must be a symptom taken seriously. Fragmentation of the continuity of sleep by brief movement arousals, electrocortical arousals, and brief awakenings typically results in diurnal symptoms that can result in performance problems and day-time difficulties. Restlessness during sleep may be due to a variety of endogenous or exogenous factors. Frequent body movements during both REM and NREM sleep can be seen in youngsters with anxiety-related sleep disorders. They may be caused by a variety of environmental factors. Importantly, restless sleep is commonly associated with periodic limb movement disorder in children (6), obstructive sleep apnea syndrome (7), high upper-airway resistance syndrome (8), narcolepsy syndrome (9), attention deficit-hyperactivity symptom complex (10), and most likely a host of other disturbances including medical and psychiatric illnesses.

Does the youngster *wet the bed at night, during sleep*? This is an important age-related symptom to identify. Many parents will not consider sleep-related enuresis a sleep disorder or sleep problem (3). Although it appears that mortality is virtually nonexistent, morbidity secondary to sleep-related enuresis is quite predictable. The underlying cause for primary sleep-related enuresis is speculative and most likely multifactorial. Possible etiologies include:

1. A maturational delay in the development of arousal response (in the presence of high arousal thresholds during childhood) from visceral afferent activity caused by bladder distension;
2. Maturational blunting of the normal antidiuretic hormone secretion peak during the sleep period resulting in water excretion during the sleep period equal to that occurring during waking hours; and
3. Uninhibited bladder contractions.

No one theory has been proven in all studies of children who suffer from enuresis. Therefore, it is most likely that there are heterogenous etiologies or a combination of etiologies. The maturational aspect of all theories is supported by the fact that the prevalence of sleep-related enuresis decreases as children age by about 15% per year in enuretic children (9).

Other treatable etiologies for sleep-related enuresis exist. Organic causes are common. sleep-related enuresis is often a presenting symptom in children with juvenile diabetes mellitus, diabetes insipidus, acute urinary tract infection, chronic/occult urinary tract infection, and anatomic urinary tract abnormalities. Other sleep-related pathologies also may present with bed-wetting as an initial complaint. Some of these include obstructive sleep apnea syndrome, high upper-airway resistance syndrome, sleep-related generalized seizure disorders, and NREM/slow-wave sleep motor disorders. In youngsters with primary sleep-related enuresis, the likelihood for significant psychopathology to be present is quite small. Less than 10% of children with primary sleep-related enuresis have a psychologic/psychiatric etiology as the underlying cause (9). It has been shown that in certain circumstances, the symptom of sleep-related enuresis secondary to psychologic distress and anxiety-related disorders (e.g., post-traumatic stress disorder) in youngsters who have suffered child abuse and/or neglect have a higher incidence of sleep-related enuresis than an age and socio-economically matched comparison population (3).

The symptom of snoring is essential to determine during the course of clinical evaluation. Loud snoring during childhood should be considered abnormal. Snoring indicates increased upper-airway resistance. The obstruction can occur anywhere, from the region of the anterior nasal valve to the glottis. All children who snore require evaluation, but this does not mean that all children who snore should be required to undergo expensive diagnostic testing in the laboratory. Only those children who manifest other historic and physical evidence that the degree of airway obstruction has resulted in or has clear potential to result in pathophysiologic abnormalities should be further evaluated polysomnographically. The clinical history and physical examination, therefore, is the key to determining which youngster requires further study.

Sleep-disordered breathing has been described in the pediatric literature for more than 100 years. Only recently has underlying physiology and pathology been somewhat understood and described. Sleep-disordered breathing in children is not a unitary phenomenon. It may present in many different ways (11). Diagnostic manifestations vary considerably suggesting either a continuum of a single disorder or a number of disorders presenting with the abnormality of the respiratory tract during sleep as the final common pathway.

Airway resistance and cessation of respiratory airflow (both nasal and oral) have a variety of etiologies that are just beginning to be understood in the adult population who suffer from sleep-disordered breathing. Three types of apneas have been described: obstructive, central, and mixed. An obstructive apnea in an adult is defined as a cessation of nasal and oral airflow for a period of at least 10 seconds with continuation of documented respiratory efforts (chest and abdomen). A central apnea is defined as cessation of nasal and oral airflow for a period of at least 10 seconds with absence of documented respiratory efforts. Mixed apneas have polysomnographic characteristics of both: an initial central component followed by a clear obstructive component. Typically the site of airway occlusion has been the upper airway, including the nasopharynx, oropharynx, and hypopharynx. Pharyngeal muscle dysfunction, excessive adipose tissue, and anatomic abnormalities have all been implicated in the genesis of upper airway occlusive respiratory events.

Much effort has been placed on identification of etiology in adults. A paucity of information is available regarding upper-airway obstruction in children. Most data on sleep-disordered breathing during childhood has been either extrapolated from adult data, preliminary observations, studies conducted with very small sample sizes, and data available from prior investigations on SIDS. Many of the data are observational. Despite these limitations of knowledge about the disorder in children, anecdotal information exists that suggests obstructive sleep apnea is a significantly different disorder when compared to adults, both in etiology and pathogenesis. Definitions are also different. For example, in order for an obstructive apneic event to be considered significant during infancy and early childhood, time criteria appear to be irrelevant. Any cessation of nasal and oral airflow despite two clear respiratory efforts can be considered a significant respiratory event, especially if cardiac and hematologic changes occur or they result in repetitive arousals (9). Central apneas of 20 seconds or longer during infancy are considered significant. Central apneas less than 20 seconds in length that are associated with bradycardia and/or hemoglobin oxygen desaturation are considered pathologic in infancy. However, criteria may be different for toddlers and older children.

Airway resistance can be increased at any point in the airway, including the anterior nasal valve; nasopharynx (adenoids); oropharynx (tonsils); hypopharynx (peripharyngeal soft tissue, musculature and pharyngeal constrictors); larynx (vocal cords and laryngeal musculature); and lower airway smooth muscles (11). A comprehensive list of all changes in function have not been elucidated and a complete understanding of the pathophysiology of abnormal increases in airway resistance is still obscure and controversial. It is most likely multifactorial in etiology. Several mechanisms may be involved. It is also unknown whether the various types of occlusive airway phenomenon during childhood are separate entities with different etiologies or various manifestations on a continuum of severity. Clearly, anatomic abnormalities (hypertrophic tonsils and adenoids) are the most common cause for upper-airway obstruction in young children. But, this does not seem to be the case in all youngsters and etiologies of upper-airway obstruction and increased airway resistance to airflow in infancy may be as different a phenomenon from childhood increased airway resistance as it is from adult obstructive sleep apnea syndrome. Much more systematic research and collaborative efforts are required in order to better describe and understand underlying pathophysiology. Other types of respiratory events exist, most of which are not clearly understood (12). For example, sighs are considered to be central respiratory pauses following an augmented breath. They are commonly seen in infants and children. These respiratory events may last only several seconds, but on occasion may be prolonged and persist for more than 20–30 seconds. Occasionally they are associated with mild to moderate changes in heart rate and oxygen desaturation. Their clinical significance is unclear and they are most likely a normal physiologic phenomenon. Post-inspiratory (expiratory) apneas have also been identified. These respiratory events appear similar polysomnographically to sighs, however, they are associated with a greater degree of change in heart rate from a sigh and bradycardia into the low 40 beat/min range has been reported. The central portion of these events appear to be a prolonged exhalation against a closed upper airway (most likely the glottis).

The history and physical examination are the most vital aspect of evaluating sleep in infants and children. Initial separation of symptoms into three major categories will greatly assist in evaluation of the problem. Disorders of excessive sleepiness, the sleepless child, and the child with parasomnias emerge. Polysomnography is required under certain circumstances. Those who require further polysomnographic testing can often be determined by further historic and clinical evaluation. However, there is no consensus regarding all indications for polysomnography during childhood. Indications also vary according to the child's age and severity of symptoms. These controversies and some suggestions regarding indications and techniques will be covered in Section II.

THE PHYSICAL EXAMINATION

The physical examination must be comprehensive and include an extensive neuro-developmental evaluation. Focus and order of the examination is generally determined by the presenting complaint as well as the order of hypotheses created and ordered during acquisition of the history (progression of the clinical problem-solving process). A complete discussion of the physical and developmental evaluation of children at various developmental levels is beyond the scope of this text and may be found in several excellent resources (13,14). Nonetheless, the following is an outline of the various systems and focus of the physical examination. It can be applicable for most age groups.

General Appearance

General appearance is considerably important in the initial evaluation of the youngster. Does the child appear well developed for chronologic age, well nourished, well hydrated, or in any acute distress? Does the youngster appear bright and alert, or sluggish and tired? Does the interaction between caretaker/parent and child appear appropriate? Is obesity present? What are the vital signs? Are they appropriate for the youngster's chronologic age? Are anthropomorphic measurements appropriate? Where does the child fall on the growth charts?

Head, Eyes, Ears, Nose, and Throat

1. Head. Where does the youngster's head circumference fall on the growth charts? Is it within two standard deviations from the mean for age and sex? Measurement of head circumference provides a highly accurate assessment of brain growth during infancy and early childhood. Is the head symmetric? Are there any malformations. Are the fontanelles open and appropriate for the youngster's chronologic age? Are there any malformations or deformities of the mid-face region.

2. Eyes. Are the extra-ocular muscles intact grossly? Are there conjugate eye movements? Is there visual fixation and is it appropriate for the youngster's age? Is it appropriate for the youngster's chronologic age? Are the pupils symmetric? Are they directly and consensually equally reactive to light (and in older children, accommodation)? Is the response to rotational nystagmus normal? Are the fundi visible? If visible, are there any abnormalities present (e.g., hemorrhage, exudate, papilledema)? If the fundi are not visible, is there a normal red reflex and is it bilaterally symmetric?

3. Mouth and Throat. Depending upon the age of the child, what are the condition of the teeth? Are there any obvious malformations? Is the tongue and its base appropriate in size? What is the shape, size, and position of the mandible? Are the mandible and maxillae symmetric? Is the oro-pharynx crowded? What are the size, shape, and position of the tonsils? Are there deformities of the hard and/or soft palate? Does the soft palate move appropriately upon phonation? What is the position and size of the uvula? Does the oral airway appear adequate in size? What is the appearance of the posterior pharyngeal walls? Does there appear to be excessive lymphoid tissue present?

4. Nose. Are the anterior nares patent? Is there narrowing in the region of the anterior nasal valve? Is there adequate, unobstructed nasal airflow? Are the nasal turbinates appropriate in size and shape? Are any nasal masses (e.g., polyps) present? Is the nasal septum deviated? Is airflow resistance decreased with manual external dilation of the anterior nasal valve region?

5. Ears and Tympanic Membranes. What are the shape and position of the pinnae (e.g., chromosomal abnormalities are often associated with low set ears)? Are the tympanic membranes intact? Is there bulging, retraction, or air/fluid levels noted (chronic serous otitis media and persistent middle ear effusions are often associated with hypertrophic adenoidal tissue obstructing the nasopharyngeal opening of the eustachian tube)?

Neck

Is the neck symmetric? Is any significant lymphadenopathy present? Are there masses which might result in extrinsic pressure (occlusion) of the airway? Is the trachea in the midline? Is the thyroid palpable? If the thyroid is palpable, is it enlarged? Is there any limitation of active or passive motion?

Chest

Is the chest wall symmetric? Is there evidence of respiratory distress (tachypnea, utilization of accessory muscles of respiration, nasal flaring, grunting, paradoxic breathing)? Is there suprasternal notch retraction with the respiratory cycle? Is there subcostal and intercostal retractions during the respiratory cycle?

Heart

What is the quality of S1? What is the quality of S2? Is the second heart sound appropriately split with the respiratory cycle? Is a third or fourth heart sound present? Are there any murmurs? What is the resting blood pressure? What is the resting pulse? Are pulses palpable in all four extremities? Are pulses equal and symmetric in all four extremities?

Lungs

Is there good air entry in all lung fields? Are breath sounds symmetric? Are there any adventitious transmitted upper-airway sounds? Are there any abnormal pulmonary sounds (e.g., rales/crackles, rhonchi, wheezing, stridor)? Is there any dullness to percussion?

Abdomen

What is the shape of the abdomen? Is it symmetric? If the patient is obese, what is the distribution of the fat pad? Is there any palpable organomegaly? Are there any masses palpable? Are bowel sounds present? What is their quality and frequency? Is there any pain, tenderness, rebound tenderness, or dullness to percussion?

Neurologic

Are the sensory and motor systems grossly intact and symmetric? What is the quality and characteristics of the deep tendon reflexes in the upper and lower extremities, and are they symmetric? Is there good muscle tone and strength? Is it symmetric? Is the patient's gait normal and appropriate for his/her chronologic age? Are any primitive reflexes present? Are there any gross abnormalities of the cranial nerves? Are there any cerebellar or vestibular findings?

Neuro-Developmental Screening

Does the youngster appear to be appropriately developed for her/his chronologic age? Have appropriate developmental landmarks been met at the correct ages? Is the assessment of fine motor, gross motor, language, and personal/social development appropriate for chronologic age? Are there isolated delays or is there global delay in all areas?

REFERENCES

1. Barrows HS, Tamblyn RM. *Problem-based Learning: An Approach to Medical Education.* New York: Springer; 1980.
2. National Commission on Sleep Disorders Research (U.S.). *Wake Up America: A National Sleep Alert.* Washington D.C.: National Commission on Sleep Disorders Research; 1993.
3. Sheldon SH, Ahart S, Levy HB. Sleep patterns in abused and neglected children. *Sleep Res* 1991;20:333.
4. Ferber R. *Solve Your Child's Sleep Problems.* New York: Simon & Schuster; 1985.
5. Sheldon SH, Garay A, Jacobsen J. REM sleep motor disorder in children. *Sleep Res* 1994;23:173.
6. Sheldon SH, Levy HB. Periodic limb movements in childhood. *Sleep Res* 1993;22:70.
7. Guilleminault C, Winkle R. A review of 50 children with OSAS. *Lung* 1981;159:275.
8. Guilleminault C, Winkle R, Korobkin R, Simmons B. Children and nocturnal snoring: evaluation of the effects of sleep-related respiratory resistive load and day-time functioning. *Eur J Pediatr* 1982;139:165–171.
9. Sheldon SH, Spire JP, Levy HB. *Pediatric Sleep Medicine.* Philadelphia: WB Saunders; 1992.
10. Sheldon SH, Irbe D, Applebaum J, Golbin A, Levy HB, Spire JP. Sleep pressure in children with attentional deficits. *Sleep Res* 1991;20A:448.
11. Sheldon SH. Diagnosis and management of upper-airway resistance syndrome in children. *RT* 1994;7:57–64.
12. Sheldon SH, Onal E, Lilie J, Spire JP. Sleep-related post-inspiratory upper airway obstruction in children. *Sleep Res* 1993;22:270.
13. Frankenberg WK, Thornton SM, Cohrs ME. *Pediatric Developmental Diagnosis.* New York: Thieme-Stratton; 1981.
14. Behrman RE, Kliegman RM, Nelson WE, Vaughan VC III, eds. *Textbook of Pediatrics*, 14th ed. Philadelphia: WB Saunders; 1992.

Development of Central Nervous System Function

The central nervous system (CNS) is the executive system that controls sleep, its components, and the sleep/wake cycle. Major changes in the CNS occur across the lifespan. An understanding of these changes is essential in evaluating CNS development polysomnographically and assessing sleep and sleep/wake cycles. This chapter addresses: (i) the developmental anatomy of the CNS and other anatomic considerations; (ii) fundamentals of analysis of EEG in the premature newborn, term newborn, infant, child, and adolescent; (iii) development and ontogenetic characteristics of the EEG and its variations; and (iv) considerations of abnormalities that might appear on EEG during polysomnography.

DEVELOPMENTAL ANATOMY OF THE CNS

Transitions from wake to sleep and sleep-state transitions are under the control of complex neural and biochemical processes. Clearly, both genetic and environmental factors are important in determining morphologic and electrophysiologic maturation of the brain. Understanding the anatomic development of the brain provides a groundwork upon which to comprehend function.

The material basis of brain and spinal cord development begins with the primitive thickened area of ectoderm called the neural plate. Very early in the development of the embryo, this initially flat, single-layer of cells rapidly becomes thickened, stratified, and begins to fold into two neural folds and a central neural groove. The thickened folds soon begin to fuse, rolling the original neural plate into the neural tube. The substance of the neural tube gives rise to all nervous elements whose cell bodies lie within the brain and spinal cord. It also furnishes all the non-nervous supporting tissues of the CNS.

Three distinct zones can be identified: the ependymal layer, the mantle layer, and the marginal layer. The ependymal layer is originally the outermost portion and contains inert supporting cells. Mitotic cells can also be found. It has been shown that these mitotic cells retract from the mantle layer into the ependymal layer when they are about to divide and temporarily lay in this zone (1). The mantle layer is composed of the majority of future neuronal cells that will ultimately form the gray matter of the CNS. The marginal layer consists of a fibrous mesh that provides a zone into which neuronal processes will eventually grow, become linked with other neurons, and connect various centers. This layer will eventually become the white matter of the brain and spinal cord.

Neurogenesis is the process in which primitive neuroblastic epithelium differentiates and specializes into neurons. As differentiation proceeds, each neuroblast becomes bipolar with outgrowths of a fiber-like process that will eventually become the axon. Shortly thereafter, the main cell body becomes multipolar due to the development of dendrites. Migration of neurons, degree of dendritic development and branching, and synaptic connections depend upon the depolarization of the neuron and neuronal networks during development (2).

Even during earliest embryonal development, the form and structure of the brain departs markedly from the simple plan that begins as the neural plate. Even before the neural groove begins to close, there is expansion of the rostral end of the neural axis in the area that will become the brain. Three points of expansion can be identified. Each point is separated by a constricted region. These expansions and constrictions define the basic subdivisions of the brain: prosencephalon (forebrain), mesencephalon (midbrain), and rhombencephalon (hindbrain). The prosencephalon and rhombencephalon subsequently subdivides into two additional secondary regions. However, the mesencephalon remains undivided.

Early in the fourth week post-conception, the prosencephalon develops a dorsal groove that subdivides the forebrain into the telencephalon (destined to become the cerebral hemispheres) and the diencephalon (the area which contain the optic vesicles). Although occurring somewhat later in embryogenesis, the rhombencephalon specializes into the metencephalon (later to become the cerebellum and pons) and the myelencephalon (primitive medulla oblongata).

As these divisions of the brain are differentiating, structural flexure begins. The primitive embryonic brain undergoes drastic angulation simultaneously in three regions: the cephalic flexure in the region of the midbrain, the cervical flexure at the junction of the brain and spinal cord, and the pontine flexure at the junction of the metencephalon and myelencephalon.

The lumen of the primitive tubular brain undergoes dramatic change corresponding to regional specialization of the walls of these cavities. The lumen in the region of the telencephalon extends into the paired future cerebral hemispheres and are destined to become the lateral ventricles. The lumen in the middle of the telencephalon and diencephalon becomes the third ventricle. A narrow canal exists within the mesencephalon that will become the cerebral aqueduct and the lumen of the metencephalon and myelencephalon becomes the fourth ventricle.

Gray matter of the brain is markedly displaced with respect to the regular alignment of cellular columns within the spinal cord. Nuclei of the brain occupy significantly different positions depending upon their particular area of specialization. Mass migration of cells in a directionally oriented response is termed neurobiotaxis and is considered to be determined by the cell bodies movement in the direction of the source from which they receive the majority of neuronal impulses (3).

Mitosis and migration continues throughout the development of the embryo and fetus. Mitosis and completion of localization of individual neurons occurs about 1 year after post-conceptional term. Neuronal activity during development appears to be responsible for migration of neurons to their appropriate position within the CNS, degree of dendritic branching, and strength of synaptic interconnection. During development, two internal processes result in a high degree of neuronal activity: the waking state and active (REM) sleep. It is possible that these two states are important during prenatal and early postnatal life for appropriate ultrastructural development of the CNS.

The myelencephalon is the most caudal portion of the CNS. It is a transitional region between the spinal cord caudally and the medulla oblongata rostrally. It is significant for being a linking pathway where typical features of the spinal cord become rearranged, displaced to new positions, and other elements not identified at lower levels are present. The one main difference between the spinal cord and medulla is the disappearance of a clear demarcation between gray and white matter by a complex merging of elements forming the reticular formation. However, certain areas in this region are spared this fusing and integration and form isolated, nuclear masses. Sensory relay nuclei and motor nuclei of cranial nerves develop within this region. Sensory relay nuclei provide correlating connection with motor nuclei of the myelencephalon through the reticular formation, descending connections with motor centers of the spinal cord, cerebellar connections, and relays with the diencephalon that ultimately end in the cortex.

The metencephalon extends from the isthmus to the pontine flexure at the caudal border of the pons. Inferior structures extend upward through this region. However, two other areas become prominent: the cerebellum dorsally and the pons ventrally. The cerebellum is responsible for coordination of stimuli related to body position and movement. The pons is the principal pathway for conduction of impulses between the cerebellar cortex and the cerebral cortex. In addition, this area contains the fourth ventricle as well as cranial nerve nuclei for the third, fourth, fifth, sixth, seventh, and eighth nerves. The pontine region will also contain executive centers required for regulation of chewing, tasting, swallowing, digestion, respiration, and circulation. The mesencephalon is also primarily associated with reflexes of the eyes and head in response to visual stimuli. It is also the principal pathway for motor fibers that unite the forebrain with lower level nuclei, important areas responsible for characteristics and epi-phenomena of active (REM) sleep.

Development of the diencephalon is essential for establishment of centers that are fundamentally responsible for the control of the sleep/wake cycle and cycling within the sleep state. The diencephalon is prominent during the second month of development, however, it becomes concealed by the greater expansion of adjacent parts of the developing brain. All neuronal impulses that eventually reach the cortex pass through the diencephalon, with the exception of those originating from olfaction. The third ventricle lies within the diencephalon. A small area in the caudal wall of the third ventricle evaginates during the seventh week of development and forms the pineal body. The pineal body eventually becomes conical, solid, and glandular. Melatonin will eventually be secreted by this structure.

After the seventh week of gestation, three main regions of the diencephalon can be identified. These regions include the epithalamus, dorsally; the thalamus, laterally; and the hypothalamus, ventrally. The thalamus rapidly outgrows the epithalamus (which ultimately becomes a synaptic region for olfactory impulses). Neuronal fibers separate the massive gray matter of the walls of the thalamus into numerous thalamic nuclei. Similarly, the walls of the hypothalamus contain various hypothalamic nuclei, the optic chiasm, suprachiasmatic nuclei, and the neural lobe of the stalk and body of the pituitary gland. The hypothalamus eventually becomes the executive region for regulation of all autonomic activity including digestion, sleep, temperature regulation, and emotional behavior.

The telencephalon is the most rostral subdivision of the brain. The two lateral outpouchings form the cerebral hemispheres, each containing a lateral ventricle. Cerebral hemispheres first begin to become prominent in the sixth week of conceptional age and expand rapidly until they overgrow the diencephalon and mesencephalon during the middle of gestation. In higher vertebrates, the telencephalon becomes the most specialized and complex portion of the brain. During development it can be divided into three distinct areas that differ in function: the corpus striatum that is directly continuous with the thalamus; the rhinencephalon; and the neopallium that represents almost all of the externally visible portions of the visible cerebral hemispheres.

ONTOGENESIS OF BRAIN ELECTRICAL ACTIVITY

Neuronal electrical activity is essential for cellular migration, dendritic branching, and synaptic facilitation. Development of EEG activity, however, is quite different from the development of single unit discharges. The EEG is the recording of summation potentials at the skin surface from underlying brain. This underlying activity is significantly influenced by distant and deeper portions of the CNS. Development of electrical activity in the fetus, newborn, child, and adult is tumultuous. Abrupt and striking changes occur between 24-weeks gestation and 3-months post-term. The EEG of the premature infant is most dependent upon conceptional age. After approximately 12-weeks post-conceptional term, the EEG patterns are replaced by different electrical rhythms in different locations. The frequency and differentiation of rhythms increase rapidly during the first year of life.

24 to 28 Weeks Conceptional Age

Although electrical activity is present prior to 24 weeks conceptional age, wakefulness and sleep cannot be differentiated by behavioral characteristics or EEG. During this time of development, the EEG reveals a discontinuous pattern (Fig. 7-1). Periods of limited electrical activity lasting up to 3 minutes are separated by a burst of activity lasting up to 20 seconds. Often this activity is symmetric, rhythmic, and may be composed of alpha, theta, and delta frequencies. Sharp waves are common at these conceptional ages and are normal when they are frontal in location or are sporadic in any location. Sporadic sharp waves and spikes may be normal up to shortly after 40-weeks gestation (4). Abnormalities should be considered if the spikes or sharp transients are repetitive, unilateral, or occur during the quiescent period of the discontinuous pattern.

28 to 32 Weeks Conceptional Age

If a discontinuous activity pattern persists, however, the bursts of activity dramatically shorten and last only about 1 to 2 seconds. Rhythmic theta waves predominate. At 28–29 weeks conceptional age, these waves are bisynchronous. Waves in the delta frequency reappear by 30 weeks. Often, 10- to 20-Hz activity is superimposed upon these slow waves and persist until conceptional term. This superimposed fast activity is termed "delta brushes" (Fig. 7-2).

32 to 36 Weeks Conceptional Age

At this time of development, two patterns of EEG maturation may be seen at different times. The first is a discontinuous pattern of slow waves in the range of 1–2 cycles per second, similar to the previous pattern, but occurring mainly over the occiput. This pattern is typically seen during quiet sleep. The second pattern is seen during wakefulness and active sleep and consists mainly of 1- to 2-Hz, continuous, synchronous, and rhythmic waves appearing diffusely over the occipital, temporal, and central regions.

36 to 40 Weeks Conceptional Age

As term approaches, three EEG patterns can be identified. The pattern of discontinuous activity continues but the pauses are short in duration and is still associated with

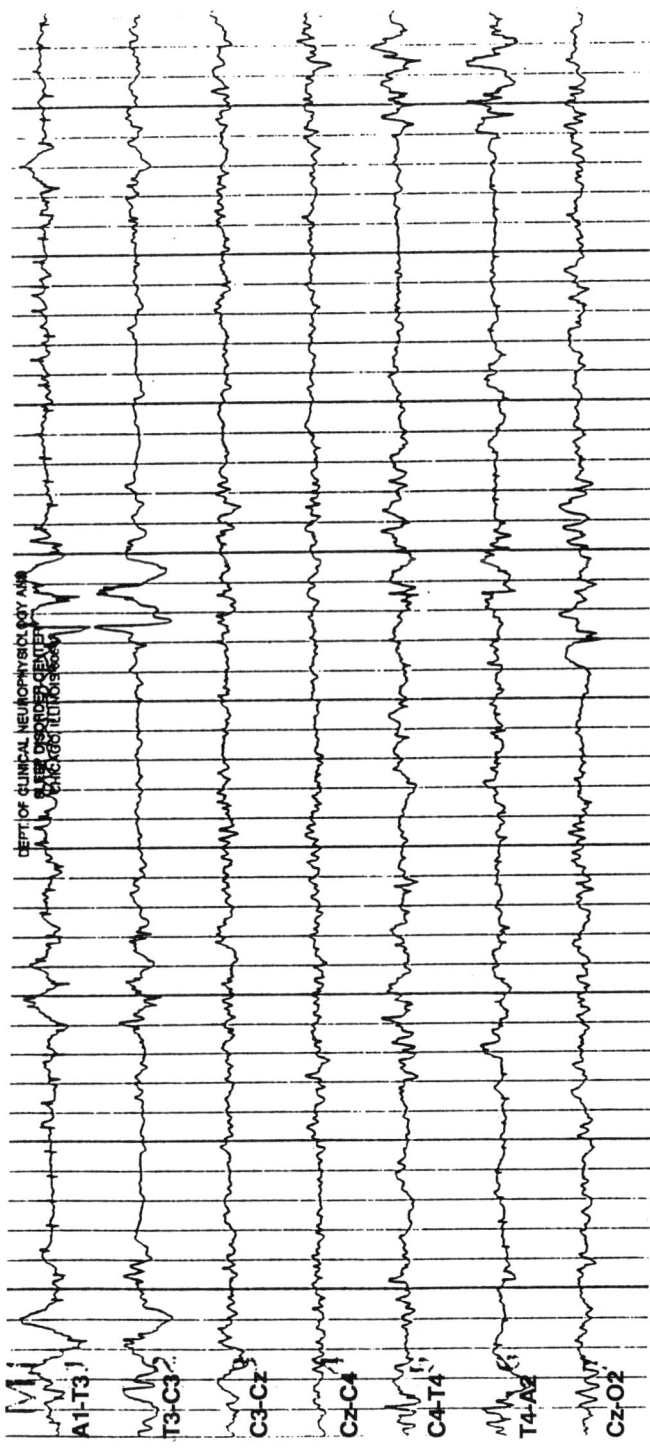

FIG. 7-1. Discontinuous EEG pattern. Periods of limited electrical activity lasting up to 3 minutes are separated by bursts of relatively symmetric alpha, theta, and delta activity.

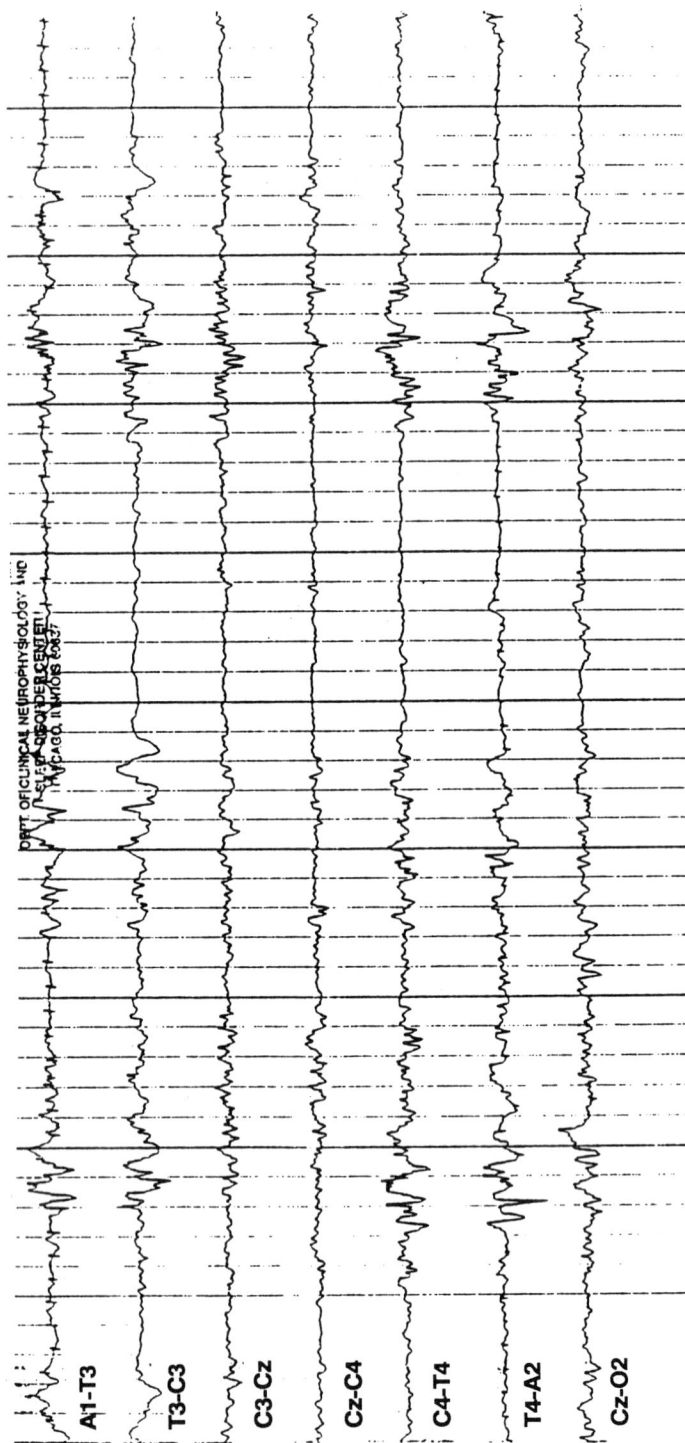

FIG. 7-2. Delta brushes. Ten- to 20-Hz activity is superimposed upon bursts of slow waves.

quiet sleep. The second pattern consists of continuous, irregular slow waves in the theta and delta frequency that appear during wakefulness and active sleep. Delta brushes are still present, but occur less often during active sleep when compared with quiet sleep. At this conceptional age, a new pattern appears that consists of diffuse, irregular slow waves of an amplitude less than 50 microvolts as an alternative to the previous pattern defining wakefulness and active sleep. At conceptional term, four EEG patterns can be identified.

Conceptional Term to 3 Months

At conceptional term, tracé alternant pattern defines quiet sleep (Fig. 7-3A–D). This is a modification of the previous discontinuous pattern and consists of bilateral bursts of high-amplitude slow waves lasting 4 to 5 seconds, alternating with periods of low-amplitude activity of similar duration. During the bursts of slow waves, frontal spikes may appear. Tracé alternant EEG pattern of quiet sleep generally disappears between 3 and 4 weeks post-conceptional term. During this developmental period, a new pattern emerges during quiet sleep that appears to represent the continued development of non-REM sleep. Continuous, high-amplitude slow waves of 0.5 to 2 Hz appear (Fig. 7-4). They are seen maximally in the posterior region of the head. Significantly faster activity of 18–25 Hz is often superimposed upon this slow-wave activity.

Continuous medium activity is the most common EEG pattern seen during active sleep and wakefulness (Fig. 7-5). This pattern consists mainly of 4 to 8 Hz, fairly rhythmic waves of less than 50 microvolts. In addition, another pattern occurs during active sleep that consists of continuous, low-amplitude, mixed slow waves with superimposed larger delta activity that are either intermittent or continuous.

Sleep/wake transitions are generally rapid during this maturational period. Certain behaviors may continue into sleep (e.g., sucking and swallowing) (Fig. 7-6A–C). *The most consistent behavior correlated to sleep in the newborn is persistent eye closure.* Sleep-state transitions are also very rapid. Sleep is entered through active sleep during this developmental period. Sleep-onset REM begins to shift to sleep onset through NREM at about 52 weeks post-conceptional age (approximately 3 months chronologic age). However, REM sleep onset may continue up to about 6 months of age. Active sleep and quiet sleep cycle at about 45 to 60 minutes. Approximately half of the total sleep time consists of active sleep and the other half quiet sleep. Prior to conceptional term in the premature infant, smooth alterations between active sleep and quiet sleep are often difficult to identify. Periods of mixed state exist and are called indeterminant sleep.

A normal sleep EEG often consists of rapid occipital rhythms of low amplitude. Sleep spindles are poorly defined and shifting, central sharp waves may begin to appear. Synchrony is variable, however, this begins to increase between bursts of discontinuous sleep pattern and is nearly completely synchronous by conceptional term.

During wake and sleep, certain EEG phenomena may be present that might be considered abnormal in older children and adults. These EEG characteristics, however, are typically normal in the neonate. Sporadic non-focal spikes, frontal sharp transients, anterior slow-wave activity, and transient asymmetries are not considered abnormal in the neonate. However, persistent phenomena (e.g., frequent focal spikes, persistent asymmetry of activity) may be abnormal, especially if associated with a history of potential abnormality or physical/behavioral findings that suggest abnormality. Under these circumstances, further investigation may be required.

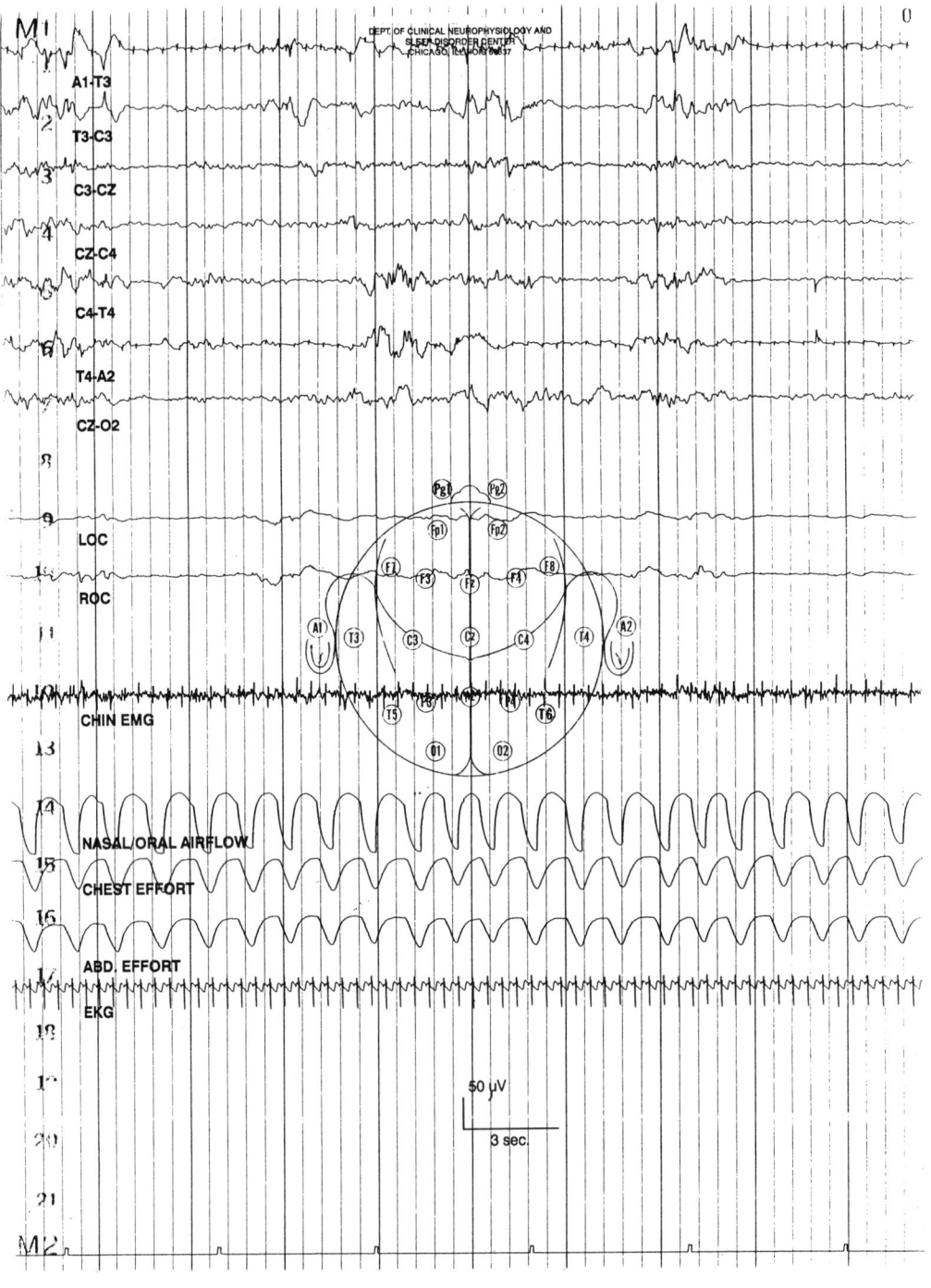

FIG. 7-3. A–D: Tracé alternant pattern of quiet sleep (4 consecutive 30-second epochs [paper speed 10 mm/second] in a term newborn). Note the discontinuous EEG pattern, absence of eye movements, tonic-chin EMG, and monotonously regular respiratory pattern. Multifocal sharp transients present in this tracing are not abnormal.

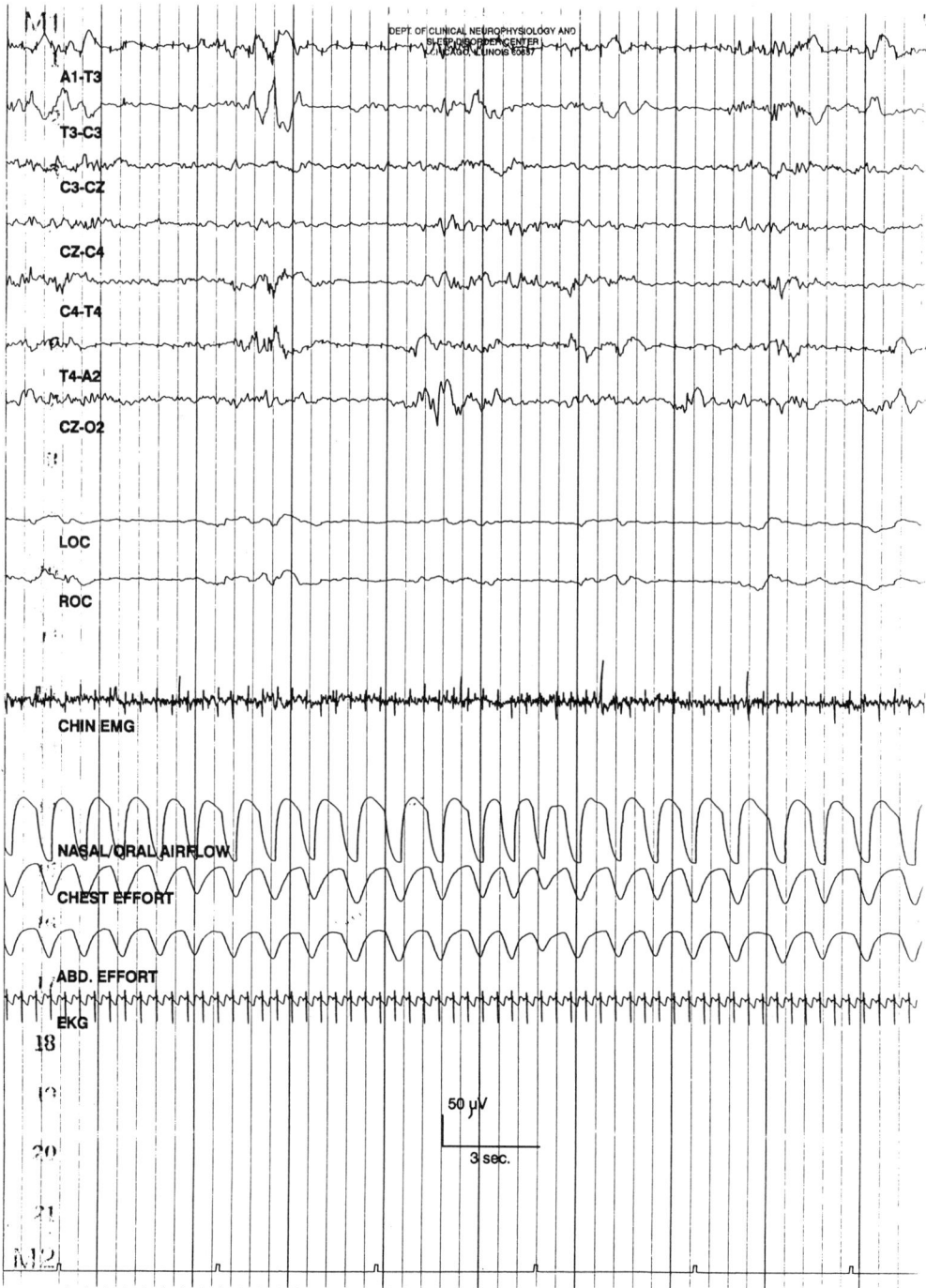

FIG. 7-3. *Continued.*

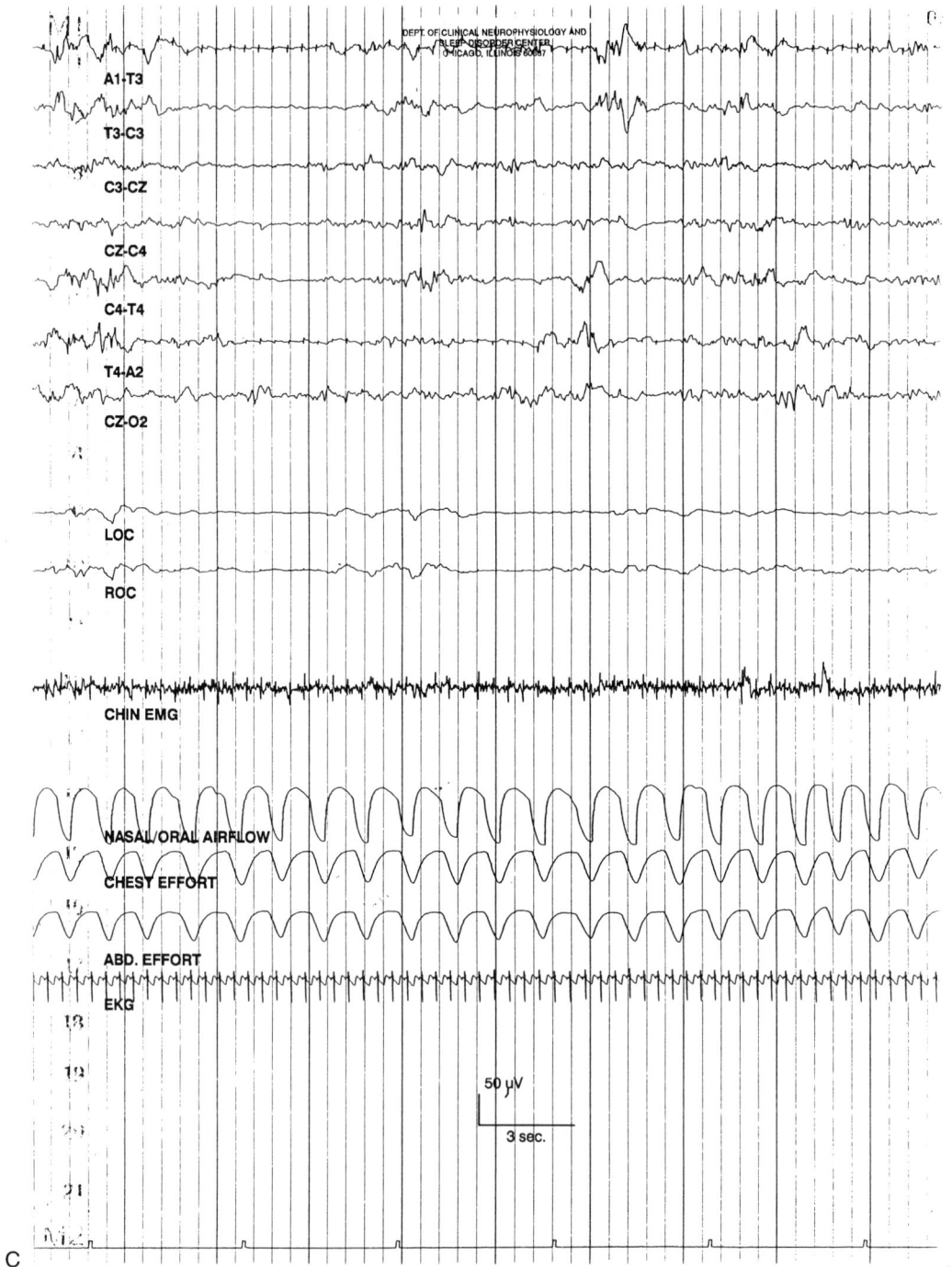

FIG. 7-3. Continued.

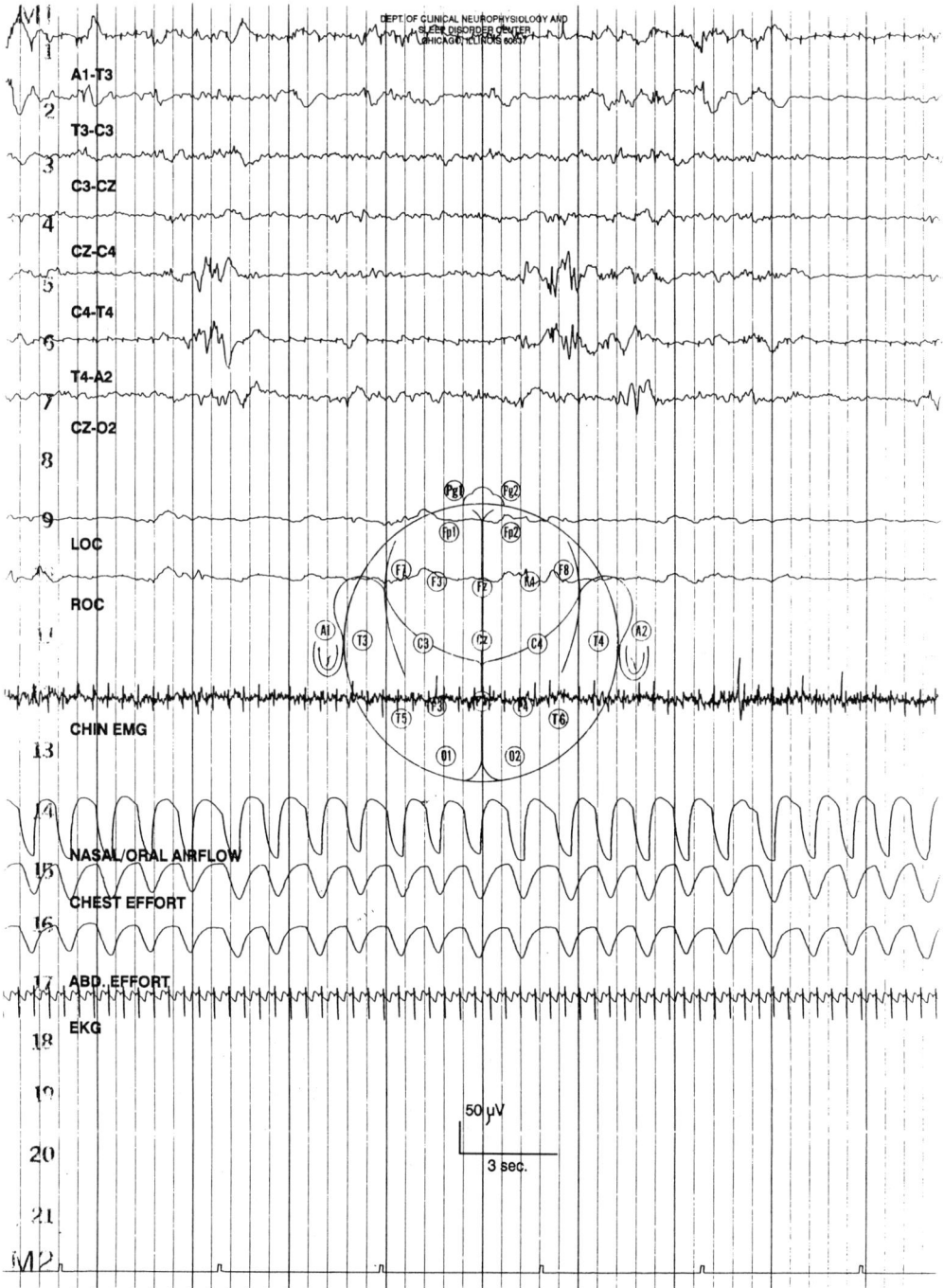

FIG. 7-3. *Continued.*

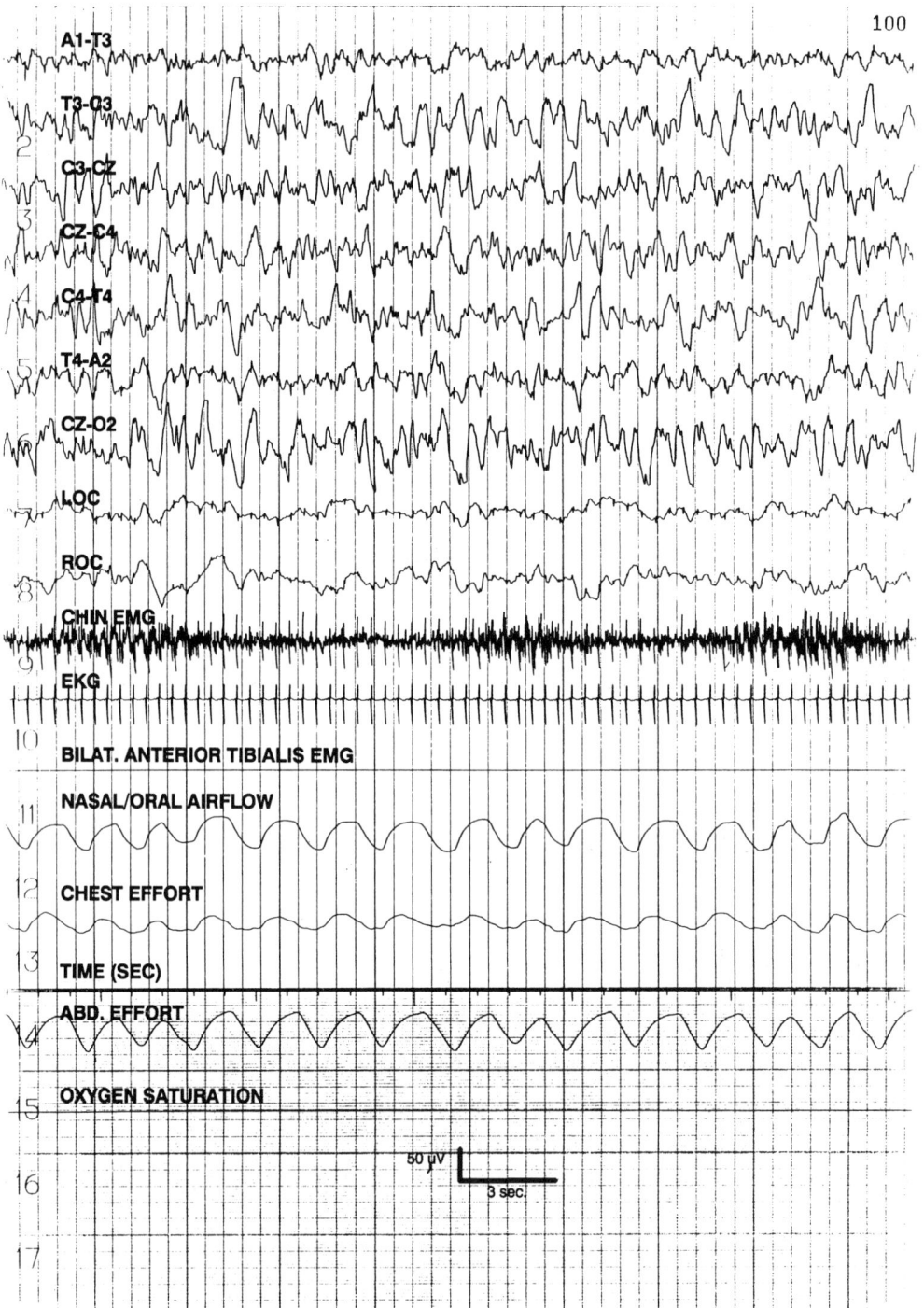

FIG. 7-4. Continuous EEG pattern of NREM sleep in a 7-week-old infant. Note the high-voltage, continuous slow activity. Clear, well-formed sleep spindles are absent. Eye movements are absent and frontal EEG activity can be seen in these channels. The chin muscle EMG is tonic. Waxing and waning chin EMG activity represents "sucking artifact." Respiratory pattern is very regular and stable.

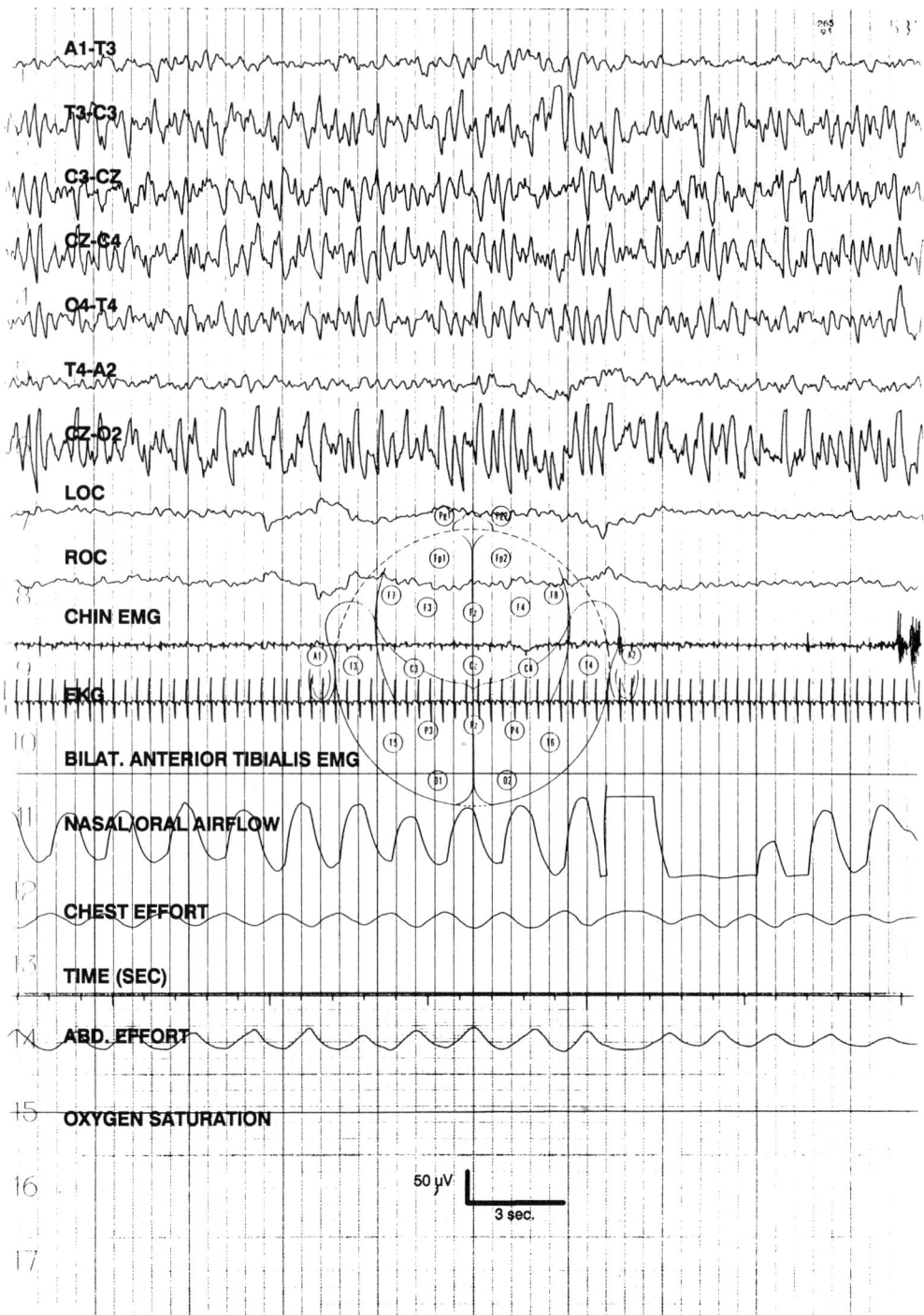

FIG. 7-5. Continuous EEG pattern of active (REM) sleep in a 7-week-old infant. Note the high-voltage, continuous slow activity (approximately 3–). However, this is considerably faster than that seen in NREM sleep (approximately 0.5–1 Hz). Rapid conjugate eye movements are present. Chin EMG reveals significant decrease in tone when compared to NREM/quiet sleep, and phasic twitches can be seen. Respiratory pattern is quite irregular and unstable.

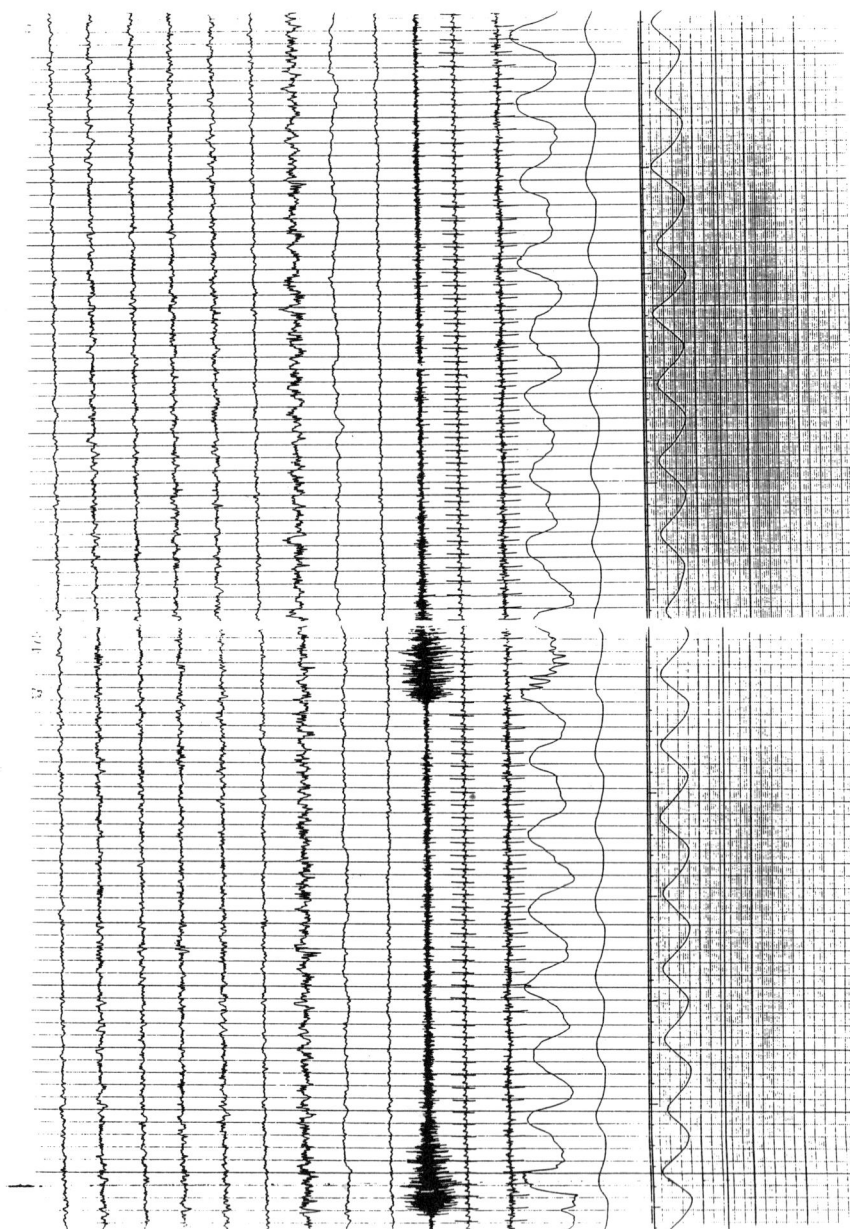

FIG. 7-6. A–C: Sucking artifact. Periodic waxing and waning of chin muscle tone is present in the chin EMG. These sucking movements can persist into transitional sleep.

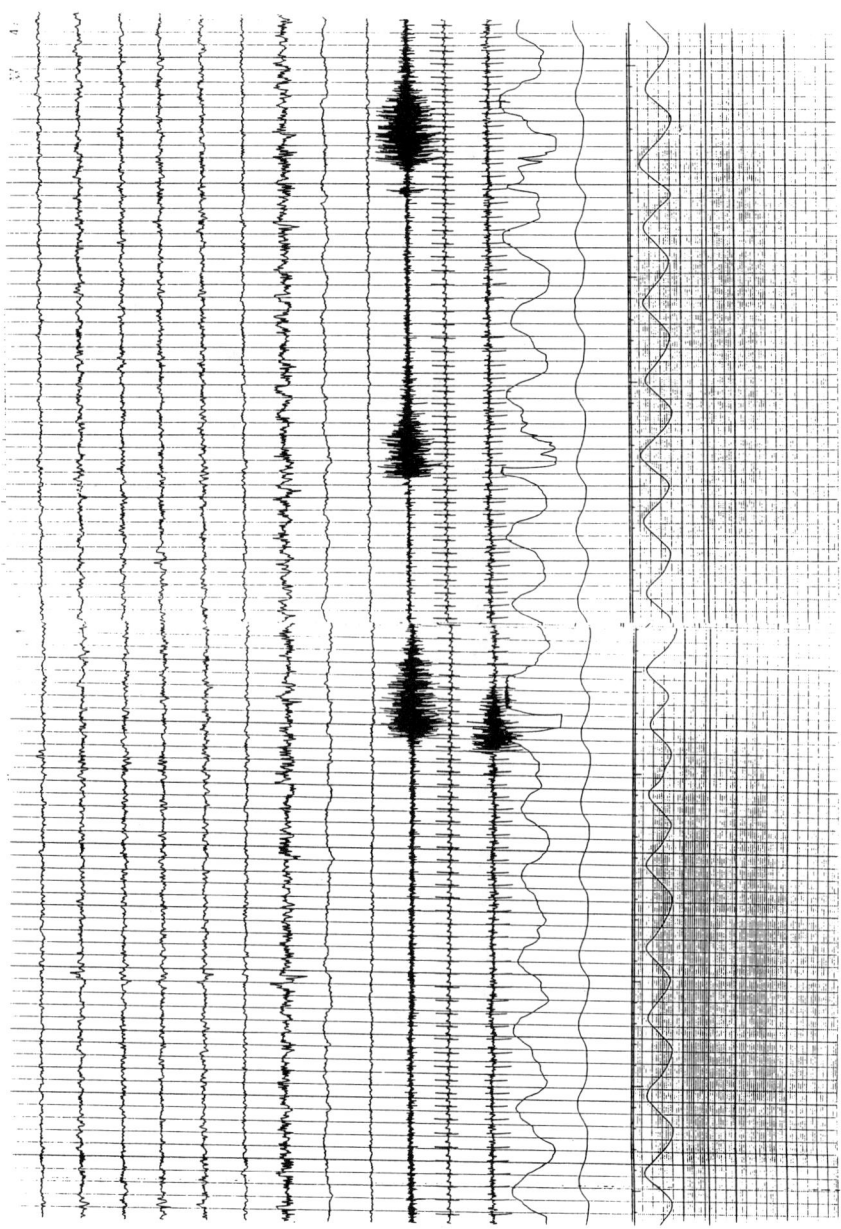

FIG. 7-6. *Continued.*

B

85

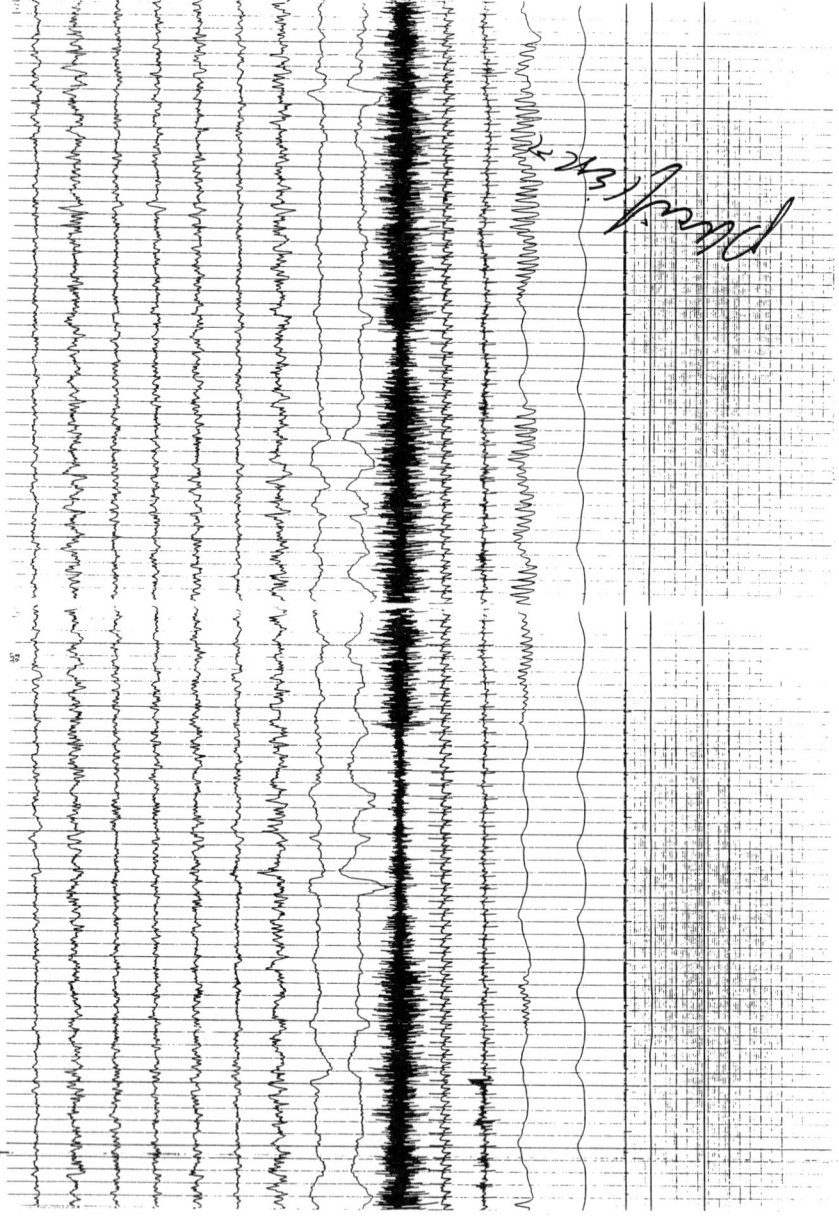

FIG. 7-6. C: Sucking artifact. Sucking on a pacifier and swallowing movements can also result in rhythmic artifact in the nasal/oral airflow channel.

C

3 Months to 12 Months of Age

This period of development of the infant reveals rapid and striking maturational changes in the EEG. Consistent waking patterns begin to emerge. Generalized delta and theta activity appear and is often more prominent posteriorly. During the first year of life, slow-wave activity during wakefulness becomes more rhythmic and diminishes considerably. From 3 to 5 months of age, theta activity increases in prominence in the central and posterior regions and becomes the dominant waking rhythm after 5 months. Absence of theta activity at this stage of development is considered abnormal (4). At 3 months of age relatively high-voltage (50–100 microvolts), 3- to 4-Hz occipital activity is present. By 5 months of age the frequency increases to about 5 Hz and continues to increase across the first year to about 6–8 Hz at 12 months of age. Voltage of this activity also decreases by about 25% over this period of time.

During this time of development, sleep-wake transitions are relatively smooth. As the transition begins, amplitude of waveforms increases and the frequency decreases. Rhythmic and synchronous 75–200 microvolts, 3- to 5-Hz activity becomes predominant.

Major changes in the sleep EEG occur over the first year of life. Tracé alternant in the newborn that is gradually replaced by the continuous slow-wave pattern by 3 months of age become more mature. Clear sleep spindles consisting of waxing and waning, medium-amplitude synchronous waves of about 12–14 Hz appear at about 6–8 weeks of age. They first appear in the central regions but then expand in distribution. Between 2–6 months sleep spindles assume mature characteristics and appear almost continuously throughout NREM sleep. Complete absence of sleep spindles between 3 to 6 months is most likely abnormal. Prior to 6 months, sleep spindles are asymmetric over the two hemispheres. They slowly become synchronous between 6–8 months. *Persistence of asymmetric spindles after 12 months of age may represent a unilateral decrease in electrical activity of the brain.*

Sleep spindles are a ubiquitous phenomenon in sleep of older children and adults. But, their physiology and the affects of neurologic disorders on their frequency and amplitude are incompletely understood. Differences in spindle frequency can be due to underlying encephalopathy, physiologic differences between partial and generalized epilepsy, as well as possible residual effects of a variety of anticonvulsant medication (5).

Spindle patterns (density, duration, frequency, amplitude, asymmetry, and asynchrony) develop quite rapidly between 1.5 and 3 months of age. This rapid development most likely reflects developmental changes in thalamo-cortical structures (6). Spindle expression varies in relation to ascending reticular activating tone, constituting a functionally inhibitory thalamo-cortical response to neurophysiologic conditions that promote central activation (7). Density of 12- to 14-Hz activity is greater in stage 2 sleep than in slow-wave sleep (6). Three months of age appears to be a significant juncture in the maturational process. Sleep-spindle evolution seems to be an accurate reflection of significant maturation of CNS processes and resultant behaviors that occur at 10 to 12 weeks of age, and in the development of NREM states and slow-wave sleep. Concordance between quantitative aspects and nocturnal organization of slow-wave sleep in infants occurs from about 4.5 months (6).

Children with CNS abnormalities and neuroradiologic and/or clinical neurologic findings frequently reveal asymmetric spindles/unilateral suppression of spindle activity (8). These EEG findings correlate as well as focal slowing in lateralizing the neuroradiologic and clinical neurologic findings.

At 3 months of age, clear demarcation of NREM states by EEG criteria is quite difficult. By 6 months, however, NREM-sleep state can typically be differentiated into three distinct states (stage 1, stage 2, and slow-wave sleep) and the EEG takes on a more mature pattern. Although rudimentary, vertex sharp transients and K-complexes can be identified in the neonatal period and typically appear for the first time between 5 and 6 months of age. Vertex waves are generally seen during lighter stages of sleep (stage 1 and 2), are of high amplitude (up to 250 microvolts), negative polarity, and last less than 200 milliseconds. K-complexes are similar to vertex waves, but are considerably slower (lasting at least 0.5 seconds). K-complexes are often followed by a sleep spindle and have a wide distribution about the vertex. Both vertex waves and K-complexes can occur in short bursts, appear spontaneously, or may occur in response to a sudden sensory stimulus.

REM-sleep EEGs also undergo transformation with a decrease in the amplitude, a slight increase in and an admixture of activity frequency. Saw-tooth waves appear and the electrical pattern gradually begins to resemble a more mature, relatively low-voltage, mixed frequency pattern. By 3–5 months of age, the percentage of REM sleep decreases and occupies about 40% of total sleep time. By the end of the first year of life, total REM time equals about 30% of total sleep time.

CHANGES DURING EARLY AND MIDDLE CHILDHOOD

Slow, consistent, and continuous change are hallmarks of early and middle childhood. However, toward the end of middle childhood, these changes are more subtle, evolve over a longer period of time, and become more consistent and reproducible.

Waking rhythms with the eyes closed gradually increase from about 5–7 Hz, relative high-voltage activity to the typical sinusoidal 8- to 12-Hz frequency of low- to medium-voltage activity characteristic of the adult pattern. It is most prominent over the occipital regions of the head. This developing alpha rhythm is characteristic of relaxed wakefulness with eyes closed. It is easily attenuated with eye opening, focusing attention, or increased vigilance. Well-developed alpha activity is present in most normal children by 8 years of age. The amplitude of alpha activity gradually increases during early and middle childhood, but remains relatively low to moderate in amplitude during puberty, adolescence, and adulthood (4).

Transitional sleep patterns of drowsiness can be identified after 1–2 years of age. This wake/sleep transition becomes more mature and alpha activity diffuses and becomes admixed with slower, mixed-frequency activity. Brief micro-sleep episodes occur and become more frequent during drowsiness and during transitional sleep (stage 1). The micro-sleep episodes become longer, consolidate, alpha activity drops out of the EEG, muscle tone may decrease slightly, and slow rolling eye movements are clearly evident.

Slow, high-voltage activity that is very prominent during infancy and early childhood decreases significantly during early and middle childhood. Diffuse synchronous theta activity is very prominent between 1 and 4 years. This activity begins to diminish after 4 years and by 5 to 6 years of age alpha activity is about equally prominent. After 6 years of age, alpha becomes the predominant waking rhythm. However, hypersynchronous theta (Fig. 7-7) activity during stage 1 and early stage 2 sleep is very common during this phase of development. Indeed, even a theta-delta pattern (Fig. 7-8) can frequently be identified during slow-wave sleep in some children.

All stages of sleep are easily discernible during middle childhood. NREM-sleep states can be clearly differentiated and become more similar to adult stages 1–4. Although fre-

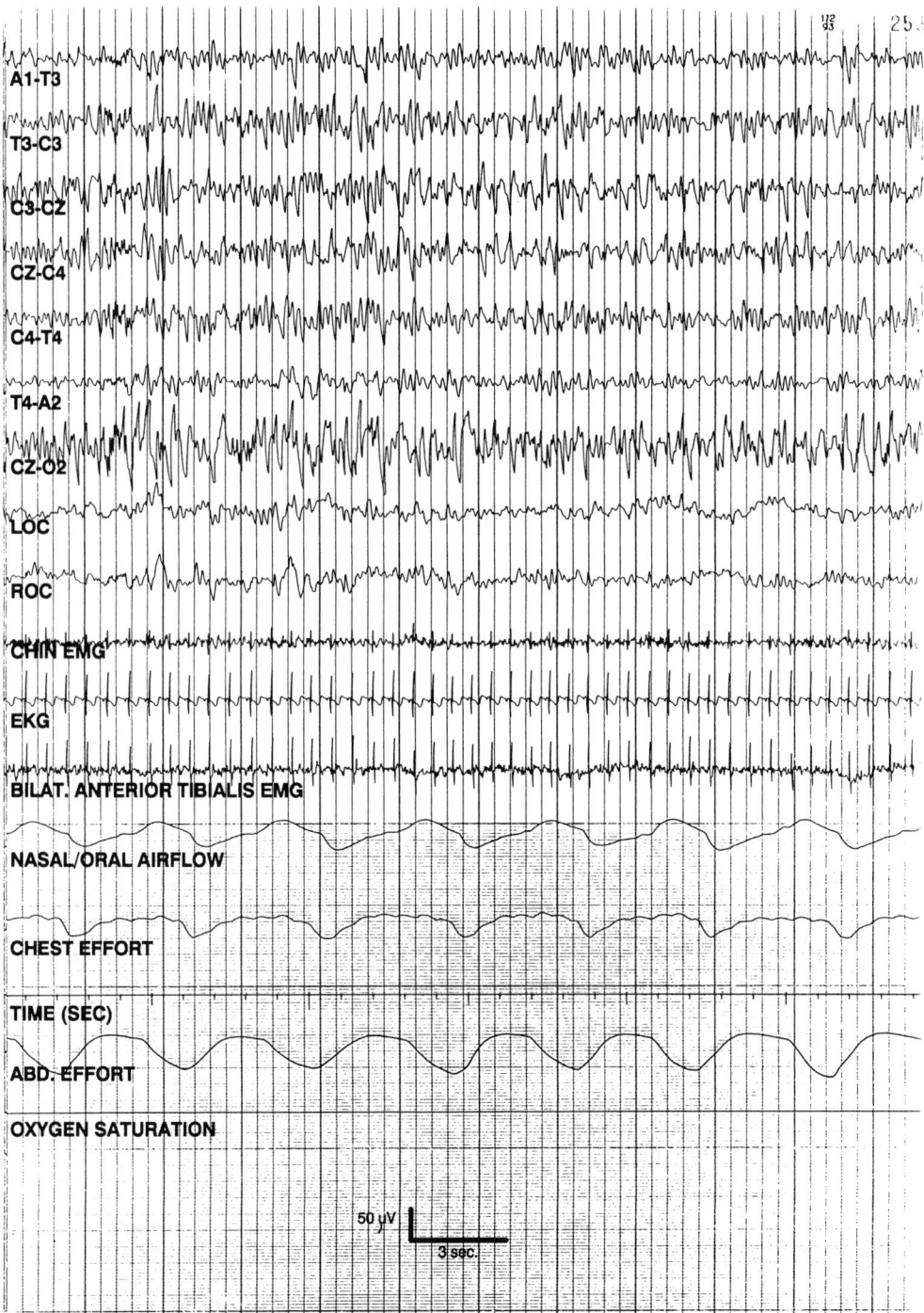

FIG. 7-7. A–B: Hypersynchronous theta activity. Intense hypersynchronous theta activity can be seen in the EEG of this 12-month-old infant. It occurs during transitional sleep as well as stage 2 NREM. However, it can be present throughout all NREM states, especially in older infants, toddlers, and young children.

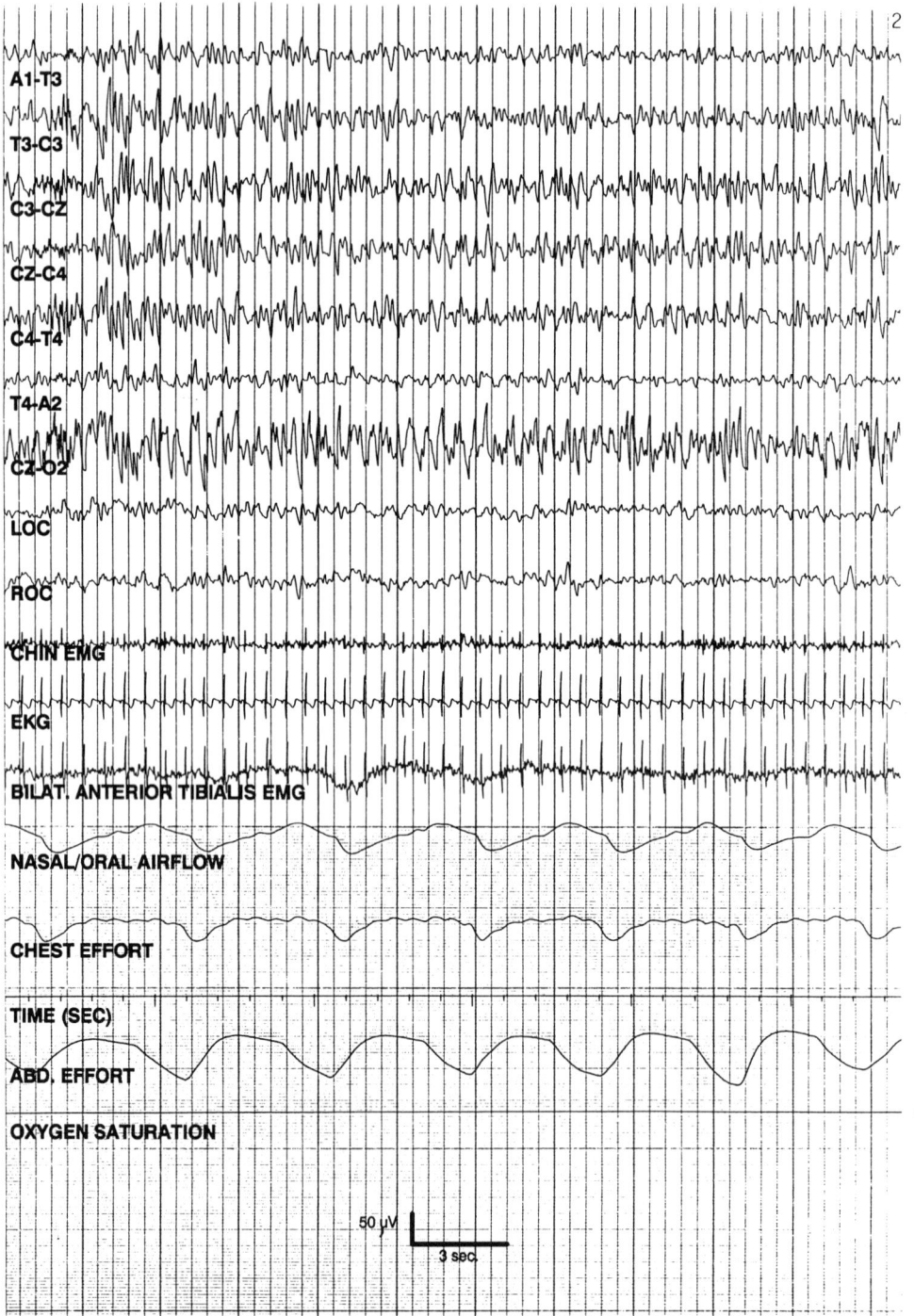

FIG. 7-7. *Continued.*

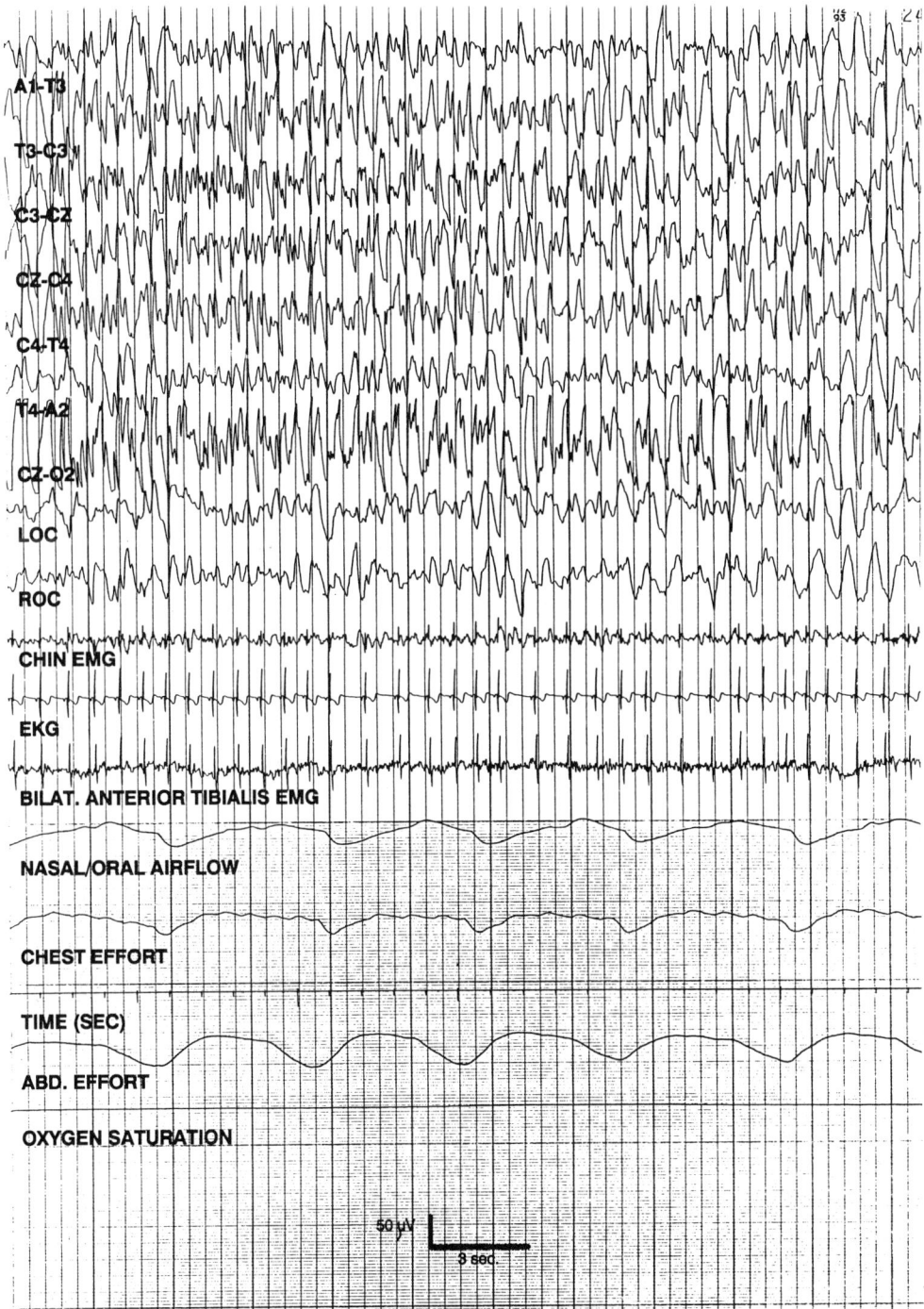

FIG. 7-8. Theta-delta pattern. At times, hypersynchronous theta activity is so ubiquitous in the EEG of some children, it may persist into slow-wave sleep and result in a theta-delta pattern. This is most likely a normal variation and the clinical significance of this finding is unknown. It can result in difficulty and underscoring of slow-wave sleep. On occasion it can be seen in older children with NREM slow-wave sleep motor parasomnias as an isolated finding.

quencies are somewhat slower in children and gradually increase to adult frequencies, the most striking difference is in the higher amplitude of wave forms at all frequencies until puberty, where a more adult pattern is notable. Positive occipital sharp transients of sleep (POSTS) begin to appear during late childhood and adolescence. This activity tends to occur during stage 1 sleep and wake/sleep transitions. Fourteen and six positive bursts are also present during transitional sleep and are more common during childhood than in adults. Both of these wave forms are most likely normal.

From early through middle childhood, structure of EEG sleep also assumes a more mature adult characteristic (8). During later infancy, sleep cycles last about 40 to 50 minutes. This cycle length increases gradually to about 60 minutes by 18–24 months and to 90 minutes by 5 years. REM-sleep EEG activity also assumes adult characteristics and cycles regularly with NREM sleep. After 3 months of age, most infants will shift from entering sleep through REM sleep to entering sleep through NREM sleep. This transition is generally complete by about 6 months to 8 months. Percent of REM sleep also gradually continues to decrease from 50% at conceptional term to 30% by 1–2 years, and 20% to 25% by 3–5 years of age.

THE ABNORMAL EEG AND POLYSOMNOGRAPHY

Traditional polysomnography involves recording one to two channels of EEG. Typically this includes one central and one occipital channel. A single channel of EEG is sufficient (when coupled with behavioral observations) to accurately *stage* sleep. Staging sleep has been considered important in evaluation of other physiologic phenomena that occur during sleep and are (or might be) state dependent. Unfortunately, a single channel of EEG recording appears to be inadequate to evaluate appropriate development of the CNS and to identify CNS abnormalities that might be *instrumental in governing the function of these other systems of interest.* In addition, development of CNS activity and function follows an orderly and exquisitely consistent progression. Although there tends to be rather wide individual variations, internal organization varies very little and state organization may be an easily distinguishable and recordable variable that can determine prognosis and outcome well before clinical evidence becomes apparent (10).

Single or dual channel EEG cannot provide all information needed to arrive at an adequate assessment of sleep in children. Therefore, multiple channels of EEG recording are recommended during polysomnography conducted on infants and children. By obtaining more comprehensive electrophysiologic data, further assessments of current and anticipated neurophysiologic problems may be made. For example, characteristic EEG patterns typify the developing infant's conceptional age (+ 2 weeks) (11). Therefore, more complete EEG evaluation during polysomnography is an excellent method for measuring brain maturation in premature neonates.

Extrauterine and intrauterine development of bioelectrical brain activity develops according to the conceptional age, regardless of variable extrauterine experiences (12). However, other categories of behavioral and neurophysiologic activities (e.g., the Moro reflex, state stability, crying, sucking) are more labile to environmental and pathologic factors.

Relationships among EEG characteristics of sleep provides significant information regarding CNS development. After neonatal illness, patterns of recovery of abnormal EEG can provide significant prognostic information (13). Comprehensive sleep analysis can significantly assist in assessing prognosis in infants who have suffered perinatal hypoxic brain injury (14). Poor prognosis has been shown to be associated with a decreased level of active sleep, sleep cycling disturbances, persistence of the tracé alternant EEG pattern of quiet sleep after 1–2 weeks of conceptional term, immaturity in bioelectrical activity of 4 weeks or more, and depression of background EEG activity. The prognosis of premature infants after hypoxic injury is improved if the EEG is normal and/or if sleep spindles are present (14). Although individual measures of consistency in maintaining waking-sleeping state during the neonatal period are variable between infants in the neonatal period, individual state concordance in the newborn period correlates quite well with long-term outcome (10).

Interestingly, a distinctive pattern of EEG termed premature temporal theta (PT-theta) can be identified in very premature infants (15). PT-theta is found independently over both temporal areas, but predominantly on the right side. It is associated with wakefulness, but mainly with active-sleep EEG. Standard polysomnography scoring channels are inadequate to identify such activity. Percentage of PT-theta increases from about 24–25 weeks conceptional age to its maximum at about 29–31 weeks. The PT-theta activity then gradually decreases during CNS maturation and is generally absent by conceptional term. Premature infants without PT-theta activity or with significantly low percentages typically have neurologic and/or other significant medical abnormalities.

Electrographic and/or clinical seizures are common in the stressed neonate. Often these seizures are occult. Almost 80% of seizures in infants with neonatal seizure disorders are subclinical (16). Clinical condition does not seem to assist in determining the frequency of seizures in these infants. Unaided visual inspection of infants seriously underestimate true seizure frequency. Long-term and comprehensive sleep EEG may be more reliable in many cases to determine true seizure frequency and to judge the adequacy of anticonvulsant treatment.

Each major epileptic syndrome in infants and children demonstrates clear relationships to sleep and wakefulness that are particular to that syndrome (17). In addition, sleep and wake alter symptomatology or type, alter distribution and composition of epileptiform wave forms, and change duration and composition of sleep stages. The latter may play a significant role in impacting development of the CNS. Although interictal, routine diurnal EEG recordings often appear normal, inter-ictal sleep records of individuals with major motor, generalized seizures often show EEG abnormalities during NREM sleep. Therefore, patients with uncertain or unknown types of seizure disorders should routinely be examined during sleep (18).

DEVELOPMENT OF EEG SLEEP CHARACTERISTICS

Comparison of EEG sleep measures vary significantly between healthy full-term and premature infants at matched conceptional age (19). When preterm infants are compared with tern newborns, the premature exhibits:

1. a longer ultradian cycle length (70 minutes versus 53 minutes);
2. increased percentage of quiet sleep and tracé alternant pattern (34% versus 28%);
3. fewer number and shorter duration of arousals;
4. fewer body movements, especially in quiet sleep; and
5. fewer rapid eye movements during active sleep.

In premature infants, the tracé alternant pattern of quiet sleep disappears earlier in the premature than in the term infant (20). In the premature infant, this pattern generally disappeared at a mean chronologic age of 21.4 days versus 33.4 days for the term infant. In addition, POSTS appeared earlier in the preterm infant. There seems to be no chronologic age difference between premature infants and term infants with respect to the age of shift from active-sleep onset to NREM-sleep onset, activity-sleep and quiet-sleep percentages of the total sleep time, and the age of disappearance of frontal sharp waves. Therefore, it appears that in clinical practice, maturational characteristics of EEG sleep can be applied to premature infants and term infants without requiring significant correction for conceptional age.

Similar patterns of EEG development can be seen during day-time sleep recordings in term infants less than 13 weeks of age. The tracé alternant pattern of quiet sleep can be identified in almost all infants up to 2-weeks post-term, but completely disappears by 6 weeks of age. Active-sleep onset occurs in 80% of day-time sleep episodes at 1 to 3 weeks of age. This decreases rapidly, however, over the next 4–6 weeks of development, but can still be present in 5% to 10% of day-time sleep episodes at 8 to 13 weeks of age (21).

Cerebral function monitoring can provide a simple addition to developmental assessment of the infant. When tracings were obtained from neonates less than 3 weeks chronologic age, significant correlations were found with the weight of the neonate at the time of the recording (22). When tracings of premature neonates were obtained at mean chronologic age of 6 weeks, a relationship was found between EEG measures and Apgar scores.

REFERENCES

1. Arey LB. *Developmental Anatomy: A Textbook and Laboratory Manual for Embryology.* Philadelphia: WB Saunders; 1966.
2. Oksenberg A, Marks G, Farber J, et al. Effect of REM sleep deprivation during the critical period of neuroanatomical development of the cat visual system. *Sleep Res* 1986;15:53.
3. Windle WF. Neurofibrillar development in the central nervous system of cat embryos between 8 and 12 mm long. *J Comp Neurol* 1933;58:643–733.
4. Spehlmann R. *EEG Primer.* Amsterdam: Elsevier; 1981.
5. Drake ME Jr, Pakalnis A, Padamadan H, Weate SM, Cannon PA. Sleep spindles in epilepsy. *Clin Electroencephalogr* 1991;22:144–149.
6. Louis J, Zhang JX, Revol M, Debilly G, Challamel MJ. Ontogenesis of nocturnal organization of sleep spindles: a longitudinal study during the first 6 months of life. *Electroencephalogr Clin Neurophysiol* 1992;83:289–296.
7. Bowersox SS, Kaitin KI, Dement WC. EEG spindle activity as a function of age: relationship to sleep continuity. *Brain Res* 1985;334:303–308.
8. Willis J, Schiffman R, Rosman NP, Kwan ES, Ehrenberg BL, Rice JC. Asymmetries of sleep spindles and beta activity in pediatric EEG. *Clin Electroencephalogr* 1990;21:48–50.
9. Sheldon SH, Spire JP, Levy HB. *Pediatric Sleep Medicine.* Philadelphia: WB Saunders; 1992.
10. Lombroso CT, Matsumiya Y. Stability in waking-sleep states in neonates as predictor of long-term neurological outcome. *Pediatrics* 1985;76:52–63.
11. Tharp BR. Electrophysiological brain maturation in premature infants: an historical perspective. *J Clin Neurophysiol* 1990;7:302–314.
12. Lombroso CT. Neurophysiological observations in diseased newborns. *Biol Psychiatry* 1975;10: 527–558.
13. Scher MS. A developmental marker of central nervous system maturation: part II. *Pediatr Neurol* 1988; 4:329–336.
14. Gyorgy I. Prognostic value of sleep analysis in newborns with perinatal hypoxic brain injury. *Acta Paediatr Acad Sci Hung* 1983;24:1–6.
15. Hughes JR, Fino JJ, Hart LA. Premature temporal theta (PT theta). *Electroencephalogr Clin Neurophysiol* 1987;67:7–15.
16. Clancy RR, Legido A, Lewis D. Occult neonatal seizures. *Epilepsia* 1988;29:256–261.
17. Donat JF, Wright FS. Sleep, epilepsy, and the EEG in infancy and childhood. *J Child Neurol* 1989;4: 84–94.
18. Wu L, Liu X, Feng Y. Sleep grand mal—all-night polygraphic EEG recordings in 20 cases. *Jpn J Psychiatry Neurol* 1992;46:395–399.

19. Scher MS, Steppe DA, Dahl RE, Asthana S, Guthrie RD. Comparison of EEG sleep measures in healthy full-term and preterm infants at matched conceptional ages. *Sleep* 1992;15:442–448.
20. Ellingson RJ, Peters JF. Development of the EEG and day-time sleep patterns in low risk premature infants during the first year of life: longitudinal observations. *Electroencephalogr Clin Neurophysiol* 1980: 50:165–171.
21. Ellingson RJ, Peters JF. Development of EEG and day-time sleep patterns in normal full-term infants during the first 3 months of life: longitudinal observations. *Electroencephalogr Clin Neurophysiol* 1980; 49:112–124.
22. Viniker DA, Maynard DE, Scott DF. Cerebral function monitor studies in neonates. *Clin Electroencephalogr* 1984;15:185–192.

SECTION II

Developmental Polysomnography

Research and clinical observations regarding sleep in the pediatric population have clearly shown that children are not just small adults. Valid laboratory techniques and evaluation procedures must be modified for the newborn, infant, and child patient. Indeed, requirements for assessment and management of children in the sleep disorders center or laboratory requires highly specialized knowledge, experience, and expertise.

The pediatric patient undergoes neurodevelopmental changes over time. Changes are both anatomic and physiologic. Transformation is sometimes very rapid, and at other times it is quite slow, stable, and monotonous. Pediatric sleep medicine must focus on this metamorphosis. It must center on differences that occur longitudinally, rather than on the steady and consistent pattern of sleep in adults. Inter-subject variability and intra-subject variation may be greater in newborns, infants, and children when compared to adults. Therefore, evaluation of pediatric patients requires a different strategy. This approach might be termed *developmental polysomnography*. Each chapter in Section II presents a paradigm developed from available literature and experience regarding clinical and laboratory considerations across various developmental stages. Focus will be placed on indications for polysomnography; polysomnographic techniques and variations at different developmental levels; scoring criteria and state determination; and interpretation of a variety of abnormalities and aberrations that might be encountered in the clinical and/or laboratory evaluation.

Because of the structure of the following presentation, resources used to develop paradigms have not been individually referenced, unless circumstances permitted or warranted. Knowledge gleaned from research, scholarly activity, observations, experience, and opinion presented in these major resource textbooks has been consolidated. The following literature was employed:

1. Ferber R. *Solve Your Child's Sleep Problems.* New York: Simon & Schuster; 1985.
2. Guilleminault C, ed. *Sleep and Its Disorders in Children.* New York: Raven Press; 1987.
3. Sheldon SH, Spire JP, Levy HB. *Pediatric Sleep Medicine.* Philadelphia: WB Saunders; 1992.
4. Kryger MH, Roth T, Dement WC, eds. *Principles and Practice of Sleep Medicine.* Philadelphia: WB Saunders; 1989.
5. Rechtschaffen A, Kales A, eds. *A Manual of Standardized Terminology, Techniques and Scoring System for Sleep Stages of Human Subjects.* Los Angeles: UCLA Brain Information Service, NINDS Neurological Information Network; 1968.
6. Anders T, Emde R, Parmelee A, eds. *A Manual of Standardized Terminology, Techniques and Criteria for Scoring of States of Sleep and Wakefulness in Newborn Infants.* UCLA Brain Information Service, NINDS Neurological Information Network; 1971.
7. Guilleminault C, ed. *Sleeping and Waking Disorders: Indications and Techniques.* Boston: Butterworths; 1982.
8. Diagnostic Classification Steering Committee: Thorpy MJ, chairman. *International Classification of Sleep Disorders: Diagnostic and Coding Manual.* Rochester, MN: American Sleep Disorders Association; 1990.
9. Spehlmann R. *EEG Primer.* Amsterdam: Elsevier; 1981.

10. Anch AM, Browman CP, Mitler MM, Walsh JK. *Sleep: A Scientific Perspective.* Englewood Cliffs, NJ: Prentice-Hall; 1988.
11. Hauri P. *The Sleep Disorders.* Kalamazoo, MI: The Upjohn Co.; 1982.
12. Cartwright RD. *A Primer on Sleep and Dreaming.* Reading, MA: Addison-Wesley; 1978.
13. Parks JD. *Sleep and Its Disorders. Major Problems in Neurology*, vol 14. London: WB Saunders; 1985.
14. Mendelson WB. *Human Sleep: Research and Clinical Care.* New York: Plenum; 1987.

8

Pediatric Polysomnographic Techniques

The most important aspect in obtaining a high-quality polysomnographic recording in the premature and term newborn infant is methodical and careful preparation. This includes preparing both the parent and child for the procedures, as well as preparing the sites for application of the variety of sensors used in the study.

Prior to the laboratory study, parents should be provided a comprehensive description of the procedure and must be given ample time to ask questions about the study, its technique, and what to expect from the night and from the results. Reassurance of parents and alleviation of fears from the unfamiliar laboratory environment and complex procedures greatly assists in parental compliance and assistance during set-up and throughout the course of the study. A comprehensive written explanation of the polysomnographic procedures may also be given to the parents prior to the study. Parents should be required to stay overnight in the laboratory with their children.

In our laboratories, we ask parents to arrive at least 1 hour prior to the anticipated time of lights-out. Lights-out should be modified to the habitual time of the youngster's time of lights-out at home. Ample time prior to lights-out provides time for acclimation to the laboratory, time for parents and infant to settle into the strange environment and time for parents or caretakers to ask any final questions prior to the investigation. Reassurance and alleviating concerns will greatly improve comfort. Parental comfort and confidence in the staff is frequently transmitted to the infant decreasing the natural tendency for tactile defensiveness in a strange environment, during set up and during the procedure.

Similar preparatory procedures are conducted whenever the infant is brought to the laboratory for polysomnography, regardless of whether the newborn is an outpatient or has not yet left the hospital. In the absence of a parent or caretaker (as frequently occurs in neonatal inpatients undergoing polysomnography), nursing care must be immediately available. It is also recommended that a one-to-one technician-to-patient ratio be utilized during the course of set-up and study.

Choice of the recording environment is extremely important. The premature infant and sick term newborn are most likely best studied in the neonatal nursery. Transport of the infant to the laboratory may pose significant risk especially if distance between the two sites is great. Neonates maintain core body temperature by non-shivering thermogenesis. In order to increase body temperature under cool environmental conditions, metabolic rate must increase. With an increase in metabolic rate, consumpton of oxygen and glucose within the Kreb cycle increases and places the tenuous infant at high risk for hypoxemia and hypoglycemia. If the recording environment is too cool, motor activity and muscle tone, therefore, increases in order to maintain core temperature at a homeothermic level (1). Variations in light and sound levels in the nursery can also increase motor activity during sleep (2).

State is related to both maturity of the central nervous system (CNS) based on conceptional age as well as environmental conditions. These state variations based on environmental conditions are more marked in the premature infant. Environmental humidity should be maintained at about 50% when the temperature is between 32° to 34° C. It is more difficult to maintain constant temperature and environmental humidity within the sleep laboratory. Temperature and humidity can be controlled fairly easily within an isolette and the study may be done within the islolette in the laboratory. Environmental light is easier to control in the lab than in the nursery, but the drawbacks of transportation and distance from the nursery and support personnel may overshadow the benefits, and a portable study within the nursery is most likely better tolerated by the infant. Variables such as constant bright light, environmental noise, and constant mechanical noise from the isolette must be recorded so that they may be kept constant and reproducible for each recording session. Disruptions of the infant's routine for medical procedures required in the nursery should be recorded and available for comparison during follow-up studies. Length and timing of the study should also be subsequently reproducible.

RECOMMENDED EQUIPMENT

Polygraph

Multichannel polygraph is required for recording of all physiologic measurements. In our laboratories, a minimum of 16 channels (13 AC and 3 DC channels) are utilized for polysomnographic recording. DC channels are utilized for recording respiratory effort and oxygen saturation. The recording equipment may be analog or digital. Resolution with analog paper output tends to be higher than digital recording output, however, digital output is acceptable and has a distinct advantage in storage of records. Digital recordings also have the advantage of automatic scoring of state and respiratory variables. Algorithms for adults have been fairly well validated. Unfortunately, algorithms for infants and children lack the same degree of validation, and because of their rapid CNS maturation, single computer programs may not be able to provide valid and reproducible information. Another practical problem tends to exist with automatic scoring. Although computer scoring is rapid and accurate, quantitative analysis is only a small portion of the assessment. Qualitative evaluation can provide information about development and progression of sleep states and can only be performed by viewing raw data.

Electrodes and Other Recording Devices

We utilize 0.6-cm diameter gold 48-inch electrodes for recording EEG, EOG, EMG, and EKG. Silver/silver-chloride electrodes may also be used, but two different types of electrodes should not be utilized together. Pre-gelled electrodes designed for prematures and newborns are available and have typically been utilized for EKG and respiratory monitoring in the neonatal intensive care unit. These electrodes may also be utilized for polysomnography (but not for EEG recordings). Pre-gelled electrodes may be used for EOG, EKG, and EMG and at times can facilitate application. Because of the fragile nature of the premature's skin, irritation, excoriation, and redness of the skin under tape and other adhesives, care should be taken in the choice of methods of application (see Technical Considerations).

Respiratory effort can be effectively monitored using piezo electric crystal effort belts specifically designed and sized for the small premature and newborn infant. These belts provide an accurate effort signal, are relatively inexpensive, and maintenance is simple. Other methods for recording effort include plesthysmography and/or strain gauges. Plesthysmography is highly accurate and can provide summation potential recording when chest and abdomen are out of phase, identifying paradoxic breathing. It tends to be more expensive and slightly more difficult to maintain than piezo crystal belts. Strain gauges are quite sensitive but can be fragile and maintenance is often difficult. Impedance pneumography has been used in the past to monitor respiratory effort. Due to the poor sensitivity and specificity (high percentage of false-positive and false-negative recordings), it is not recommended for prolonged polysomnographic recordings in the laboratory. Intercostal surface EMG has also been utilized for determination of respiratory effort. As with impedance pneumography, this method of measuring respiratory effort lacks sensitivity and specificity and should be discouraged in premature and term newborns.

Monitors to continuously measure respiratory airflow must be available. Although some oral breathing can occur, neonates are considered obligate nasal breathers. Therefore, measurement of oral airflow is less critical in the premature and/or term infant than in older infants and children. Several methods for measurement of airflow are available and many laboratories utilize at least two methods simultaneously. Utilizing two simultaneous airflow measures provides back-up since artifact and problems with maintenance of sensors are quite common. Measurement of airflow by thermistry is reliable and very cost effective. On occasion, sensitivity is not as great as other methods in determining very small and slow changes in airflow. It does, however, provide very specific information regarding airflow, but not on CO_2 retention.

Capnography provides close estimation of end-tidal CO_2, is as noninvasive as thermistry, and is somewhat more sensitive to small changes in CO_2, which is an estimate of airflow. However, capnography continues to be significantly more expensive than thermistry and technical problems with maintenance of patency of tubing are very common and technically frustrating. Some laboratories utilize both thermistry and capnography simultaneously. Maintenance of both sensors is very difficult, but having two operational systems provides back-up if one fails. Each also provides slightly different information, providing more specific technical data to assist in interpretation. Capnography provides an estimate of end-tidal CO_2, since mixing of expired air and environmental air occurs. Accurate measurement of end-tidal CO_2 requires the use of a tight-fitting mask that covers both the mouth and nose. This technique is often quite intrusive, and the mask is more frequently displaced than the nasal cannulae for capnography.

Continuous determination of oxygen saturation is typically accomplished by noninvasive pulse oximetry. Standard pulse oximeters may be utilized and interfaced with polygraphic equipment. On occasion in seriously ill neonates, allowances will need to be made for the percentage of fetal hemoglobin, core body temperature, and the infants' arterial pH since these factors can affect the position of the hemoglobin-oxygen dissociation curve. Appropriate size and position of probes for optimal measurement of oxygen saturation should be stressed. Measurement of transcutaneous oxygen content and transcutaneous CO_2 content has been utilized in some laboratories (3,4). These methods are quite sensitive, accurate, and reproducible in continuously monitored blood gas concentrations. Unfortunately, they are not benign procedures and complications and adverse reactions are common. Probes require heating and blistering burns of infants' skin is not uncommon. However, transcutaneous CO_2 measurement may be important in determining the presence of alveolar hypoventilation and the risk and benefits of utilizing this technique may outweigh the risks of continuously disrupting the sleep-wake continuum in order to draw arterial blood gases.

Instrumentation to determine and record body movement and body position is important to add to the comprehensive polysomnographic recording. Limb muscle EMG may be added to continuously evaluate limb muscle movements. Motion detectors and position monitors are commercially available, but many are quite expensive. There is no substitute for an alert technician who is constantly monitoring the patient and documenting and describing the newborn's activity, movements, and body position (as well as position changes). *Timed synchronization of video, audio, and the polysomnographic record* is often indispensible in making polysomnographic assessments and interpretations. Technician notes added to video/audio playback with polygraphic synchronization provide optimal information. This is of particular importance in patients manifesting unusual motor behaviors (and sounds) reported to occur during sleep that may require EEG correlation. Respiratory sounds and efforts can be visually, audibly, and polygraphically coordinated for interpretation. Video/audio taping and split-screen recording also allows for characterization of sleep-related movement disorders and the determination of artifacts that may cause misinterpretation.

Optional equipment might include esophageal pH monitoring devices, esophageal manometer to measure intrathoracic pressure, surface microphones for sonographic recording of snoring and other sleep-related vocalizations, actigraphs/accelerometers to measure and record body movements and/or position changes, as well as any other equipment that the laboratory might feel useful in the polysomnographic analysis of individual patient's needs.

In any facility performing investigations on newborns (premature or term) equipment should be available for *maintenance and monitoring of the neonate's body temperature.* As previously described, neonates maintain core body temperature by non-shivering thermogenetic mechanisms. It is, therefore, essential to assist in the maintenance of a neutral thermal environment for the sick or tenuous newborn. If the infant is in the normal newborn nursery and is otherwise stable, continuous monitoring of temperature is typically not necessary. Sick newborns are best studied in the neonatal unit in order to avoid the trauma of transportation to the laboratory. Therefore, portability of equipment and appropriate technical staffing is essential.

Facilities for parents are mandatory. The laboratory should be organized to accommodate not only the infant in a crib or isolette, but also to provide room for the parent to remain with their child. It is important, however, for technical personnel to clearly document the parent's sleep-related activities, since they may modify the infant's sleeping environment and bias the polysomnogram (e.g., parent's loud snoring resulting in frequent arousals, awakenings, and body movements).

Equipment used for data analysis and storage must have neonatal and infant software available. Drawbacks of these computer programs have already been presented. Simple modification of adult software is inadequate. The capability of computer analysis of digitized data provides for post-hoc manipulation of information and is cost effective for storage. The computer equipment should have the capability to produce hard copies of epochs.

TECHNICAL CONSIDERATIONS

Polysomnography should provide accurate and reproducible information to determine:

1. Sleep/wake states, including determination of latencies, cycle lengths, percent of active sleep, percent quiet sleep, percent indeterminate sleep, percent wake, length of longest uninterrupted sleep episode, and maturation of architecture;
2. Characteristics of the EEG, including symmetry and maturation;
3. Characterization of cardiorespiratory function;
4. Characterization of body movements, behaviors, and recording of body position during recording;
5. Characterization and integration of other parameters, such as gastroesophageal reflux with sleep/wake-related parameters and body position; and
6. Correlation of various physiologic parameters with progression of sleep/wake states across the recording and several sleep/wake and feeding cycles, as well as correlation with EEG activity.

Techniques, protocols, and equipment should be available to handle special situations in the laboratory, e.g., evaluation of the need for supplemental oxygen, assisted respiration (i.e., nasal CPAP, controlled ventilation), evaluation of the need for and follow-up of home monitoring, and evaluation of tracheostomy flow.

EEG

Standard International 10-20 system of electrode placement should be utilized. Standard sleep laboratory polysomnographic montage requires only 1 to 2 channels of EEG recording to identify sleep state. These channels are typically one central channel (C3-A2 or C4-A1) for scoring and one occipital channel (O1-A2 or O2-A1) for identification of sleep onset. These widely spaced channel recordings, however, do not appear to be adequate in recording polysomnographic EEG for premature and/or term newborn infants (especially the ill neonate). A more complete or bipolar screening montage should be standard. Specific modification to the EEG electrode recording array may be chosen depending upon the clinical situation. Premature and term newborn infants often require a "double distance" electrode selection because of the small cranial size (Fig. 8-1). A recommended montage might be:

Fp1-T3
T3-O1
Fp2-T4
T4-O2
A1-C3
C3-C4
C4-A2
Cz-O2

Paper speed is recommended at 10 mm/second. This provides for economy of paper and interpretation of EEG characteristics is still possible. Slower speeds are sometimes utilized to more clearly document respiratory patterns, but the ability to adequately interpret EEG characteristics is lost at these slower speeds. If seizure activity is suspected, paper speed should be increased to 30 mm/second for an adequate length of time for

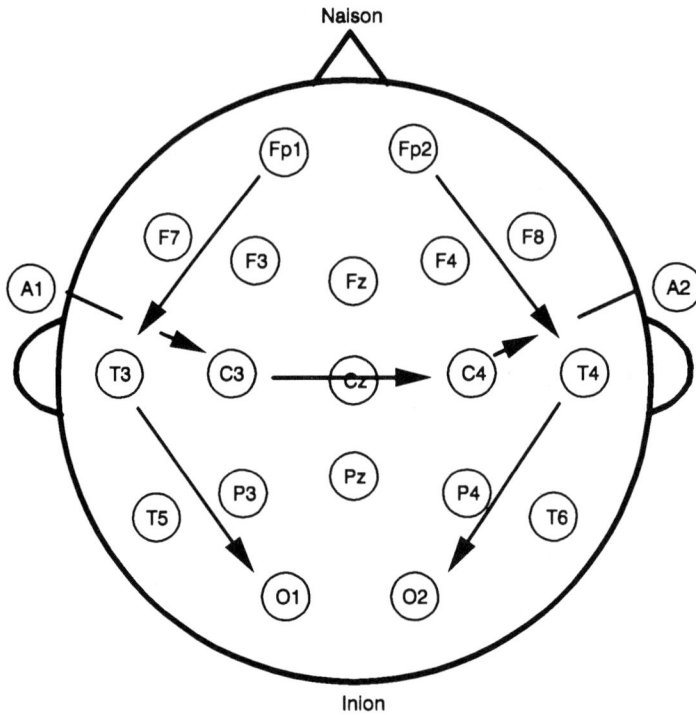

FIG. 8-1. Double-distance parasagittal montage.

more accurate interpretation of the activity to be possible (at least 2–5 minutes) before returning the paper speed to 10 millimeter/second. Digital recording equipment permits the playback at a variety of speeds and montage settings, obviating the need to change paper speed.

EOG

Standard electro-oculographic activity may be monitored using two electrodes placed approximately 0.5 to 1.0 centimeters lateral to the outer canthus of each eye. The electrodes should also be offset from the horizontal by a distance of about 0.5 to 1.0 centimeters. Offsetting the electrodes from the horizontal assures that vertical and oblique eye movements can also be recorded. A difference in potential of up to 100 µV exists between the cornea (positive) and retina (negative) making the globe of the eye a functional dipole. The polarity of the electrical field changes as the eye moves. Grossly, eye movements are synchronous, abrupt, and coordinated (saccadic eye movements) during wakefulness and active sleep. In the premature and term newborn, however, eye movements may be dysconjugate.

Two channels recording eye movements are generally recommended. This will allow for the differentiation of the eye movement potentials and other signals that may appear similar to conjugate eye movements. Under certain circumstances, however, a single channel may be used to record the EOG and both left-outer canthus and right-outer canthus electrodes may be referred to each other, rather than to a reference electrode.

EMG

Standard chin muscle EMG should be used as one criterion for sleep-state identification. Proper placement of the electrodes can provide not only information regarding skeletal muscle tone during various states, but in the presence of obstructive apnea, can provide information regarding activity of glossopharyngeus muscle. Three electrodes should be placed in the mental and submental regions. Only two electrodes are required, however, placement of the third provides a back-up for one electrode pair in the event that one of the electrodes is lost. One electrode is placed at the apex of the chin, in the region of the insertion of the glossopharyngeus muscle at the junction of the right and left mandibular bone. The second and third electrodes are placed in the region of the belly of the digastric muscle just to the right and left of the infant's trachea. These areas can be easily identified by palpating the area of greatest muscle retraction during the act of sucking and swallowing (3). Two of the chin muscle electrodes are referred to each other and are recorded on one channel of the polygraph. If there are technical difficulties with one of the electrodes during the study, the remaining functional electrode may be referred to the back-up electrode and the infant will not have to be disturbed in order for replacement of the electrodes.

Recording of Respiratory Effort

Respiratory efforts should be measured with either peizo crystal electrode belts specifically fitted for the premature and term infant, appropriate pneumatic transducers, or plethysmography. Each method will provide reliable results. Chest effort and abdominal effort should be measured on separate recording channels and should be calibrated in phase when the child is awake (assuming no persistent respiratory distress is present resulting in paradoxic breathing during the waking state). Measuring respiratory effort only by chest wall and abdominal impedance has poor sensitivity and specificity and should be avoided during comprehensive polysomnography.

When belts are utilized (either strain gauge, peizo crystal, or pneumatic), placement for chest effort should be either 1-cm above or below the nipple line. This provides for monitoring chest movement at the point of greatest excursion. Abdominal belts should also be placed at the point of maximal excursion. This can be identified by monitoring the infant's breathing prior to placement. It may be either at the level of the umbilicus or somewhat higher, half way between the umbilicus and the xiphoid process.

Monitoring Nasal/Oral Airflow

"Airflow" may be measured/monitored by thermistor or thermocouple. Although thermocouple measurements have been utilized in the past, it is somewhat less sensitive than measurement of airflow by thermistry, and thermistry is generally considered better procedurally. Nasal and oral airflow may be recorded on separate channels. Recording nasal airflow and oral airflow on separate polygraph channels can provide information regarding whether the patient is breathing through the nose, mouth, or both. Nasal and oral airflow may also be coupled on a single channel. This provides for adequate measurement of airflow as well as freeing up a channel for measurement of another physiologic parameter. Although not universal, most newborns are obligate nasal breathers and measurement of nasal airflow alone may be adequate in most studies.

End-tidal CO_2 measurement is a highly accurate method of measuring expired CO_2 at the nose and mouth. In order to accurately measure true end-tidal CO_2, a tight-fitting mask covering the nose and mouth is required. These masks may be intrusive to the sleep of the neonate and masks are easily displaced. Close estimation of end-tidal CO_2 can be accomplished with capnography. Capnography requires the placement of small cannulae (placed similarly to thermistors/thermocouples) by the nose and mouth. Capnography provides a fairly accurate determination of expired CO_2, which may be more sensitive than thermistry in identifying small changes in airflow and increased expired CO_2 during hypopnea, obstructive hypoventilation, and situations involving increased upper-airway resistance. Unfortunately, technical problems are frequent with capnography and displacement and occlusion of the cannulae are common. These difficulties may be major limiting factors. Some laboratories utilize both thermistry and capnography simultaneously to monitor airflow and expired CO_2 at the nose and mouth.

When capnography is utilized, the appropriate-size cannulae are placed a short distance into each nostril. An additional projection is typically placed in front of the mouth in order to sample air expired through the mouth. The cannulae are taped to the lateral aspects of the upper lip and cheek. Thermistors are placed on the upper lip in a similar manner, however, they are not inserted into the nostrils. The sensors are interposed into the airstream in front of the nostrils and the mouth and taped in a similar manner. Infants may often drool and loosen the tape. The tape may be better secured, and irritation from the adhesive minimized by placement of tincture of benzoin on the skin prior to application of the tape.

Monitoring Hemoglobin-Oxygen Saturation

Continuous monitoring of SpO_2 by pulse oximetry should be standard for all neonatal polysomnographic procedures. Placement of the oximetry probe is dependent upon the size of the infant. In small premature infants, the foot is typically the most stable and reliable location of placement. However, it may be placed on the hand, finger, or toe if the infant's size permits. Because pulse oximetry is sensitive to movement and movement artifact is common, a method to differentiate physiologic oxygen desaturation from movement artifact should be utilized. This typically involves addition of a pulse signal to the montage. If the pulse signal is strong and regular, desaturations recorded are due to physiologic hemoglobin oxygen desaturation. If the pulse signal is absent, recorded decrease in SpO_2 is most likely artifact. Some laboratories depend on the recording of these pulse wave forms, while other laboratories utilize dual oximeters to ensure that recordings are accurate. Movement recorded by limb EMG and/or accelerometers may assist in differentiating artifact from physiologic oxygen desaturation. Videotape review may also be helpful. Probably the most helpful information can be provided by the vigilant technician/technologist who very frequently documents the infant's behavior on the recording.

In the sick neonate and/or the premature infant, the infant's arterial pH and temperature should be known at the time of the study and documented. Arterial pH and temperature can result in a shift in the hemoglobin-oxygen dissociation curve. Changes in SpO_2 will vary with changes in actual oxygen tension. The type of oximeters utilized in each laboratory should be identified. Oxygen saturation measurements can vary between oximeters at the same oxygen tension in the same patient (5,6). It is imperative that the appropriate probe be used with each oximeter. *Oximetry probes cannot be interchanged.* Complications (burns) can occur when probes are interchanged (7,8).

Oxygen content can also be accurately monitored transcutaneously. *Transcutaneous oxygen concentration* ($TcPO_2$) and *transcutaneous CO_2 concentration* ($TcPCO_2$) had been commonly used in the neonatal intensive care unit. Unfortunately, the complication rate (burns) from the heated probes are greater than seen with continuous monitoring of SpO_2. Therefore, continuous monitoring of TcPO2 and $TcPCO_2$ should be reserved for specific circumstances (e.g., assessment of congenital central hypoventilation syndrome, ventilatory failure).

Measurement of Heart Rate and Rhythm

Continuous monitoring of heart rate and rhythm may be accomplished by using standard EKG lead-2 placement. Disposable pre-gelled electrodes may be utilized for continuous monitoring of the EKG. Alternatively, EKG may be recorded by an electrode placed in the middle of the chest (mid-sternal region) and referenced to A1 or A2. This would require utilization of an electrode of the same composition as the EEG electrodes and pre-gelled electrodes would not be recommended. Heart rate is determined by the frequency of QRS complexes. Beat-to-beat variability should be evaluated by comparison of R-R intervals. Beat-to-beat variability should be assessed during wakefulness, quiet sleep, active sleep, and indeterminate sleep. In its absence, problems with autonomic control of heart rate may be present. This cannot be diagnosed polysomnographically by a single EKG lead alone, and other variables must be taken into consideration along with the EKG.

Monitoring Movement and Behavioral Observations

Body and limb movements and activity during polysomnography may be accomplished by limb EMG (upper and lower), direct observations by technician with notations on the record, and/or split-screen video/audio recordings. Actigraphy may also be considered for monitoring movements. Behavioral observations and technician notations are vital for accurate analysis of neonatal polysomnograms.

Behavioral observations by the technician/technologist are best recorded directly on the polygraph paper when they occur. With digital recordings, these behavioral citations may be typed directly onto the record. We have found that video/audio tape recording of the entire polysomnogram (using split-screen technique) is quite helpful in post-hoc analysis of the recording. Behavioral observations written directly on the record are cued to the videotape recording so that the polysomnographer may view the behaviors cited by the technician. It is essential that video and polygraphic synchronization occurs so that finding specific epochs is facilitated. In some instances, it is quite useful to summarize behavioral observations at regularly spaced time intervals.

Standard Timing and Duration of Study

Neonatal polysomnograms should last a minimum of 6 hours, but optimally 8 hours. The recording should last a sufficient amount of time to allow for appropriate characterization of all physiologic parameters within the context of both a weak circadian and strong ultradian sleep-wake-feeding cycle in the newborn. Two (2) sleep-wake-feeding cycles should be monitored. Although many laboratories will perform diurnal studies on newborn infants, this is typically done for the convenience of the staff rather than for appropriate identification of physiologic abnormalities. Under ideal circumstances, polysomnographic studies on premature and term neonates should include late evening and early morning cycles (e.g., 2200 to 0600). In the immediate neonatal period, because of the large amount of the 24-hour continuum spent in the sleeping state, it is often not necessary to do an overnight study (depending upon the abnormality being evaluated). During a diurnal study, sufficient time should be provided to evaluate the infant both awake and asleep over two cycles. Because of the occurrence of some problems (e.g., movement disorders, unusual behaviors, seizures), a prolonged study of 12 to 24 hours may be indicated. When this is not possible (e.g., infants whose underlying medical problems preclude them from being moved from the NICU), modification of the standard protocol may be required.

Electrode Application and Techniques

The most important aspect in obtaining a high-quality, reproducible polysomnogram in the premature and term neonate is meticulous preparation of the patient and the sites of electrode application. Persistent monitoring of the quality of signals being recorded and maintenance of electrodes relies on the presence of a caring and diligent technician.

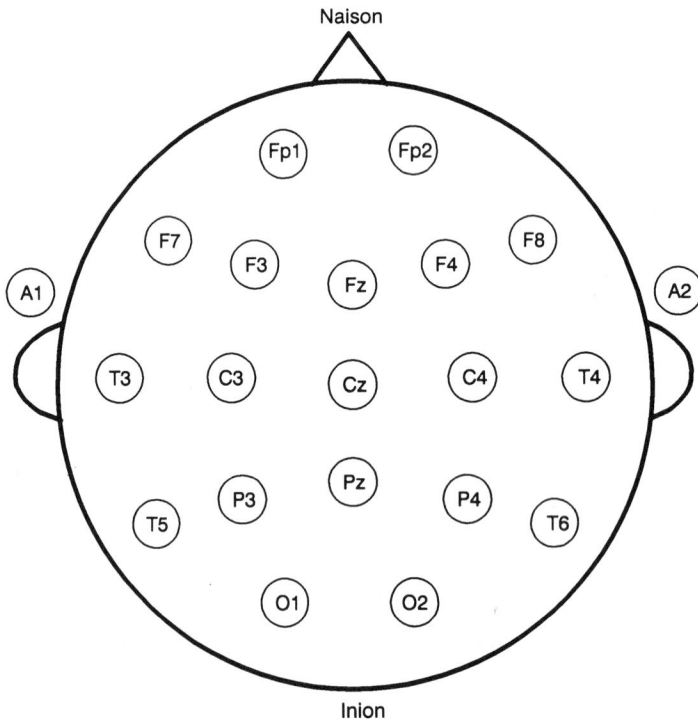

FIG. 8-2. International 10–20 System of Electrode Placement is based on precise location of scalp points by measurement from 4 clearly identifiable landmarks (naison, inion, and the left and right preauricular points). It uses the distances between these landmarks to generate a system of lines which run sagittally and coronally. These lines intersect at intervals of 10% and 20% of their total length. All electrodes are placed at the intersection of these lines.

EEG

The head is measured according to the International 10-20 System of electrode placement (Fig. 8-2). In the small premature infant and the term newborn, a double-distance montage is often selected. If the electrode site falls over a fontanelle or an over-riding suture line, the location may be slightly modified in order for the electrodes to be placed over an intact cranial surface. If modification of placement is required, it must be done bilaterally and symmetrically. Notation must be made on the polysomnographic record montage as well as in the laboratory medical record. Hair must be washed of oils, cleaned, and dried prior to the study. Parents can provide assistance in holding the infant during set-up. If a parent or caregiver is not present, an assistant is essential in order to best provide for the infant's needs and comfort. The scalp should be prepared in a standard manner, with Omniprep or acetone-alcohol preparation. Although best preparation of the site requires abrasion of the skin, care must be taken in the premature and term newborn since too vigorous preparation of the site might result in significant injury to the underlying skin. Electrodes may be applied with electrode paste and gauze covering or may be affixed to the scalp with collodion. Collodian provides for more secure attachment of electrodes to the scalp for prolonged recordings, however, in small premature infants and term newborns, this may not be ideal. In premature and term newborns collodian can result in irritation to the skin and scalp electrodes should be applied with paste and gauze coverings.

EOG

Electrode sites are selected approximately 0.5- to 1.0-cm lateral and 0.5- to 1.0-cm superior to the left outer canthus, and 0.5- to 1.0-cm lateral and 0.5- to 1.0-cm inferior to the right outer canthus. Sites are prepared with either Omniprep or alcohol and the skin is vigorously scrubbed. Care must be taken to not instill alcohol into the eye. Electrode gel or paste is applied to the electrode and it is affixed to the site with hypoallergenic tape. It is unusual for there to be difficulty in adhesion of the tape in these sites.

EMG

Three electrodes are placed to record chin muscle EMG. One electrode is located in the submandibular region immediately beneath the apex. Two electrodes are symmetrically placed at the belly of the digastric muscles on either side of the submandibular region. Skin is prepared in a similar manner to the EOG. The site is vigorously scrubbed with an alcohol swab or Omniprep. Again, care must be taken to not significantly injure the skin. Electrode paste is applied and the electrodes are secured to the sites with hypoallergenic tape. Because of moisture at these sites, maintenance of the tape adhesive may occasionally be difficult and tincture of benzoin applied to the skin prior to taping may assist in maintenance of the tape. Tincture of benzoin may also assist in protecting the skin from irritation from the adhesive on the tape.

Head Wrapping

It is often advisable to wrap the head in premature and term newborns who are undergoing polysomnography. Head wrapping will assist in placing even pressure on all covered electrodes and will help protect the electrodes from displacement during the course of the study. We utilize Kerlix wrap. It is important to wait approximately 15 minutes after electrode application. There must be enough time for drying of collodion to occur (if air compressor drying was not done) or for the conductive electrode paste to harden. Care must be taken not to create a "gel bridge" between electrodes. If this occurs, the head must be unwrapped and the electrodes reapplied or the inter-electrode space appropriately cleaned. Head wrapping can include the chin muscle electrodes, EEG electrodes, and a portion of the electro-oculogram electrodes. Wrapping begins under the chin and over the crown of the head. The wrap is then extended around the forehead of the infant. Layers should not be so thick as to result in sweating, but should be sufficient to protect the electrodes. After wrapping is complete, electrode impedance is checked. If the impedance of electrodes is below 5000 ohms, the study may proceed. If greater than 5000 ohms, electrodes should be checked and most likely reapplied. Wrapping with firm even pressure is important in achieving a high-quality, overnight recording.

Patient Calibrations

In the premature neonate, standard patient calibration is impossible. However, prior to the onset of the study, behavioral observations can be made and recorded on the polysomnogram that can provide the polysomnographer important information in further interpretation of the study. The infant's state should be documented. For example, it should be stated whether the infant appears awake or asleep; if the eyes are opened or closed; if the infant is squirming or moving (but quiet); if the infant is crying; if the infant is sucking; facial grimacing; muscle/limb twitching; parental intervention; or other behavioral manifestations which can assist in interpretation of the study after lights-out.

Initial Polygraphic Parameters

EEG

Initial EEG settings can vary according to the type of polygraphic equipment and amplifiers utilized. The manufacturer's manual should be carefully read and recommendations incorporated into the laboratory's protocol. High-frequency filter setting might begin at *35* and adjusted to assure optimal instrument response. Low-frequency filter setting (time constant) might begin at *1*. This also should be adjusted to assure the most reliable recording. Sensitivity might begin at 7 µV/mm. In premature and term newborns, amplitude of waveforms is typically very high; if this gain is too high, it results in pen blocking which renders the EEG tracing very difficult to interpret. After the beginning of the recording, the sensitivity may be decreased to 10 µV/mm or lower in order to obtain the most interpretable recording. Once optimal sensitivity is obtained, it should remain constant for the remainder of the study.

Electro-Oculogram

Initial recommended amplifier settings for recording the electro-oculogram are as follows: sensitivity, 7 µV/mm; high-frequency filter setting of 35; and low-frequency filter (time constant) setting of 0.3. The lowest low-frequency filter setting that does not result in amplifier blocking should be used. With an initial sensitivity of 7 uV/mm, frontal EEG artifact is typically obtained. Although a gain of this magnitude provides large pen excursions with eye movements and can assist in detecting small eye movements, EEG interference may provide unacceptable artifact. In our laboratories we utilize a sensitivity beginning at 20 uV/mm. This provides for ample detection of even small eye movements and eliminates a significant portion of frontal EEG artifact (except during periods of constant high-voltage, slow-wave activity).

Chin Muscle EMG and Limb EMG

Initial recommended amplifier settings are as follows: Low-frequency filter 5; high-frequency filter 70; sensitivity 3–5 uV/mm or higher. Sensitivity can be adjusted during patient calibrations/observations and initially adjusted during the first REM period in order to obtain the best recording. Once modified during this first active-sleep period, EMG sensitivity should not be changed unless there are compelling reasons. Relatively high sensitivities should be chosen in order to more clearly identify low-tonic EMG activity during active sleep. Minimal high-frequency filtering should be done since EMG frequency recording range should be the highest possible on the particular amplifier. Sixty-cycle interference may be blocked by using the 60 Hz notch filter. Low-frequency filtering may be utilized to eliminate slow potentials generated from other sources, e.g., respiratory artifact.

EKG

Initial amplifier settings should be: high-frequency filter 70; low-frequency filter 1; sensitivity 2 μV/mm. The gain should be adjusted prior to beginning the study so that there is no pen blocking and specific characteristics of the EKG can be identified. Polarity should be adjusted so that the P waves and T waves are upright.

Respiratory Variables

If using AC amplification, initial settings should be: high-frequency filter 35; low-frequency filter 0.3; sensitivity 30 uV/mm. Often DC amplification is utilized to record respiratory variables. In these cases, sensitivities and balancing voltages should be adjusted in order to obtain maximal pen excursion during normal respiration without pen blocking.

REFERENCES

1. Parmelee AH Jr, Bruck K, Bruck M. Activity and inactivity cycles during the sleep of premature infants exposed to neutral temperatures. *Biol Neonate* 1962;4:317.
2. Murray B, Campbell D. Sleep states in the newborn: influence of sound. *Neuropadiatrie* 1971;2:335.
3. Hoppenbrouwers T. Electronic monitoring in the newborn and young infant: theoretical considerations. In: Guilleminault C, ed. *Sleeping and Waking: Indications and Techniques.* Boston: Butterworths; 1982: 17–59.
4. Hoppenbrouwers T, Geidel S, Ruiz ME, Judson L. Electronic monitoring in the newborn and young infant: technical guidelines. In: Guilleminault C, ed. *Sleeping and Waking: Indications and Techniques.* Boston: Butterworths; 1982:61–125.
5. Poets CF, Southall MD. Noninvasive monitoring of oxygenation in infants and children: practical considerations and areas of concern. *Pediatrics* 1994;93:737–746.

6. Thilo EH, Andersen D, Wasserstein ML, Schmidt J, Luckey D. Saturation by pulse oximetry: comparison of the results obtained by instruments of different brands. *J Pediatr* 1993;122:620–626.
7. Murphy KG, Secunda JA, Rockoff MA. Severe burns from a pulse oximeter. *Anesthesiology* 1990;73: 350–352.
8. Sobel DB. Burning of a neonate due to a pulse oximeter: arterial saturation monitoring. *Pediatrics* 1992; 89:154–155.

9

Premature and Term Newborns

Sleep-related abnormalities in the premature infant are most frequently overshadowed by medical problems. Attention is typically focused on preservation and maintenance of ventilation, and protection of the integrity of the developing but fragile central nervous system (CNS). Polysomnography done on the sick premature infant will often be difficult to interpret and may be replete with artifactual information due to the need for medical intervention. Polysomnography is often deferred until stabilization of all medical and/or surgical illnesses. However, polysomnography can provide information during treatment, especially in those neonates requiring assisted ventilation and those who experience seizures.

MOST COMMON INDICATIONS FOR POLYSOMNOGRAPHY

Apnea of Prematurity

Apnea of prematurity is defined as periodic breathing with pathologic apnea in a premature infant. Periodic breathing is present in almost all prematures less than 28-weeks gestation (1) and almost half of prematures during the neonatal period (2–4). Pathologic

TABLE 9-1. *Indications for polysomnography*

Most common indications	Indicated under certain circumstances	Potential indications
Apnea of prematurity	Congenital hypotonia	Intrauterine-drug exposure
Sibling of SIDS victim	S/P intraventricular	Bronchopulmonary dysplasia
Congenital central hypo-	hemorrhage	after ventilator weaning
ventilation syndrome	S/P intracranial	Abnormal feeding/swallowing
Apparent life-threatening	infection	Congenital malformations of
event	Hypertonia	the head, neck, and chest
Unexplained sleep-	Infantile spasms	CNS abnormalities (e.g.,
related hypoxemia	Gastroesophageal	hydrocephalus)
Mid-face congenital	reflux	State discordance and lack
anomalies		of circadian/ultradian
Seizures		organization
Stridor		
Decanulation of		
tracheostomy		

apneas are respiratory pauses of 20 seconds or longer or respiratory pauses less than 20 seconds, but associated with significant oxygen desaturation and bradycardia. Most of these respiratory pauses are central in origin, but obstructive and mixed events commonly occur (5–7).

Siblings of SIDS Victims

Premature newborns are at higher risk for SIDS. Presence of a history of a previous sibling who has died of SIDS greatly increases the risk of sudden unexpected death during sleep. Although there are no clear polysomnographic data that can predict the increased likelihood, the sleep study can rule out certain types of abnormalities that can be associated with apnea or sleep-related deterioration during this delicate time of life (e.g., seizures, obstructive apnea). Although infants with documented apnea rarely die of SIDS, there are certain subtle polysomnographic changes that have been identified in infants who have subsequently died of SIDS. Some of these include, but are not limited to: prolonged, uninterrupted sleep states (particularly quiet sleep); increased percentage of periodic breathing during sleep (particularly active sleep); decreased beat-to-beat variability of heart rate.

Congenital Central Hypoventilation Syndrome

Congenital central hypoventilation syndrome may present in the premature infant shortly after birth. Spontaneous breathing during sleep does not occur and resuscitation is often required. Difficulty weaning from mechanical ventilation is common. Unexplained cyanosis during sleep may be the only presenting symptom. Congenital central hypoventilation syndrome may also present as an apparent life-threatening event. The infant may not breathe spontaneously or respiratory efforts may be erratic and cease at sleep onset. Progressive pulmonary hypertension, cor pulmonale, and cerebral hypoxic encephalopathy may occur.

Apparent Life-Threatening Events

Apparent life-threatening events (ALTEs) occurring in the premature infant are more frequent at home after discharge from the nursery. Episodes are frightening to the caretaker and there is generally a belief that the infant would have died if there was no caretaker intervention. Polysomnography should be part of the comprehensive evaluation of all premature infants who have suffered an ALTE.

Unexplained Sleep-Related Hypoxemia

Unexplained hypoxemia during sleep may be identified in the nursery after delivery or may be noted at home after discharge as an ALTE. In the nursery, hypoxemia is most often identified by either a significant fall in the SpO_2 during sleep in the infant who is being monitored by pulse oximetry. Fall in $PaO2$ during sleep may be an indicator of congenital central hypoventilation syndrome. In addition, unexplained hypoxemia during sleep in the premature infant may be due to sleep-related seizures, congenital central hypoventilation syndrome, septicemia, positioning with neck flexion, anemia, metabolic abnormalities, right-to-left shunts (cardiac and extra-cardiac), or other congenital abnormalities.

Mid-Face Congenital Anomalies

Congenital anomalies of the mid-face region are often associated with breathing abnormalities (mostly obstructive) during wakefulness and sleep. Choanal atresia is often associated with an inability to breathe due to the fact that newborns are generally obligate nasal breathers. Premature newborns with congenital abnormalities, such as Pierre Robin syndrome, Treacher Collins syndrome, and Crouzon's disease are frequently associated with physiologically significant obstructive sleep apnea. Newborns with cleft palate after repair and children with syndromes associated with macroglossia are also associated with obstructive apnea in the newborn period.

Seizures

Suspected seizure disorders are clear indications for polysomnography in the premature infant. Seizures may indicate an acute (e.g., CNS infection) or chronic problem (e.g., metabolic abnormality). Seizures in the premature neonate are often secondary to hypoxic encephalopathy or intraventricular hemorrhage. Polysomnography can significantly assist in determining the severity of the seizure disorder, its course, as well as its control after anticonvulsant therapy has been instituted (when indicated).

Stridor

Stridor in the premature infant may be secondary to a number of causes. If resuscitation and endotracheal intubation was required, trauma to the larynx might have resulted in edema or vocal cord injury causing airway obstruction. Some congenital causes for stridor include laryngomalacia and tracheomalacia. Other congenital abnormalities of the trachea and/or larynx may also result in airway obstruction exacerbated by normal sleep-related hypotonia. Polysomnography can provide information regarding the degree of airway obstruction and the possible hemodynamic significance.

Decanulation After Tracheostomy

Polysomnography can provide considerable information regarding the patency of the upper airway after tracheostomy. Monitoring airflow at the nose and mouth, as well as at the tracheostomy site can provide valuable information regarding the patency and function of the tracheostomy when open. In addition, with the tracheostomy capped, patency of the upper airway can be determined and the safety of decanulation assessed.

POLYSOMNOGRAPHY INDICATED UNDER CERTAIN CIRCUMSTANCES

Congenital Hypotonia

Congenital syndromes that are associated with skeletal muscle hypotonia in the newborn (e.g., Down syndrome, Hoffman-Werdnig syndrome) are often associated with upper-airway obstruction and clinically significant obstructive sleep apnea. Anatomic abnormalities may contribute to the presence or degree of sleep-disordered breathing, however, a lesser degree of anatomic occlusion may be more clinically significant in children with neuromuscular hypotonia. Nocturnal polysomnography is indicated to determine the affect of nocturnal sleep-related pathology to diurnal function or functional impairment.

Status-Post Intraventricular Hemorrhage

Intraventricular hemorrhage is not uncommon in the extremely premature newborn infant. Prognosis is often poor. Polysomnography can provide a fairly clear assessment of the degree of EEG and state development with respect to conceptional age. Although the need for rehabilitative intervention is determined by clinical indication, serial polysomnography may provide insight into prognosis and response to treatment in these fragile youngsters.

Status-Post Intracranial Infection

Systemic infection is common in premature infants due to immaturity of the immune system and the inability to localize infection. Neurologic damage can be caused by such intracranial infections (e.g., group B, beta hemolytic streptococcus). Intracranial infection may be associated with apnea of prematurity and apnea of infancy. Polysomnography may be able to assist in characterizing apnea secondary to intracranial infection (e.g., central/brainstem-mediated, seizure-related, upper-airway mechanical obstruction). Other clinical and laboratory data will also be important. Polysomnography may also be important in determining the effect of the infection on CNS development and/or the probability of neurologic sequelae and neurodevelopmental outcome. Evaluation of respiratory status, EEG development, maturation of state, and state organization can be determined polysomnographically and provide clues to prognosis.

Hypertonia

Symptom complexes associated with neonatal hypertonia are likely to be indications for polysomnography. Increased skeletal muscle tone associated with cerebral palsy are usually associated with initial neonatal hypotonia. Conditions associated with hypertonia are varied and have a wide heterogeneity of etiologies. Generalized hypertonia may be associated with apnea during the neonatal period. The apnea may be directly related to CNS (cortical and/or brainstem) dysfunction or may be due to abnormal peripheral pharyngeal/laryngeal muscle performance. Gag reflex may be affected resulting in sleep-related breathing difficulties secondary to gastroesophageal reflux or an inability to protect the airway against pharyngeal secretions.

Infantile Spasms

Infantile spasms are associated with a poor long-term prognosis and may be identified by a hypsarrhythmia pattern on EEG in the newborn. Sleep-related EEG changes and identification of abnormal EEG patterns may be available polysomnographically. Lack of state concordance may also reflect the poor prognosis in newborn infants with infantile spasms.

Gastroesophageal Reflux

Gastroesophageal reflux (GER) has been considered to be one possible etiology of sleep-disordered breathing in premature and term infants. Clearly, if there is reflux into the pharynx associated with reflex glottic closure (laryngospasm), apnea can occur. Apnea secondary to GER-related laryngospasm can present as an ALTE in the premature or term newborn. Glottic closure in response to a pharyngeal stimulus might be considered a normal response (rather than an abnormal phenomenon) if it prevents pulmonary aspiration. It has been shown that proximal esophageal reflux in newborn infants is not associated with apnea, but instead, with arousal.

Several other important variables must be considered during polysomnography. Many laboratories and centers have included esophageal pH monitoring as a standard variable in sleep studies performed on premature and term newborns. Concurrent esophageal pH monitoring can provide information regarding the presence or absence of reflux, but it is quite controversial whether simple reflux without regurgitation into the pharynx is a common etiology of apnea of prematurity and/or apnea of infancy. The pH probe itself may confound the investigation. First, the placement of the pH probe introduces a foreign body into the pharynx. It is not known whether the presence of a pharyngeal foreign body changes the pattern of the visceral afferent limb of pharyngeal reflexes essential for the maintenance of pharyngeal patency in the premature or term newborn. Second, it is difficult to determine whether reflux identified with an esophageal pH probe meter is directly or indirectly associated with respiratory events. Third, there is evidence in the literature that even proximal esophageal reflux during sleep in newborn infants is associated with arousal, but not with apnea (8). Fourth, gastroesophageal reflux is present in most premature and term newborns to some extent. Cause and effect relationships are extremely difficult to determine. Finally, although relatively benign, placement of an indwelling esophageal catheter carries certain risks (e.g., unintentional tracheal intubation, esophageal perforation) and these risks (although small) may not be warranted during routine polysomnography.

Patterns of abnormal respiratory events associated with GER also appear to be different than obstructive apneas due to anatomic or neuromuscular dysfunction. Obstructive episodes associated with GER tend to be more sporadic and paroxysmal, rather than the typical periodic respiratory events seen with classical upper-airway obstruction (unless there is a positional component, which can easily be determined in the laboratory). Occlusive respiratory events associated with pharyngeal reflux are often associated with coughing and choking. Significant oxygen desaturation may or may not occur. In spite of its limitations and the presence of controversy, polysomnography will frequently be able to differentiate apnea secondary to gastroesophageal reflux from other forms of sleep-disordered breathing in the premature and term newborn.

Potential Indications for Polysomnography

Intrauterine-Drug Exposure

Some controversy exists regarding the need for polysomnography on all babies exposed to drugs (especially cocaine) in utero. There had been speculation that there is an increased frequency of sleep-disordered breathing/central sleep apnea in premature babies born to cocaine-using mothers. In addition, an increase in the frequency of ALTE has been suggested. Conflicting data does exist, and these hypotheses remain to be proven. However, a wide variety of effects on the CNS occurs when the fetus is exposed to drugs during gestation. Polypharmacy and alcohol are frequently involved. The effect of alcohol on the developing CNS is clear and the fetal alcohol syndrome has been well described. Unfortunately, many infants exposed to cocaine in utero may reveal abnormalities, such as apnea, early in life but these seem to resolve as the youngster matures. At age 3 years, the IUDE children may appear remarkably normal. Although not yet clearly established, significant abnormalities can be identified in cognition and performance in some drug-exposed children once school begins. Longitudinal polysomnography may be able to provide accurate assessment of apnea during the neonatal and subsequent periods. It may also provide insight into developmental aspects of EEG and state organization. This may provide useful information regarding the development of CNS function as well as the long-term effects of intrauterine-drug exposure.

Bronchopulmonary Dysplasia After Ventilator Weaning

Bronchopulmonary dysplasia is primarily a result of oxygen toxicity in the young premature infant undergoing standard ventilator therapy. Symptoms relate to chronic obstructive pulmonary disease. Some infants become oxygen dependent, and oxygenation occasionally is worse during sleep. Polysomnography can provide useful information regarding the degree of state-dependent respiratory impairment with this complication of prematurity.

Abnormal Feeding/Swallowing

Many premature newborns lack coordination of sucking and swallowing. This is often due to immaturity of reflexes and autonomic responses associated with these tasks. Feeding difficulties are the most prominent features. Often these youngsters have to be tube fed or require parenteral nutrition. Lack of organization of sucking and swallowing involves the muscles of the tongue, face, pharynx, and esophagus. Barium swallow radiographic studies can provide information on the coordination of the many muscles involved, but these tests cannot provide information regarding the effect on the coordination of state-dependent respiratory function. Lack of balance between pharyngeal muscles may affect organization of upper-airway reflexes required for maintenance of airway patency during the respiratory cycle, resulting in obstructive respiratory events.

Congenital Malformations of the Head, Neck, and Chest

Any malformation of the head, neck, or chest may result in improper balance of pharyngeal and upper-airway muscular activity resulting in obstructive respiratory events and/or sleep-disordered breathing. Polysomnography is the most accepted technique for evaluation of preoperative airway patency during sleep as well as monitoring and follow-up post-operatively (when surgery is indicated and undertaken).

CNS Abnormalities

Polysomnography may aid in the diagnosis and management of significant abnormalities resulting from CNS anomalies (e.g., hydrocephalus, Arnold-Chiari malformation). Symptomatology can range from behavioral sleep disorders, circadian rhythm/sleep-wake schedule abnormalities, to cardiorespiratory disorders due to autonomic nervous system dysfunction. Sleep architecture and maturation determined polysomnographically can aid in assessment and follow-up. Prognosis might also be possible. Response to treatment interventions may also be identified polysomnographically by improvement in structure and content of sleep and maturation of EEG variables.

State Discordance and Lack of Circadian Organization

Infants who are recovering from significant medical illnesses and who have been in the neonatal nursery for prolonged periods of time may be exposed to an abnormal circadian environment. Although more attention is being paid to cycling light within neonatal nurseries and attempts are being made to minimize noise and intrusive medical interventions, most neonatal units are brightly lit 24 hours a day. Noise is almost constant, and because of the fragile nature of the premature newborn, medical interventions are typically frequent. The potential for development of state discordance and disruption of appropriate ultradian and circadian organization is significant. Sleep evaluation, actigraphy, and polysomnography may provide insight into the degree of disruption and the presence of CNS integrity in those infants in the nursery who appear to be delayed in development of state concordance and sleep-wake cycling structure at appropriate conceptional ages.

EVALUATION AND SCORING OF PREMATURE AND TERM NEWBORN POLYSOMNOGRAMS

All polysomnograms should be recorded and scored for state determination in an epoch-by-epoch manner. Each standard epoch should extend 20 seconds or 30 seconds (comparable to paper speeds of 10 mm/seconds and 15 mm/seconds, respectively). Paper speed should be maintained for the entire study unless seizures are suspected. If sleep-related seizure activity is being evaluated, standard EEG paper speed of 30 mm/seconds should be utilized.

Behavioral Observations

Behavioral observations are exceedingly important in evaluating sleep of premature and term neonates. Notations should be made directly on the polygraphic record and should include comments regarding the eyes, mouth, facial expressions, body movements, vocalizations, and caretaker interventions. *Eyes* should be recorded as open, closed, blinking, and their appearance. *Mouth* activity should include movements of the lips, sucking, and chewing. Rhythmic movements of the jaw and mouth should also be recorded. Grimaces, smiling, frowning, and other *facial expressions* should be identified and described. Crying, whimpering, grunting, and other *vocalizations* are important variables in differentiating state and assisting in interpretation of the record. *Caretaker's interventions* may include feeding, diaper changing, soothing, breast feeding, bathing, or other unforseen interventions.

Active Wake

During active wake, the neonate may be crying or moving. The polysomnograph is most often filled with muscle and movement artifact, muscle tone is high, and pen blocking is frequent. EEG is often uninterpretable. Eyes are open and blinking can be demonstrated on the EOG. Conjugate eye movements might be identified. Limb EMG is high,

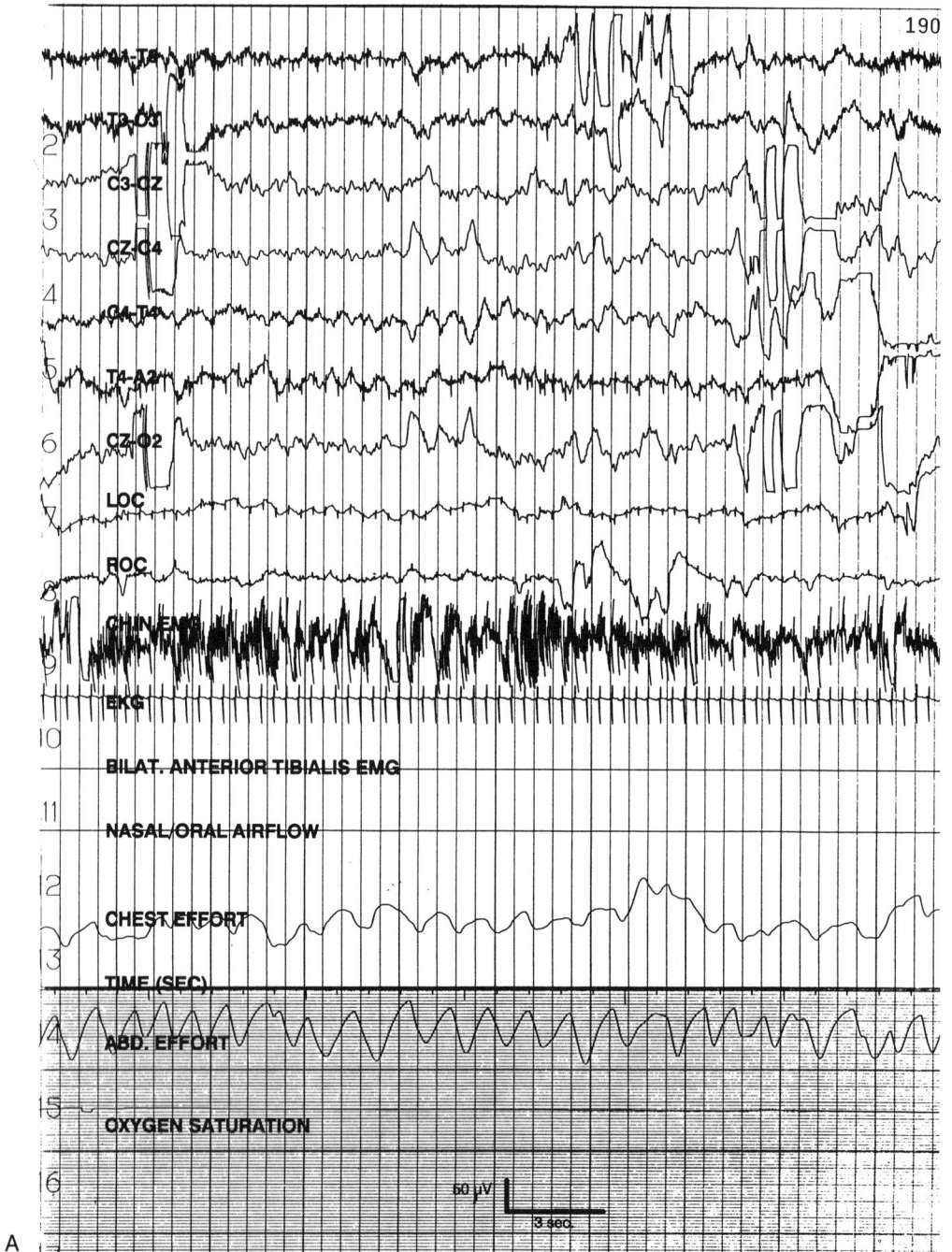

FIG. 9-1. A–B: Active wake in a newborn infant. A waking background rhythm of medium frequency (4–8 Hz) and relatively low-voltage (> 50 μV) activity is present in the EEG. Movement/ muscle artifact is also present. Conjugate eye movements can be seen in the EOG and just prior to these epochs the technician reported that the baby was "awake, moving, with eyes

Continued.

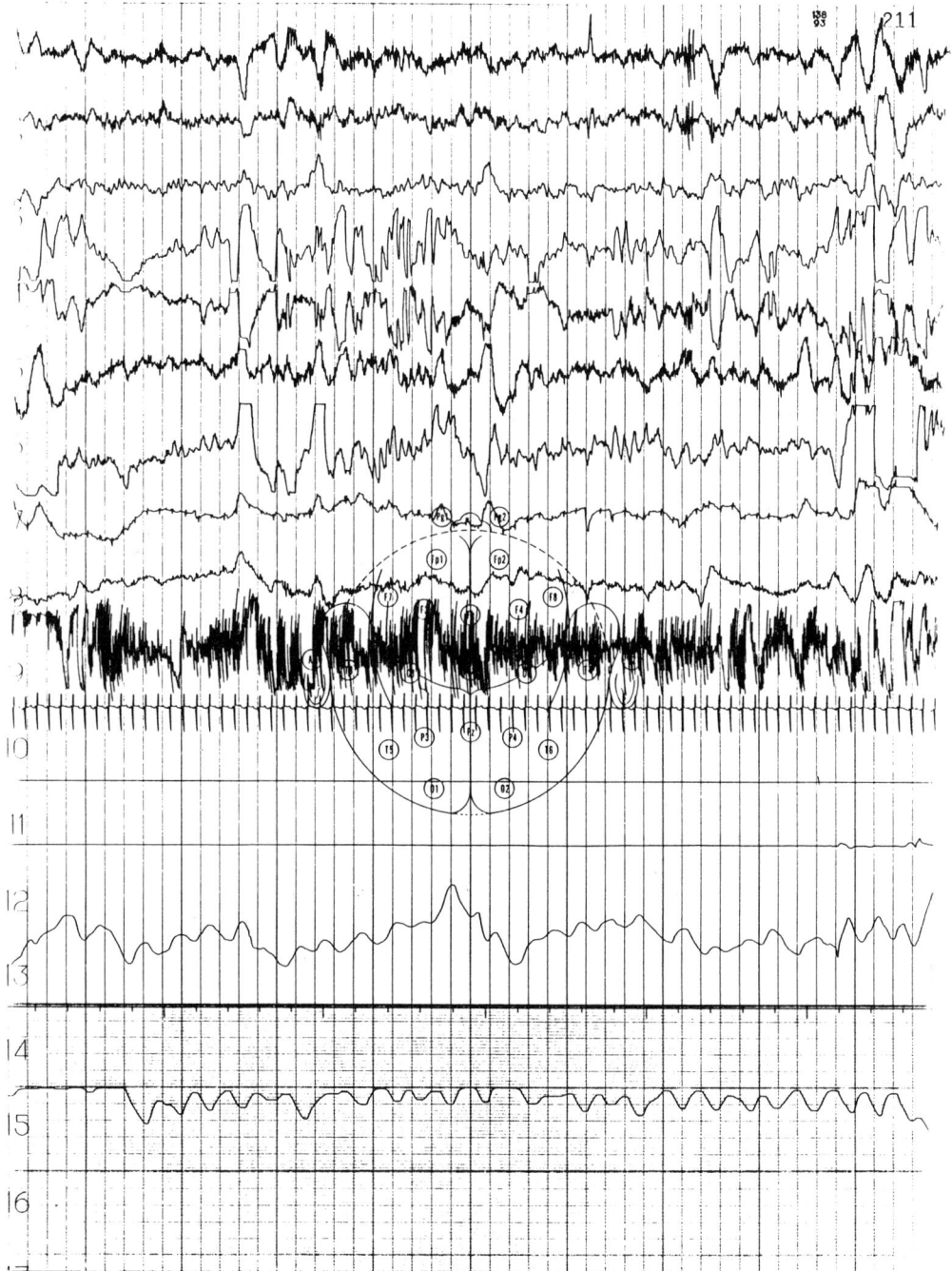

B

open." Chin muscle tone is high and sucking movements can be seen. Nasal/oral airflow is not yet being monitored. Often, young patients do not tolerate placement of the airflow sensor during wakefulness. The appropriate recording device can be properly positioned during the first episode of quiet sleep.

movement commonly noted. EKG is variable and typically rapid. Respiration is rapid and variable. It may be difficult during periods of active wake to obtain a high-quality airflow signal. Respiratory efforts are very irregular and efforts may be associated with pauses, cries, vocalizations, and periods of tachypnea, especially during episodes of crying. Oximetry may be reliable if a good pulse signal is obtained, however, desaturations associated with movement and poor pulse signal are most likely artifact and not physiologic (Fig. 9-1).

Quiet Wake

During quiet wakefulness, the newborn is observed lying quietly in the crib with eyes open. There may be small movements of the limbs, minor vocalizations, head movements, or mouth movements (e.g., sucking, smiling, grimacing). EEG reveals a relatively low-voltage, mixed-frequency rhythm. *Prior to 28 weeks* conceptional age, wakefulness cannot be clearly determined by EEG pattern alone (9). Typically, only a discontinuous EEG pattern occurs. This consists of periods of up to 3 minutes with minimal activity separated by bursts of bi-hemispheric activity (mostly slow-wave activity and activity in the theta and alpha range that is not bilaterally synchronous) lasting up to 20 seconds. Sharp transients are normal in the frontal regions and sporadic spikes are common in any location. They should be considered abnormal if they occur from a single location or during the discontinuous period. *Between 28 to 31 weeks* conceptional age, the single discontinuous pattern continues but the bursts of activity last 1–2 seconds with 4- to 6-Hz rhythmic waves that are typically bisynchronous. At about 30 weeks, high-voltage slow waves reappear and fast activity of about 10–20 Hz becomes superimposed on these slow waves and is termed "delta brushes." These delta brushes may be present until shortly before conceptional term. By *32 to 35 weeks*, a pattern of continuous, rhythmic, and often synchronous slow-wave activity in the 1- to 2-Hz region appear in a wide distribution and are seen during wakefulness (and active sleep, see below). At *36 to 40 weeks conceptional age*, a new pattern appears, consisting of diffuse, irregular, continuous slow waves of relatively low amplitude (generally less than 50 μvolts) during wakefulness (and active sleep). EOG may reveal conjugate eye movements that occur in bursts or may reveal the infant tracking slowly moving objects (especially faces). EMG may reveal similar movements to active wakefulness, including sucking, chin quivering, vocalizations, etc. Heart rate remains relatively rapid when compared to sleep. Because of the rate, it may be difficult to visually identify beat-to-beat variability and a normal sinus arrhythmia. *Respiration* is irregular, but more stable than during active wakefulness. *Oxygen saturation* remains quite stable and movement artifact is minimal during quiet wakefulness.

Feeding

Polysomnography during feeding is similar to that of quiet wakefulness and drowsiness (sleep/wake transitions). The EEG initially reveals clear patterns of wakefulness that may change as the infant continues feeding. Transition to sleep may be apparent. EOG may show slow, rolling, and/or dysconjugate movements. The eyes are often closed, but may be open and reveal conjugate eye movements. EMG reveals suck and swallow artifact. This may continue into the initial stages of sleep (throughout transition).

Sleep Onset

Sleep onset is much more difficult to identify in the premature and term neonate than in the older child and adult. In adults, the presence of clear alpha rhythm during relaxed wakefulness and its diffusion and disappearance is a clear indication of the transition to sleep. In neonates, without the presence of well-developed alpha activity, the transition from wake to active sleep is generally through a period of drowsiness identified by both behavioral and polygraphic criteria. During this transition state, the eyes may be open but close more frequently, for longer periods of time. The eyes do not appear focused and may look glassy. Eyes will not follow slowly moving objects or faces. Eye movements may be absent. The newborn may not have any body movements, or may have intermittent writhing movements. Facial activity may be similar to quiet wakefulness. During the transition, these brief periods of drowsiness may alternate with periods of active sleep.

Active Sleep

Active sleep appears quite similar to wakefulness polysomnographically in the premature and term neonate. There is considerable behavioral activity intermixed with short periods of quiescence. Since newborns enter sleep through active sleep, it may be difficult to identify the exact transition. A period of drowsiness typically intervenes. At about 32 weeks of conceptional age, *EEG* characteristics differentiate active from quiet sleep. However, patterns of wakefulness and active sleep are more difficult to differentiate. During active sleep, there is a pattern of continuous 1- to 2-Hz activity. There is a wide distribution of this slow-wave activity, it is considerably rhythmic and synchronous. Differentiation between active sleep and wakefulness may require behavioral observations. *EMG* may be helpful in differentiation of active sleep and wakefulness (as well as quiet sleep). There is tonic muscle activity during wakefulness, drowsiness, and quiet sleep. Muscle tone is decreased during active sleep. However, movements and phasic activity are frequent and more prolonged than in older infants and young children. Major movements are also more common in younger neonates, making simple polygraphic differentiation difficult. *EOG* reveals clear saccadic eye movements. In addition, some slow, rolling eye movements may be noted. *Heart rate* is variable during active sleep and beat-to-beat variability is accentuated. *Respiration* is irregular. Periods of tachypnea and bradypnea are present. Hypopnea and brief central apneas are frequent. Periodic breathing is more common during active sleep. The younger the conceptional age, the greater percentage of periodic breathing is present. Although it is unclear and somewhat controversial what percentage of active sleep and total sleep time is normal, and in which state periodic breathing may occur, it generally signifies immaturity of central control of breathing. The greater the percentage of periodic breathing as conceptional term is reached (as well as during the neonatal period), the greater the likelihood there are problems with the central control of respiration (Fig. 9-2).

Quiet Sleep

Quiet sleep is characterized by closed eyes, quiescence, and monotony of physiologic activity. Occasional muscle twitches can occur, but for the most part, there is no motor activity during quiet sleep. *EEG* is characterized by one of several patterns, depending upon the conceptional age of the newborn. At approximately 32 weeks conceptional age,

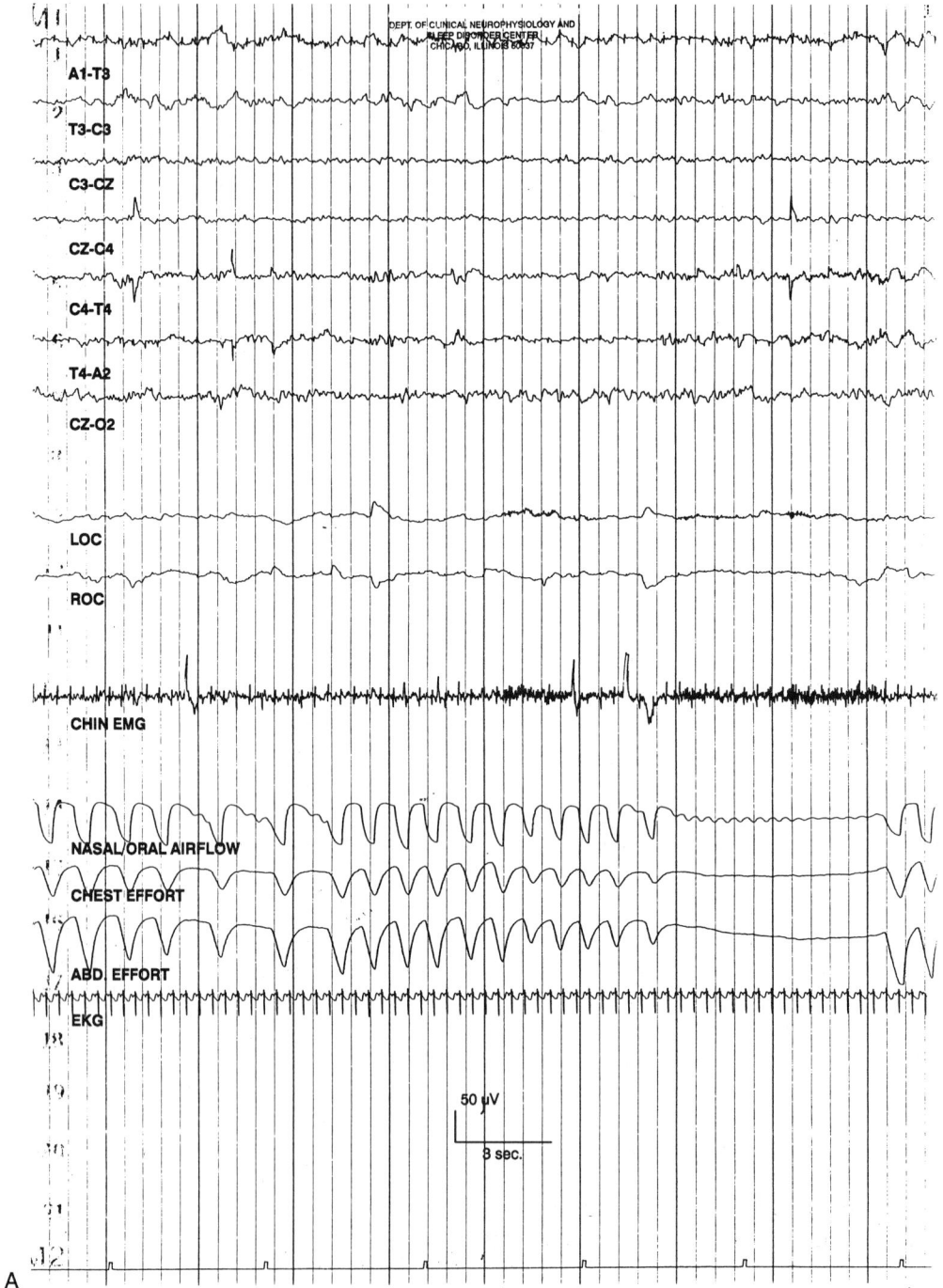

FIG. 9-2. A–D: Active sleep in a 2-week-old infant. The EEG reveals relatively low-voltage (> 50 μvolts), continuous activity at about 4–7 Hz. Rapid conjugate eye movements are present and chin muscle tone is low, but interrupted by phasic muscle activity. Periodic breathing is also present. The ripples seen during the respiratory pauses in the airflow channel represent "pulse artifact" with the appearance of small expiratory puffs during ventricular diastole. This artifact typically indicates a widely patent and unobstructed airway.

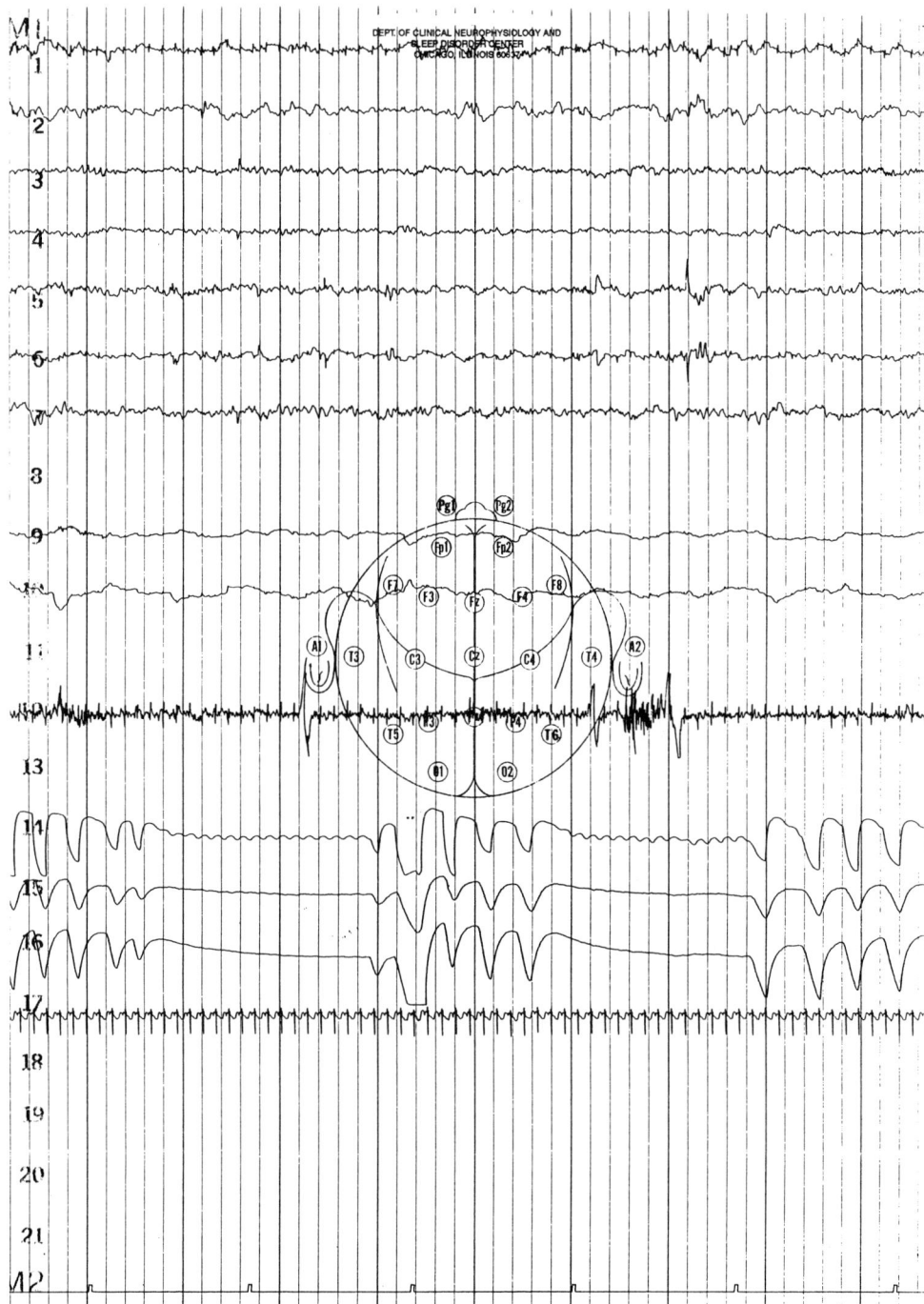

FIG. 9-2. *Continued.*

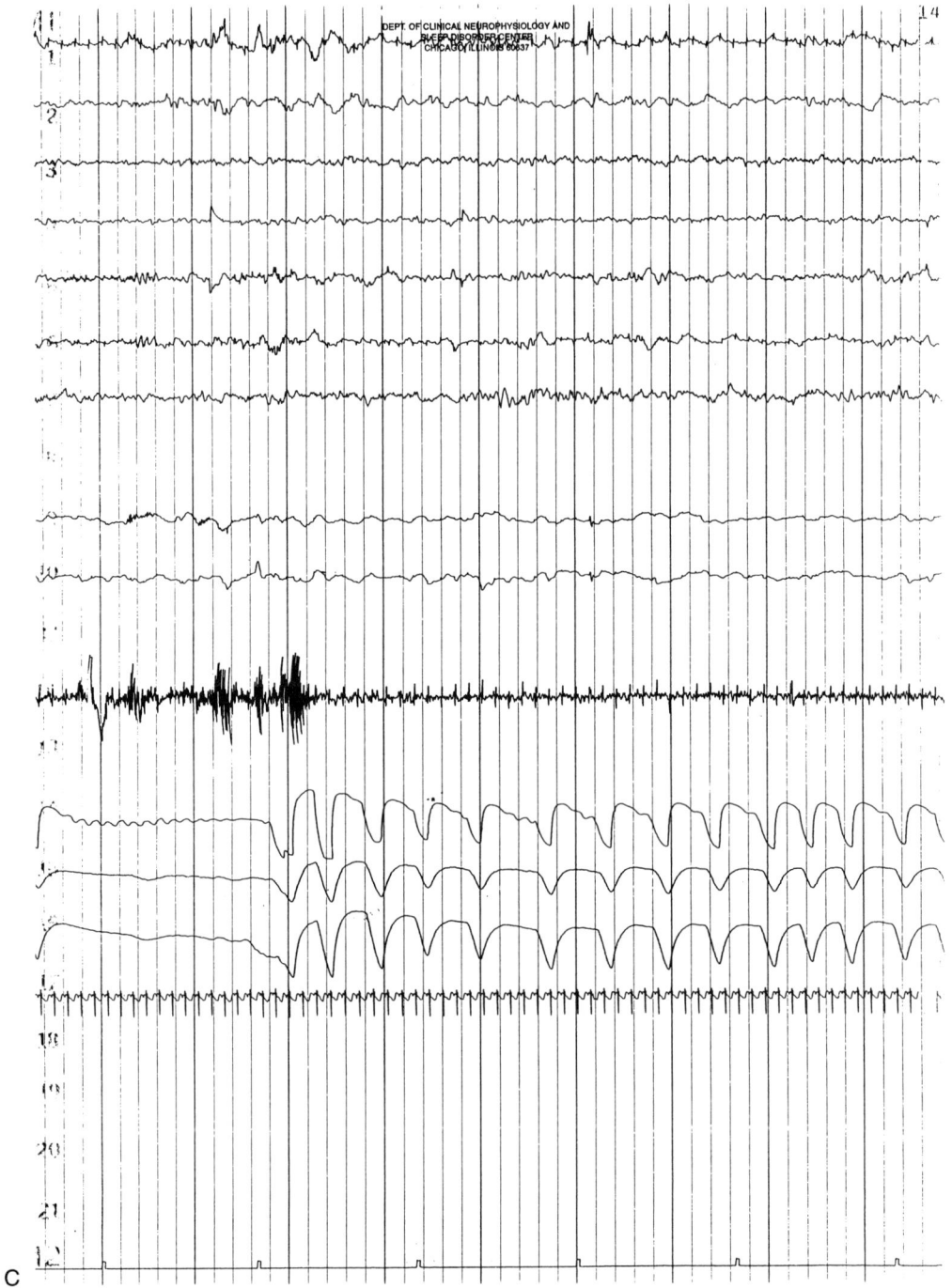

FIG. 9-2. *Continued.*

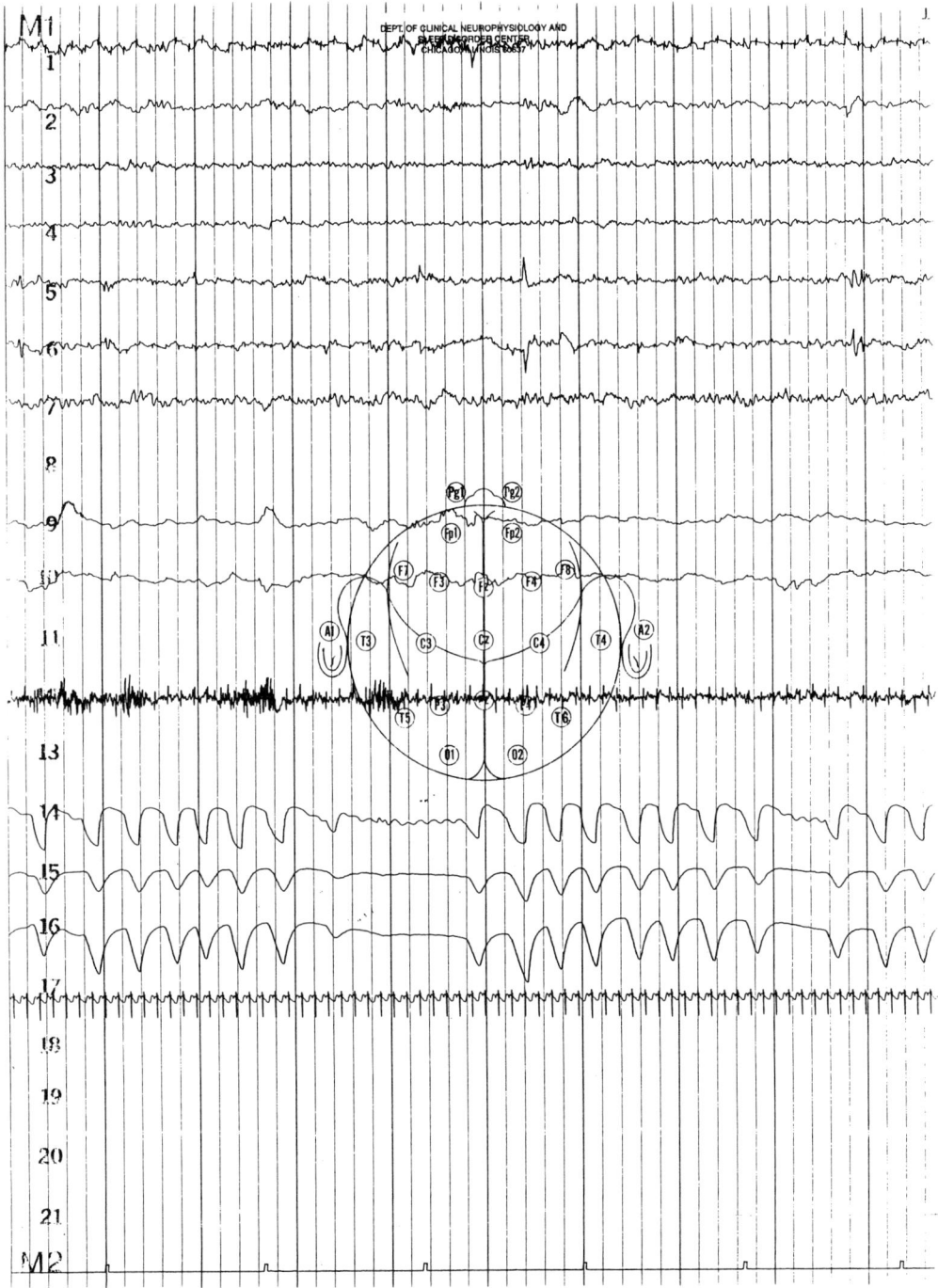

FIG. 9-2. Continued.

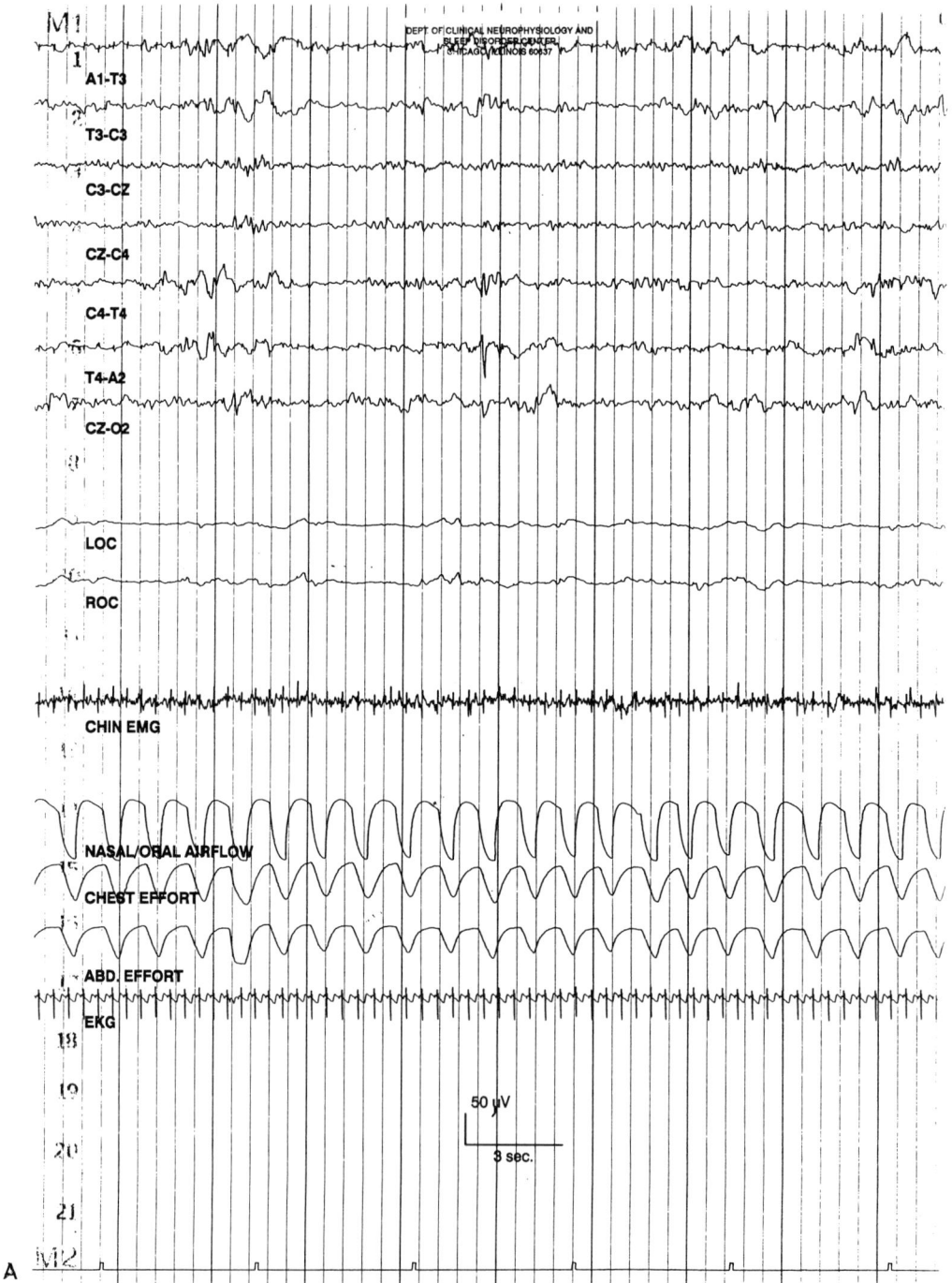

FIG. 9-3. A–D: Quiet sleep in a 2-day-old infant. A clear tracé alternant EEG pattern is present. Eye movements are absent in the EOG. Chin muscle tone remains tonic. Respiratory pattern is monotonous and regular.

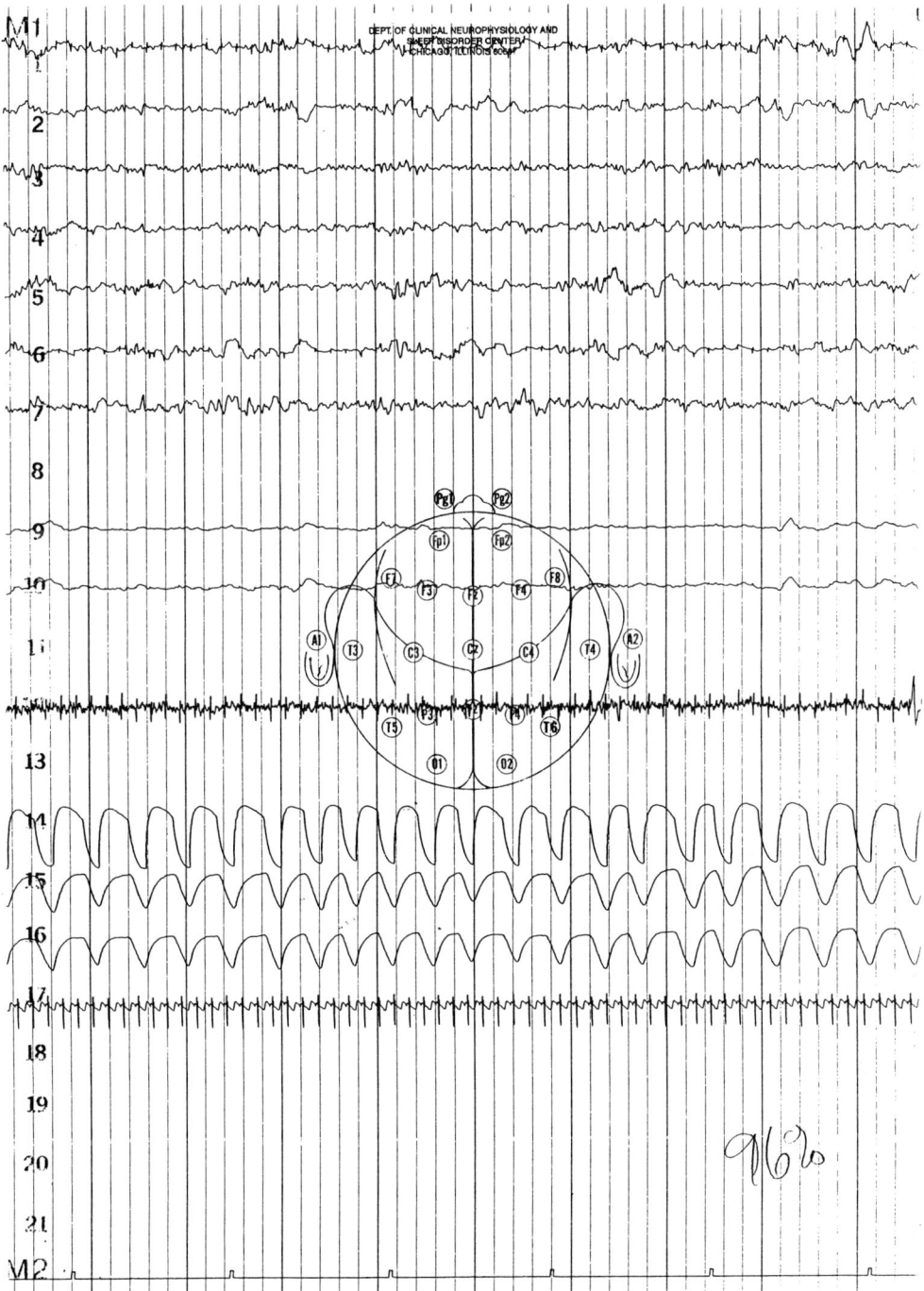

FIG. 9-3. *Continued.*

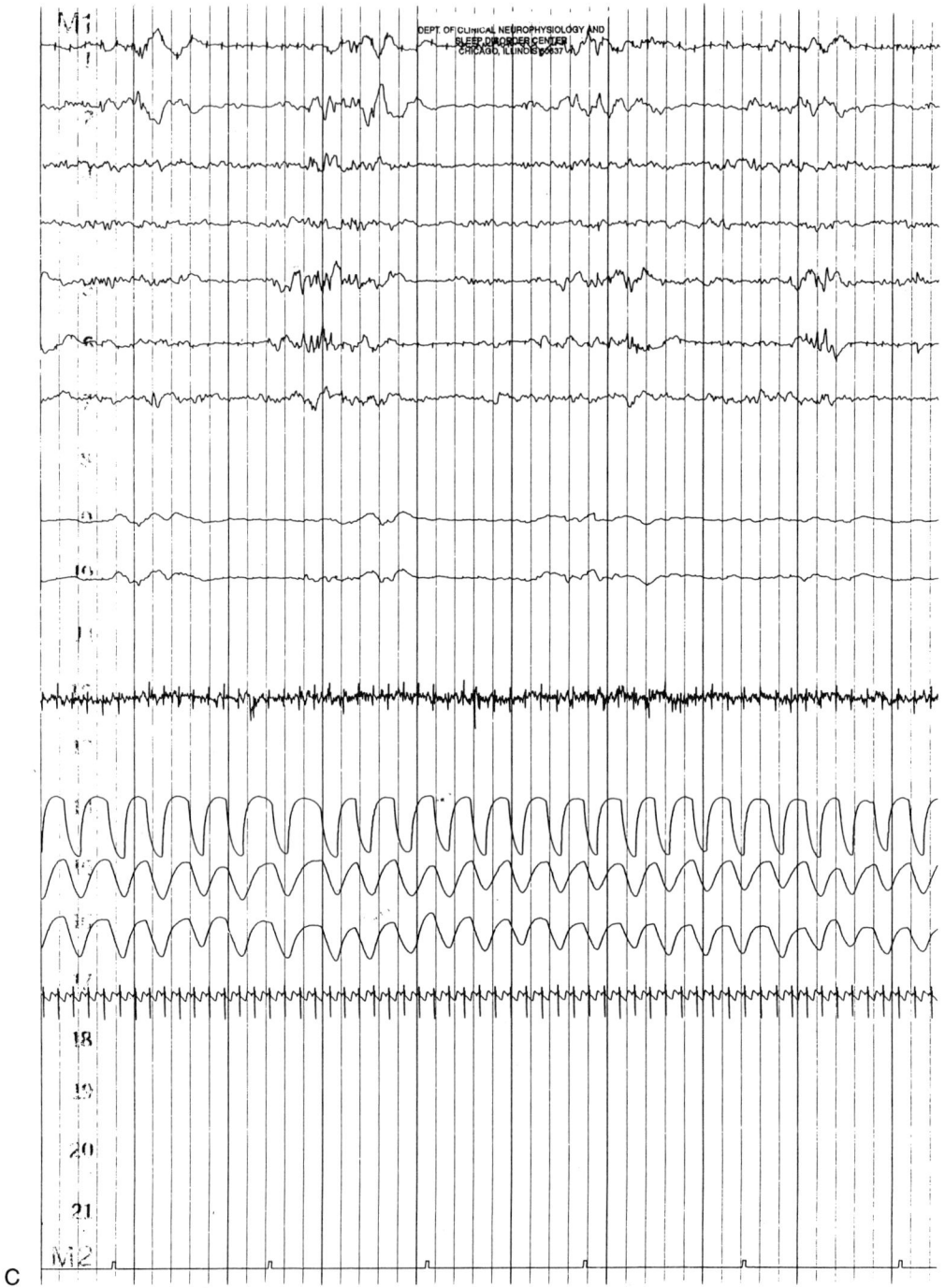

FIG. 9-3. *Continued.*

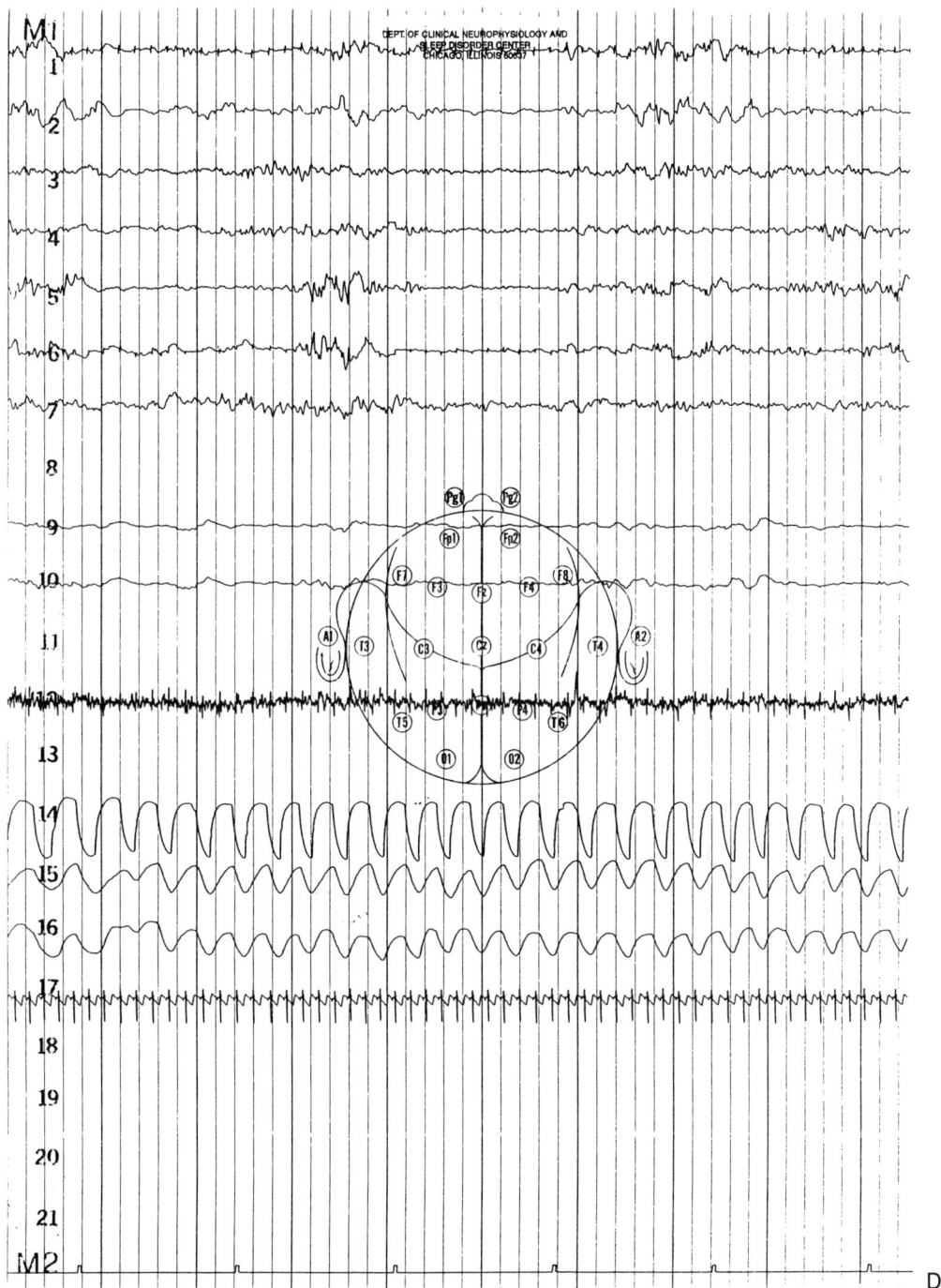

FIG. 9-3. *Continued.*

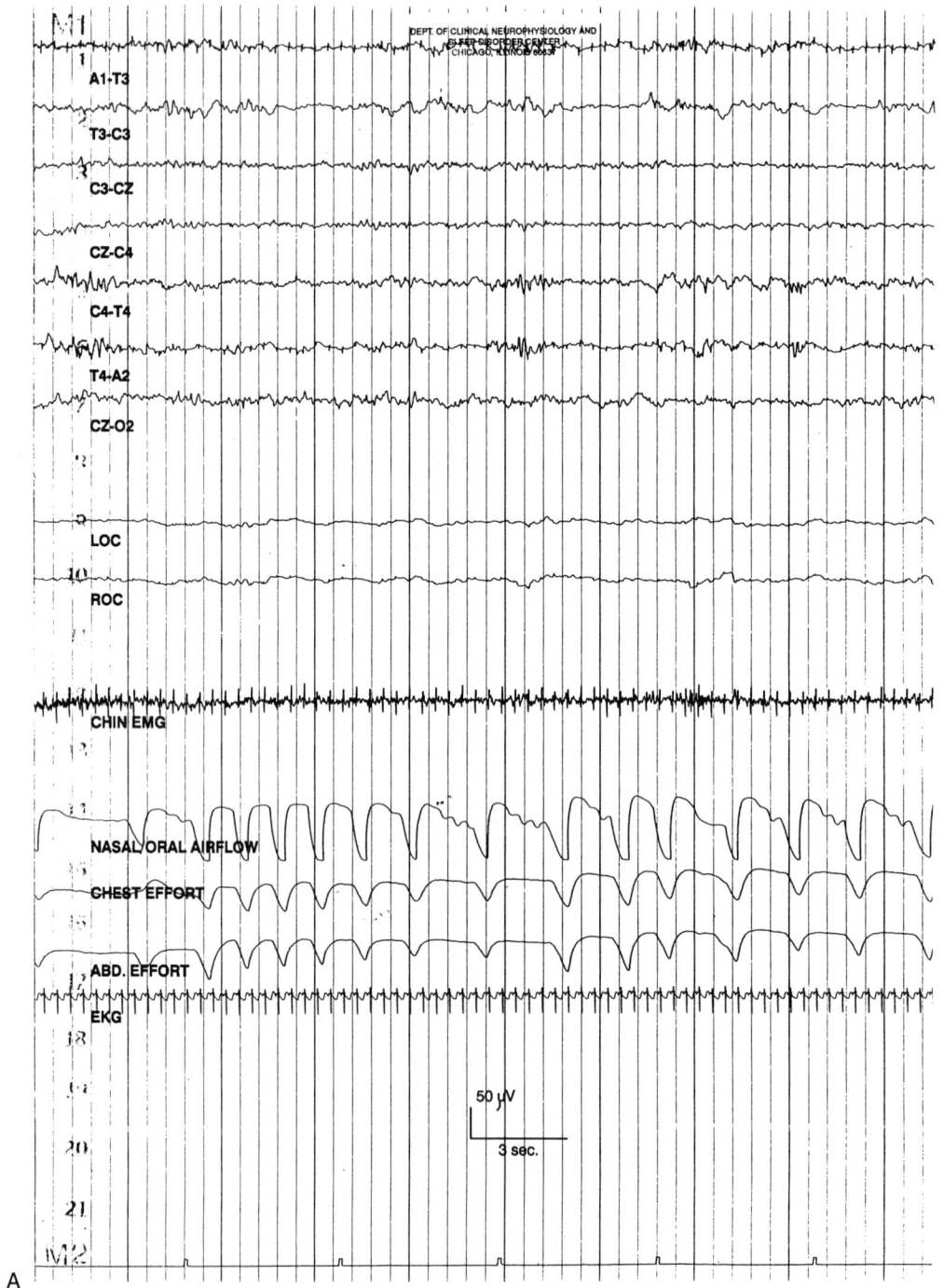

FIG. 9-4. A–C: Indeterminant sleep in a 2-day-old infant. The EEG reveals a variable and mixed pattern. Eye movements are absent in the EOG. Chin muscle tone is low and there are phasic twitches seen. Respiration is variable and occasionally unstable.

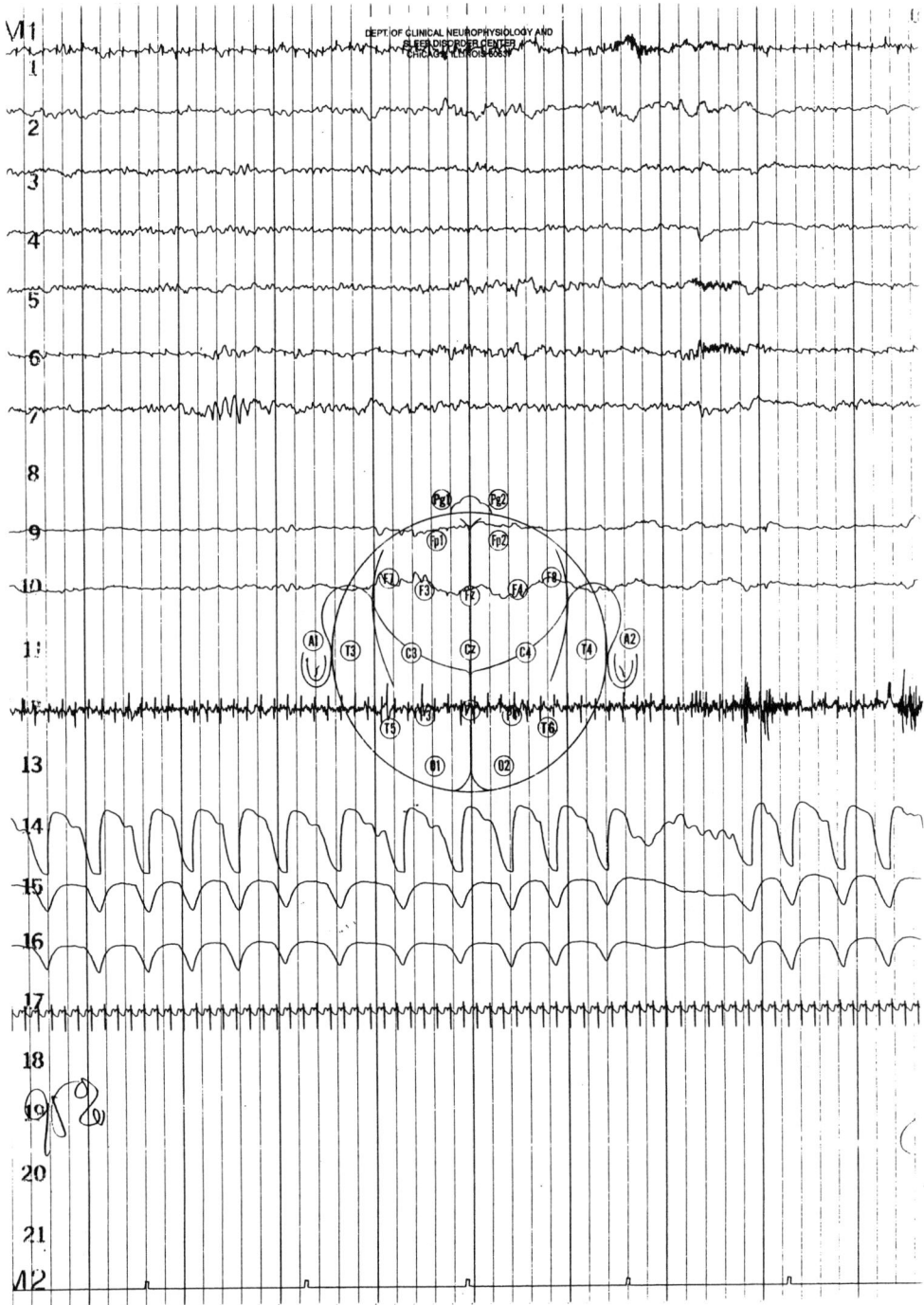

FIG. 9-4. *Continued.*

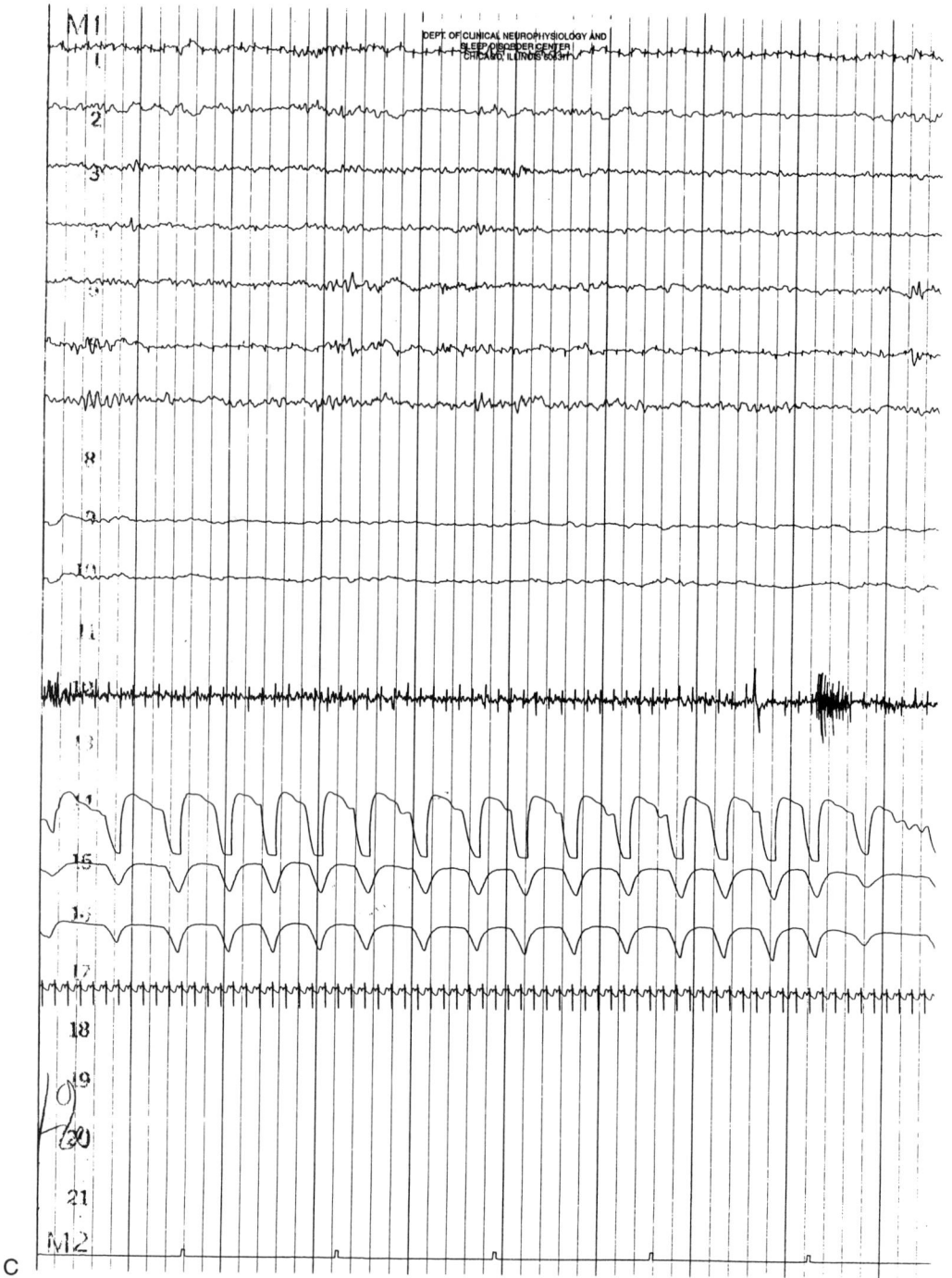

FIG. 9-4. *Continued.*

a discontinuous pattern of activity is predominant, There are bursts of slow waves in the frequency range of 1–2 Hz that are most clearly localized over the posterior head regions. By 36 weeks, EEG activity of quiet sleep may consist of a tracé alternant pattern. Bursts of high-voltage waves with frequencies between 0.5 to 3 Hz occur. There is occasional superimposition of rapid low-voltage waves and sharp waves interspersed. The bursts generally have a duration of 3–8 seconds and are separated by the discontinuous pattern of a relatively low-voltage, mixed-frequency pattern lasting about 4–8 seconds. In addition, a high-voltage, slow-wave pattern consisting of continuous rhythmic activity may occur. A mixed pattern is also identified that consists of both high-voltage slow waves and relatively low-voltage, mixed-frequency patterns.

EMG tone is high during quiet sleep and only rare phasic activity is present. *Eye movements* are absent during quiet sleep and the eyes are persistently closed. *Respiration* is monotonously regular during quiet sleep. Occasional post-sigh respiratory pauses may be present, but are not associated with oxygen desaturation nor with EKG changes (Fig. 9-3).

Indeterminate Sleep

Indeterminate sleep has been termed transitional or intermediate sleep (10–12). It may also be thought of as a dissociated state or a mixture of various components of two or more states. A certain number of epochs do not meet the standard criteria that defines specific states. Anders, Emde, and Parmelee suggested that these epochs be termed indeterminate sleep (13). In neonates, these epochs occur most often during transitions from wake to sleep and during state transitions. They also occur when the infant is arousing. The change from active sleep to quiet sleep is much more likely to manifest indeterminate sleep than the transition from quiet sleep to active sleep. The percentage of mixed states and indeterminate sleep may provide useful information regarding prognosis for infants who do not show normal state organization (Fig. 9-4).

REFERENCES

1. National Institutes of Health Consensus Development Conference. *Infantile Apnea and Home Monitoring.* Bethesda, MD: US Department of Health and Human Services, Oct 1, 1987, NIH Pub No 87-2905.
2. Rigatto H. Apnea. *Pediatr Clin North Am* 1982;29–1105.
3. Bouterline-Young HJ, Smith CA. Respiration of full-term and of premature infants. *Am J Dis Child* 1953;80:753.
4. Daily WJR, Klaus M, Meyer HBP. Apnea in premature infants: monitoring incidence heart rate changes, and effect of environmental temperature. *Pediatrics* 1969;43–510.
5. Dransfield DA, Spiter AR, Fox WW. Episodic airway obstruction in premature infants. *Am J Dis Child* 1983;137:441.
6. Thach BT, Stark AR. Spontaneous neck flexion and airway obstruction during apneic spells in preterm infants. *J Pediatr* 1979;94:275.
7. Milner AD, Boon AW, Saunders RA, Hopkin IE. Upper airways obstruction and apnoea in preterm babies. *Arch Dis Child* 1980;55:22.
8. Kahn A, Rebuffat E, Sottiaux M, Dufour D, Cadranel S, Reiterer F. Arousals induced by proximal esophageal reflux in infants. *Sleep* 1991;14:39–42.
9. Spehlmann R. *EEG Primer.* Amsterdam: Elsevier; 1981.
10. Parmelee AH Jr, Akiyama Y, Schultz MA, Wenner WH, Schulte FJ, Stern E. *The Electroencephalogram in Active and Quiet Sleep in Infants.* In: Kellaway P, Petersen I, eds. *Clinical Electroencephalography of Children.* New York: Grune & Stratton; 1968.
11. Parmelee AH Jr, Schulte FJ, Akiyama Y, Wenner WH, Schultz MA, Stern E. Maturation of EEG activity during sleep in premature infants. *Electroencephalogr Clin Neurophysiol* 1968;24:319.
12. Petre-Quaden O. Ontogenesis of paradoxical sleep in the human newborn. *J Neurol Sci* 1967;4:153.
13. Anders T, Emde R, Parmelee A, eds. *A Manual of Standardized Terminology, Techniques and Criteria for Scoring of States of Sleep and Wakefulness in Newborn Infants.* Los Angeles: UCLA Brain Information Service, NINDS Neurological Information Network; 1971.

10

One Month to Twelve Months

A wide variety of changes occur during the first year of post-natal life. It is a period of rapid growth and/or development of many organ systems. Central nervous system (CNS) development during this early stage of life is complex and is sensitive to both internal and environmental factors. The structure of sleep and the sleep-wake cycle closely mirrors these neurodevelopmental changes. Dendritic branching in the brain is occurring at a rapid pace. Neuronal migration occurs early, and synaptic connections and myelination are progressing. EEG development, development of state organization and circadian cycling are important parameters that can be assessed polysomnographically.

MOST COMMON INDICATIONS FOR POLYSOMNOGRAPHY

Apparent Life-Threatening Events

Apparent life-threatening events (ALTEs) are episodes observed by parents in which apneic events are thought to be present and some intervention is attempted. Events are frightening to the observer and often result in resuscitative efforts. They should not be termed "near miss SIDS" or "aborted SIDS" (1) since such labels imply a misleading association between ALTEs and SIDS. Most infants with ALTEs do not die of SIDS and infants who die of SIDS most frequently do not have a history of ALTEs (1,2).

TABLE 10-1. *Indications for polysomnography*

Most common indications	Indicated under certain circumstances	Potential indications
ALTE	Gastroesophageal reflux	Intrauterine-drug exposure
Seizure disorder	Developmental delays	Colic
Loud snoring	Hypertonia	State disorganization
Stridor	RSV pulmonary infection	CNS abnormalities
S/P Cleft palate repair	Failure to thrive	Nocturnal wakings without
Mandibular hypoplasia	S/P prematurity	behavioral etiologies
Macroglossia		Abnormal feeding/
Frequent apnea alarms		swallowing
Unexplained bradycardia		Congenital malformations
Unexplained hypoxemia		
Movement disorders		
Hypotonia		

ALTE describes a clinical syndrome. A variety of identifiable conditions can cause such episodes (e.g., GER, systemic infection, CNS tumors, seizures, upper-airway obstruction, anemia, and central hypoventilation syndrome).

ALTEs are probably the most common indication for conducting polysomnography in infants from 1 to 6 months of age. Infants who have suffered from an event that could be life threatening require comprehensive evaluation. Polysomnography can provide information regarding maturation of respiration, stability of autonomic nervous system function, maturation of the respiratory system, maturation of the CNS, and present (or absence) of abnormalities of state organization. Presence of prolonged uninterrupted sleep states can be determined by polysomnography. Percentages of indeterminate sleep and periodic breathing are important determinants in the assessment of infants who have suffered an ALTE. In addition, assessment for the presence of other abnormalities that may result in ALTE can be determined polysomnographically (e.g., gastroesophageal reflux, cardiac arrhythmias, seizure disorder).

Decisions regarding whether to prescribe a home monitor *should not be determined by polysomnography.* Prescriptions for home cardiorespiratory monitoring of an infant after an ALTE is based on clinical evaluation and criteria. Polysomnography is utilized primarily to evaluate victims of ALTEs for the presence of treatable conditions.

Apnea of Infancy

Apnea of infancy is defined as respiratory pauses of 20 seconds or more, or apneic events lasting less than 20 seconds that are associated with a significant fall in heart rate and/or decrease in hemoglobin-oxygen saturation (with or without cyanosis). Apnea of infancy appears to be a different disorder than apnea of prematurity. It occurs in term infants (rather than premature infants) and response to administration of methylxanthines is variable. Apnea of infancy is also apparently not associated with an increased risk of sudden unexpected nocturnal death. It seems to be a common cause of ALTE in apparently otherwise normal newborns.

Two different types of physiologic respiratory events (4) can result in respiratory events that appear graphically similar to pathologic apneas. Sleep-related breath-holding spells (SRBH) and post-sigh respiratory pauses can last 20 seconds or longer. SRBH are often associated with a profound decrease in heart rate. However, bradycardia occurs *during the first 9 seconds of the event* (similar/identical to performance of a Valsalva Maneuver), compared to a pathologic obstructive apnea or central apnea where there is a progressive decrease in the heart rate during the event. Post-sigh pauses are generally not associated with a decrease in the heart rate. Neither is associated with significant fall in oxygen saturation. Polysomnography can clearly differentiate between these various types of respiratory pauses (4). It is unclear whether longitudinal cardiorespiratory monitoring is advisable in infants with SRBH and post-sigh respiratory pauses. Prescription of monitors should be based upon clinical criteria.

Congenital Central Hypoventilation Syndrome

Although congenital central hypoventilation syndrome is often diagnosed in the newborn period, it may present later during infancy as an ALTE or as unexplained cyanosis (or oxygen desaturation) during sleep. Typically, the infants appear completely normal during wakefulness. Polysomnography reveals hypoventilation during sleep rather than periods of occlusive apneic events. $PaCO_2$ and/or $TcPCO_2$ is typically elevated. Periodic arousals may occur. Polysomnography is necessary for accurate characterization of respiratory events as well as longitudinal monitoring of progress and for follow-up. Sleep-related ventilator management, bi-level CPAP, or diaphragmatic pacing is typically required.

Seizure Disorders

Sleep-related seizures are a clear indication for comprehensive polysomnography between 1 and 6 months of age. Comprehensive sleep EEG can assist in determining seizure control and assessment of functional status in infants who are suffering from sleep-related ictal events. Since seizure may be one cause of ALTEs, polysomnography may provide useful information in ruling out seizure as the cause of ALTE.

Snoring

A history of loud snoring during infancy, especially if the snoring is associated with perceptible pauses and snorts, is a clear indication for polysomnography. Polysomnography is the most widely accepted method for determination of the presence of obstructive sleep apnea syndrome. During early infancy, snoring associated with upper-airway obstruction may signify an anatomic abnormality such as micrognathia, macroglossia, choanal stenosis, or pharyngeal masses. It may signify the presence a neuromuscular abnormality. These possibilities should be carefully evaluated during the initial clinical assessment. Polysomnography may reveal the presence of obstructive, mixed, or expiratory apnea, or high upper-airway resistance. Polysomnography can assist in determining both the presence and severity of upper-airway obstruction.

Sleep-Related Stridor

Inspiratory stridor suggests airway obstruction at the level of the glottis. Sleep-related stridor can occur under a number of circumstances: laryngospasm secondary to GER into the pharynx, laryngo-tracheomalacia, idiopathic sleep-related laryngospasm, laryngeal dystonia, and seizure disorders. Polysomnography can help differentiate etiology and degree of airway obstruction as well as clinical implications.

Cleft Palate Repair

Sleep-related occlusive airway disease frequently occurs after repair of cleft palate. Creation of a pharyngeal flap can occlude the airway enough to result in high-airflow resistance and obstructive sleep apnea. A wide range of symptoms can occur. The degree of airflow resistance depends upon airway patency, diameter, and function. Significant morbidity (ranging from typical diurnal symptoms associated with OSAS to pulmonary hypertension and cor pulmonale) is seen secondary to the airway occlusion during sleep after surgery.

Mandibular Hypoplasia and Macroglossia

Syndromes with features of mandibular and/or maxillary hypoplasia are often associated with OSAS. A narrow airway with abnormal muscular origins and insertions resulting in dysfunctional muscle motion are the typical causes. Severe sequelae can occur. Syndromes commonly associated with mandibular hypoplasia include Treacher Collins and Pierre Robin syndrome. Syndromes associated with macroglossia might include Beckwith syndrome. Polysomnography can provide information regarding severity of airway obstruction as well as provide a method of monitoring patients longitudinally after therapeutic intervention.

Frequent Home Apnea Monitor Alarms

Cardiorespiratory alarms are common in infants being monitored at home after an ALTE or for apnea of infancy, apnea of prematurity, and other indications for home monitoring. It is often difficult to determine whether alarms are real or artifactual based on parental reports. Home-event recorders provide some information regarding the presence of pathologic apneas. However, raw data from each event recording requires close analysis prior to determination of whether an event is artifact or pathologic.

Polysomnography can clearly differentiate between true and false alarms. Home monitors should be brought to the laboratory and utilized during the course of the polysomnogram. All apnea/bradycardia alarms must be directly recorded on the polysomnographic recording.

Unexplained Sleep-Related Bradycardia

Sleep-related bradycardia may be identified during monitoring in the neonatal nursery or may be first noted during home monitoring after an ALTE. Holter monitoring may or may not provide adequate information regarding the cause of the bradycardia. Measuring multiple physiologic parameters simultaneously during polysomnographic recording can provide more significant information into the cause of unexplained decreases in heart rate during sleep. Episodes may be associated with pathologic apnea, benign sleep-related breath-holding (physiologic expiratory apnea), laryngospasm, intrinsic cardiovascular abnormalities, or autonomic nervous system dysfunction.

Unexplained Sleep-Related Hypoxemia

Sleep-related hypoxemia may also be identified in the neonatal nursery during the newborn period while the infant is being monitored during the course of acute medical illness. Cyanosis during wakefulness may be a result of primary underlying pulmonary or cardiac disease/disorders. Sleep-related hypoxemia may be first noted as an ALTE by parents at home. It may signify alveolar hypoventilation during sleep, congenital hypoventilation, sleep-related seizures, autonomic nervous system dysfunction, sleep-related cardiac arrhythmia, or obstructive sleep apnea syndrome. Polysomnography is a valuable tool in assessing the underlying cause for sleep-related hypoxemia in the infant with normal oxygen concentrations/saturations during wakefulness.

Sleep-Related Movement Disorders

Motor activity during sleep is common during infancy. Phasic movements, major body movements, vocalizations, facial movements, twitches, and writhing type activity is typically seen. Most of these movement behaviors are normal. Even rhythmic movements of the body and head are frequently seen during state transitions. These types of movements are most likely maturational phenomena during this age group. The most common are body shuttling, body rocking, head banging, head rolling, and other rhythmic movements. Benign rhythmic movement disorders tend to occur during sleep-wake transitions and may persist into sleep for brief periods of time. Those rhythmic and/or stereotypic behaviors occurring exclusively during sleep (apparently unrelated to sleep-wake transitions) are less likely to be benign and sleep laboratory evaluation is most likely warranted.

Conditions Associated with Hypotonia

Generalized neuromuscular diseases (e.g., Werdnig-Hoffman disease, type II spinal muscular atrophy, Down syndrome) associated with hypotonia are often indications for polysomnography. Generalized hypotonia affects all skeletal muscles. Hypotonia can have a profound effect on pharyngeal muscles resulting in an inability to maintain pharyngeal patency during sleep and obstructive breathing. Generalized hypotonia can also be associated with nocturnal oxygen desaturations, and assessment of the ability to sustain ventilation by diaphragm and accessory muscles of breathing can also be evaluated in the sleep laboratory.

POLYSOMNOGRAPHY INDICATED UNDER CERTAIN CIRCUMSTANCES

Gastroesophageal Reflux

Gastroesophageal reflux (GER) is *very* common during early infancy. Almost all newborn infants will reflux to some degree. Cardioesophageal sphincter tone and esophageal coordination mature quite rapidly during early infancy but approximately one third of infants will still reflux at 6 months of age (5,6). Reflux into the esophagus typically results in arousal, not apnea (7). Obstructive apneas occur when there is reflux into the pharynx during sleep. The occlusion is typically due to laryngospasm. Clinical symptoms include frequent regurgitation or vomiting after feedings, nasal regurgitation, inconsolable crying secondary to esophageal irritation and pain (symptoms resembling colic), choking, gagging, coughing, and stridor during feeding. Similar symptoms can occur during sleep. Coughing, choking, gagging, and/or apneic events associated with gastroesophageal reflux tend to be sporadic, only occurring several times during the entire sleep period. *They are not periodic* as seen in classical obstructive sleep apnea.

Developmental Delays

Developmental delays and unexplained failure to thrive can be evaluated in the sleep laboratory to provide assessments of cross-sectional functional status and may be able to provide prognostic (neurodevelopmental outcome) information under certain circumstances. Longitudinal evaluations may be able to provide more reliable and sensitive data regarding functional, behavioral, and environmental causes for the developmental delay, compared with a purely physiologic abnormality.

Unexplained Failure to Thrive

Polysomnography can assist in the evaluation of unexplained failure to thrive. Failure to thrive is commonly associated with disease and obstructive sleep apnea syndrome during infancy. Upper-airway obstruction may be due to a variety of causes and polysomnography can identify secondary pathophysiologic changes associated with the primary etiology.

Neurologic Conditions Associated with Hypertonia

The presence of a neuromuscular disorder is an indication for polysomnography when diurnal symptoms and/or control are at question. Characterization of EEG, its maturation, and state organization can be assessed. Hypertonia can be associated with abnormal function of the pharyngeal musculature, and when clinically indicated, the presence of sleep-related breathing disorders can be best evaluated polysomnographically.

Respiratory Syncytial Virus (RSV) Infections

RSV infections are common causes of apnea during early infancy. The infection is most prevalent during the late fall and winter months. In small infants, the infection presents as a pulmonary infection. Apnea can occur at any time during the acute phase or recovery phase of the illness. It can be associated with ALTE and sudden unexpected nocturnal death. In the presence of infection, consideration should be given to obtaining polysomnography to assist in determination of the infant's pulmonary status during sleep and the possible need for monitoring.

Premature Infant with Complications of Prematurity

Older premature infants who had complications during the neonatal period (e.g., intraventricular hemorrhage, intracranial infection, bronchopulmonary dysplasia, apnea of prematurity) can benefit from polysomnography. Polysomnography can provide information regarding the functional status of the infant (by evaluation of state development), degree of morbid complications from the primary medical disease/disorder, and monitoring of the improvement of status by rehabilitative efforts and recovery.

POTENTIAL INDICATIONS FOR POLYSOMNOGRAPHY

Intrauterine-Drug Exposure

Although during this time of life apnea may be more common in infants exposed to drugs (especially cocaine) during gestation, it is not a universal phenomenon and all infants who have experienced intrauterine-drug exposure (IUDE) need not be tested in the laboratory for apnea. Infants positive for drugs at birth should be evaluated clinically. Developmental aspects of EEG and state concordance can provide both functional and prognostic information. Therefore, a baseline study for physiologic neurodevelopmental landmarks may prove in the future to be a more sensitive indicator for early and intensive intervention.

Colic

Episodes of colic begin at 2 to 3 weeks of age in normal, healthy term newborns. Colic paroxysms are of extreme irritability, which are typically inconsolable by parents. Episodes last for more than 3 hours per day and more than 3 days per week, associated with uninhibited motor activity, hypertonia during the episodes, and violent screaming. Attacks typically occur during late afternoon and evening hours. Episodes of colic must be differentiated from NREM motor disorders/parasomnias, seizures, GER, apnea, and pain syndromes/conditions. Polysomnography may be helpful in sorting out paroxysmal disorders, especially if symptoms are present after 4 months of age.

State Disorganization and Circadian Rhythm Abnormalities

Significant changes occur in biologic rhythm development between 1 and 6 months of age. Ultradian rhythm begins to fade and a circadian rhythm becomes predominant. In the absence of emergence of appropriate rhythms between 8 and 12 weeks of age, a sleep disorders evaluation is most likely indicated. A sleep log is the first step in evaluation. Behavioral etiologies are most common. If these do not seem to be the primary underlying cause (the most important suggestive symptom is an inability of the infant to sleep anywhere, even when suspected behavioral correlates are present), polysomnography can be helpful in differentiating behavioral and environmental causes from an underlying physiologic abnormality.

CNS Abnormalities

Clinically diagnosed CNS abnormalities may be associated with sleep-related symptoms that can further compound developmental problems. Primary CNS disorders (e.g., Arnold Chiari malformation, seizure disorders, cerebral palsy) can be associated with sleep-related respiratory impairment, electrical seizure activity isolated to sleep, fragmentation of the continuity of sleep, state discordance, and autonomic nervous system dysfunction. Each has particular polysomnographic characteristics that can assist in diagnosis and management.

Nocturnal Wakings Without Identifiable Behavioral Cause

Nocturnal wakings during the first 10 weeks of life are normal and reflect dominant ultradian cycling of the infant. By 8 to 10 weeks of age, sleep begins to consolidate at night with the longest sleep period being during nocturnal hours and the longest wake period occurring during the day. By 12 to 16 weeks, sleep begins to consolidate at night without waking for feeding and diurnal sleep consolidates into discrete nap periods. If this does not occur, the causes may be behavioral (e.g., environmental sleep disorder, inappropriate parental expectations, etc.) or physiologic (e.g., obstructive sleep apnea, gastroesophageal reflux). If the etiology is unclear, polysomnography can assist in the diagnosis.

Abnormal Feeding and Swallowing Syndromes

Syndromes associated with pharyngeal incoordination and swallowing defects may be associated with neuromuscular abnormalities. This incoordination may also be associated with abnormal movements of the pharyngeal airway during sleep. This may result in occlusive airway events. These conditions may be due to underlying CNS abnormalities, intrinsic pharyngeal disorders, esophageal abnormalities, congenital anatomic defects, or autonomic nervous system disorders.

Congenital Malformations of the Head, Neck, Face, and/or Chest

Any malformation of the face, head, neck, or chest can result in airway obstruction during sleep. During all evaluations possible sleep abnormalities should be considered. When sleep dysfunction appears to be present based on historic information, polysomnography should be considered.

TECHNICAL CONSIDERATIONS AND TECHNIQUES

The most important aspect in obtaining a high-quality and reproducible polysomnographic recording is proper preparation of the parents and the infant. Parents should be provided with a comprehensive description of the polysomnographic procedure both verbally and in writing. Since these studies are most often performed as outpatients, parents should be offered an opportunity to visit the laboratory prior to the study. This can provide time for the center staff to answer questions and assuage any parental anxieties or fears.

Parents are asked to arrive at the center about 1 hour prior to the beginning of the study so that acclimation to the sleeping environment may occur. This also allows the infant time to acclimate to personnel.

After 1–2 months of age, body temperature regulation has matured to a point where warming units are not necessary. Humidity in the sleep laboratory can be centrally controlled. The temperature of the sleeping environment should be comfortable for the parents. Infants should not be over-dressed for sleep. They should wear bed-clothing similar to that in which the parent feels comfortable. In younger infants, swaddling may be necessary. Choice of bed-clothing should take this swaddling into consideration so as not to over-heat the infant.

A crib of the sort used in the home setting should be available for the infant. Hospital cribs are not necessary. Parents should sleep in the room with the infant.

Length of the study should include at least 2 sleep-wake cycles (including one feeding during the middle of the study). Nocturnal studies seem to be required because of the emerging circadian rhythms. Circadian rhythms exist not only for the sleep-wake cycle, but also for abnormal respiratory events and abnormal CNS electrical activity. In the older infant who has consolidated sleep into a single nocturnal sleep period, a minimum of 10 hours of sleep recording should be sought. Diurnal nap studies should be discouraged. Because of the change in emerging biologic rhythms, presence and severity of respiratory and CNS abnormalities cannot be appreciated during diurnal naps.

Recommended Equipment

Recommended equipment is identical to that required for conducting polysomnography in premature and newborn infants. A 16-channel polygraph and appropriate electrodes and recording devices for electroencephalography, electro-oculography, electromyography, electrocardiography, respiratory effort, respiratory airflow, and oximetry must be available. Video monitoring (especially split-screen video/audio) is extremely helpful in assessment and documentation of polysomnography. Instrumentation to determine and record body movement and position can be helpful. The most helpful aspect of polysomnogram analysis is the provision of almost continuous technician notation directly on the recording.

Technical Considerations

During this developmental period, polysomnography should provide accurate and reproducible information regarding: (i) EEG maturation and development; (ii) state concordance and development of sleep architecture; (iii) characterization of cardiorespiratory function including airflow, effort, oxygenation, and cardiac rate and rhythm; (iv) characterization of body movements and position; and (v) integration of all physiologic parameters. As with premature and term newborns, techniques, protocols, and equipment should be available to handle special situations in the laboratory, including but not be limited to the need for supplemental oxygen, assisted and/or controlled ventilation, nasal CPAP, need for follow-up home monitoring, and evaluation of tracheostomy flow.

EEG

Standard International 10-20 system of electrode placement should be utilized. Montage selection should be determined by the needs of the diagnostic study. A complete bipolar screening montage should be standard. Specific modification of the electrode array should be based on the needs of the infant and the presenting clinical situation. A recommended standard montage might be:

A1-T3
T3-C3
C3-Cz (Fig. 10-1)
Cz-C4
C4-T4
T4-A2
Cz-O2

Paper speed is recommended at 10 mm/second. For prolonged monitoring EEG, a paper speed of 15 mm/second might be chosen. If ictal activity is suspected, the paper speed should be increased to 30 mm/second. Digital technology provides the ability to record the EEG parameters at one speed, but choose playback at a variety of speeds and in a variety of montage selections. What is particularly lost during digital/paperless recordings is resolution of EEG activity.

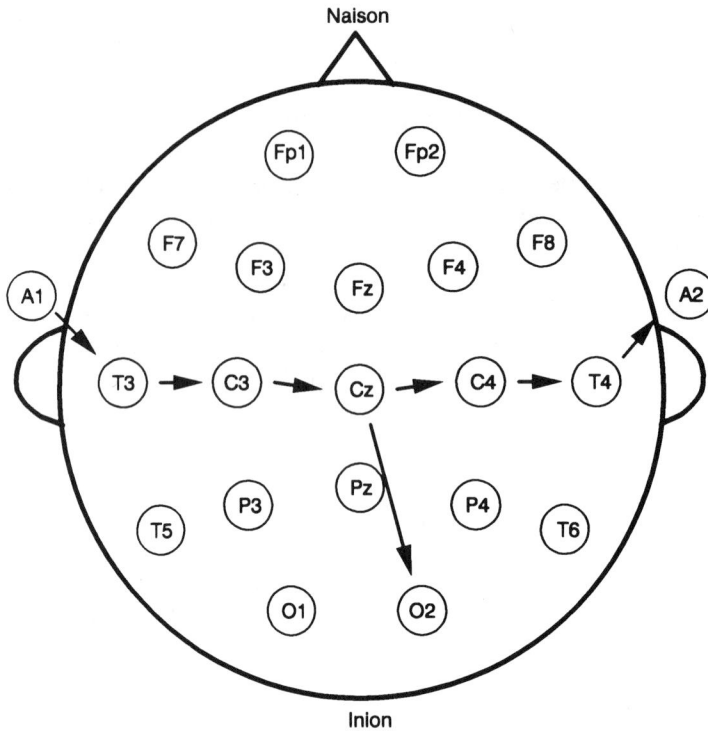

FIG. 10-1. Bipolar, transcoronal montage. The occipital channel (Cz–O2) may be used for sleep-state scoring as well as assistance in identifying wake-sleep transitions (alpha activity which is generally most preponderant over the posterior head region).

Other Physiologic Parameters

EOG, EMG, EKG, limb movements, and respiratory efforts should be measured according to the standard protocol established at the beginning of this section.

ELECTRODE APPLICATION AND TECHNIQUES

The most important aspect in the recording of a high-quality polysomnogram is preparation of the infant (and parents) for the study. Most studies will be performed on an outpatient basis and patients and parents should be appropriately prepared and introduced to the procedure. Meticulous and careful preparation of the electrode sites are essential. Persistent monitoring of signal quality and maintenance of electrode placement requires the presence and tenacity of a caring, competent, and diligent technician.

Head Wrapping

Head wrapping is advisable during this age group. Wrapping the head with Kerlix will assist in placing even pressure on all covered electrodes and protects the electrodes during frequent head and body movements during the study. The head should be wrapped using the procedure presented on pages 109-110.

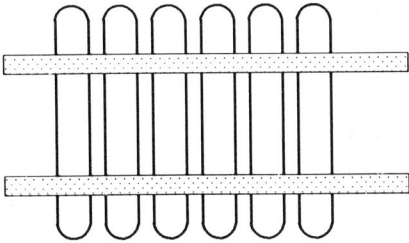

FIG. 10-2. Armboard restraint for smaller infants. Attach several tongue blades together with tape.

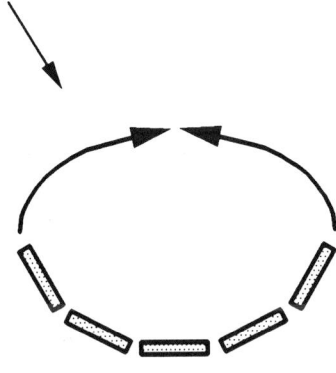

FIG. 10-3. Armboard restraint for smaller infants. Form a loose tube around the infant's elbow.

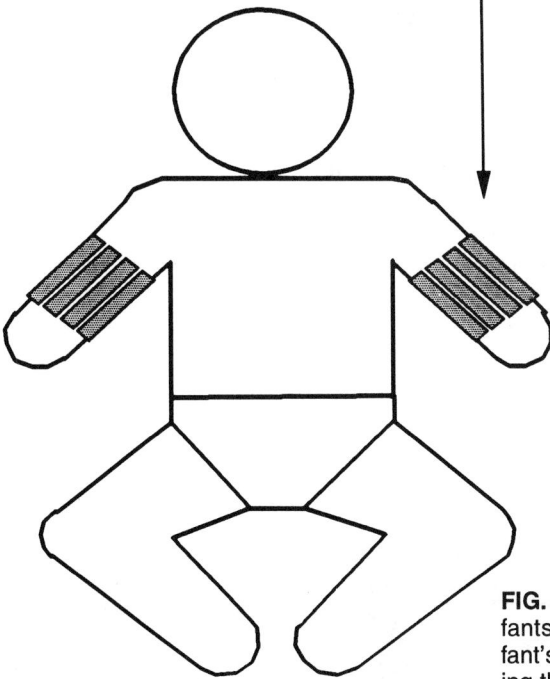

FIG. 10-4. Armboard restraint for smaller infants. Join the tongue blades around the infant's arm with tape in order to prevent bending the arm at the elbow. The infant will have the freedom to move his arms, but will be unable to reach the electrodes.

Arm Restraints

During this age period, frequent arm and leg movements during the course of the study are common. Frequently, during arousals electrodes become displaced by older infants swiping and pulling at the electrodes. It is advisable to prevent the infant's arms from reaching the electrodes. Full restraint of the arms is not advisable since it can disrupt the study and establish an artificial situation. Full arm and leg restraint will also limit the older infant's movements and ability to roll and change body position. Arm restraints, however, can be applied in a sensitive manner without causing disruption of the study and giving the infant mobility but still limiting arm movements so that electrodes can be maintained.

Arm restraints can be created for small infants by taping tongue blades together, gently wrapping the arm (including the antecubital fossae and elbow), and encircling the wrapped region with the taped tongue blades (Figs. 10-2–10-4).

Tongue blades are often too small for older infants, but, the same restraint may be accomplished by using a padded arm board placed at the elbow in order to prevent movement of the arms (Fig. 10-5).

Patient Calibrations

As in the premature and term infant, standard patient calibration cannot be performed. Prior to the onset of the study, behavioral observations must be recorded on the polysomnogram. The technician's behavioral observations and notations should be frequent since they can provide the polysomnographer vital information regarding activity during the course of the study that is important for interpretation.

Initial Polygraphic Parameters

Initial parameters should be set as described on pages 110-111. Since equipment varies considerably, manufacturers' recommendations and modifications should be incorporated into the laboratory calibration and recording procedures. During the initial portions of the study, parameters should be adjusted to record the most reliable and interpretable tracings. Adjustment and modification of digital equipment is considerably different from analog machines. Each laboratory should establish its own guidelines for modification of the recording of each physiologic parameter.

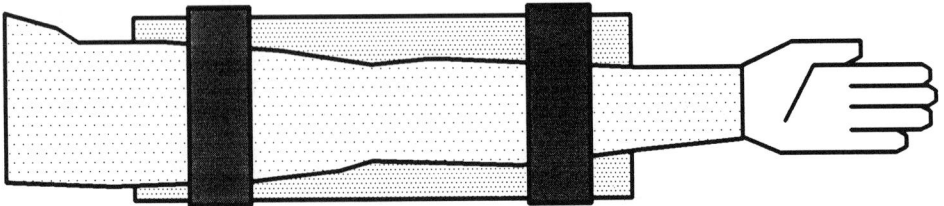

FIG. 10-5. Armboard restraint for older infants and toddlers.

EVALUATION AND SCORING OF POLYSOMNOGRAMS OF INFANTS ONE TO SIX MONTHS OF AGE

All polysomnograms should be recorded and scored for state determination in an epoch-by-epoch manner. Although epochs of 30 seconds are standard, epochs of 20 seconds are acceptable for clinical studies. Paper speed may be varied according to the clinical situation. With paperless systems, recording speed is standard. Playback can be modified depending upon the interpretation needs.

Between 1 and 6 months of age, a wide variety of changes occur in the development of the infant's state. EEG undergoes maturational changes. NREM-sleep states begin to become identifiable and distinct. Total sleep time decreases from about 17 to 18 hours during the neonatal period to about 14 to 15 hours by 16 weeks and 13 to 14 hours by 8 months (7).

During this time period, clear age demarcations do not exist. There is gradual change and transition is the rule rather than the exception. Therefore, rules for scoring state and determination of sleep stage are less important than identification of maturational issues related to EEG, sleep structure, and state development.

EEG development, on the other hand, appears to follow a maturational pattern that is quite exact and reproducible according to conceptional age. Variations in EEG maturation during the first 6 months of life may provide more information regarding development than behavioral evaluations during the waking state. Indeed, the development of state also follows a pattern with fairly reproducible internal and external validity. However, state changes require the evaluation of multiple physiologic variables that may mature at different times making state determination more difficult than identification of specific EEG characteristics.

Behavioral Observations

Recording infant's behaviors during the course of the study is essential for interpretation. Notations should be made directly on the record. Comments about twitches, facial movements, vocalizations, body movements, limb movements, and caretaker's interventions should be included. Technician's notations regarding artifacts and attempts to correct them should also be recorded directly on the polysomnogram.

Wakefulness

Between 1 and 6 months of age *EEG* of wakefulness is characterized by regional differences in electrical activity. Amplitude is relatively high (50 to 100 µV), background rhythm is rather slow (when compared to more mature states) and reaction to stimulation is generally present. Waking background rhythm consists of rhythmic and mixed frequencies in the delta and theta range. Posterior slow-wave activity is common. Before 5 months of age, rhythmic occipital activity develops from the diffuse theta activity. This diffuse theta activity may be most prominent over the central and posterior regions. Absence of generalized rhythmic theta activity during wakefulness should be considered abnormal. Occipital EEG rhythms can be clearly distinguished from the background by 3 months of age. Frequencies range from 3–4 Hz and amplitude is reduced when the eyes are open. They become more regular and increase to about 5-Hz frequency by 5 months of age.

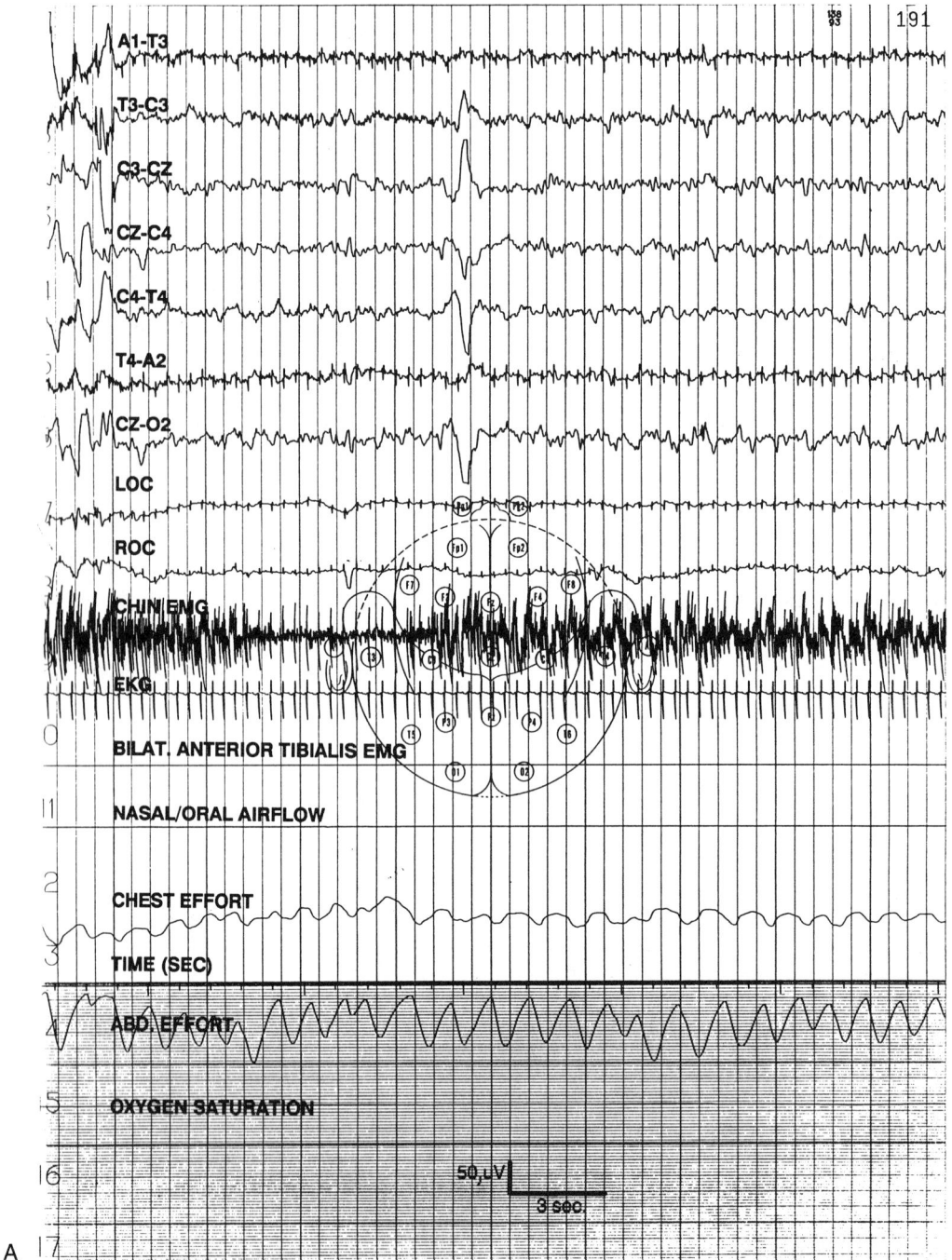

FIG. 10-6. A–B: Quiet wakefulness in a 2-month-old infant. A relatively low-voltage, mixed-frequency EEG with occasional movement artifact. Although there are minimal eye movements noted on the EOG, the technician's notes confirm that the patient is awake. Chin tone is high

Continued.

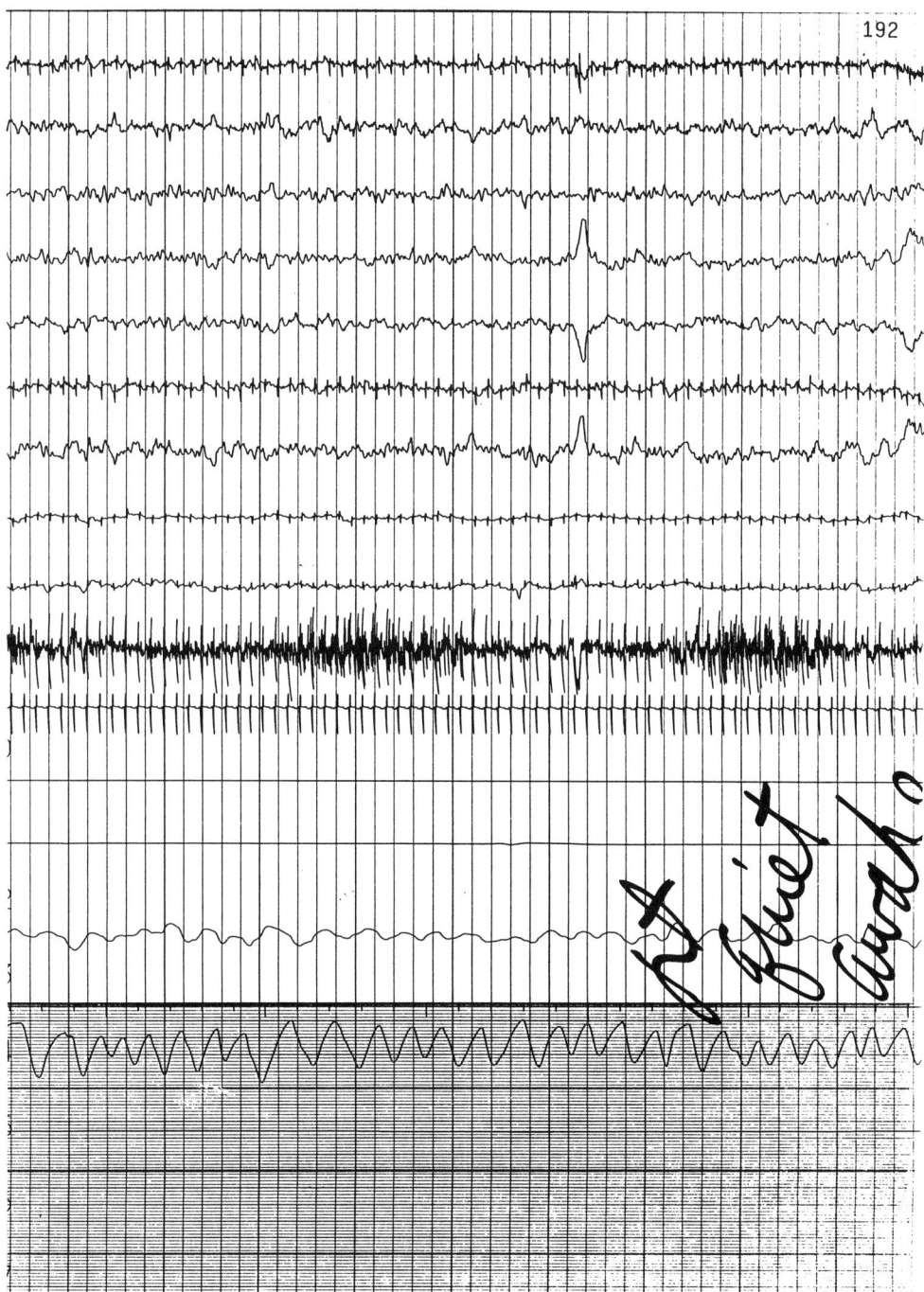

and there is sucking artifact noted. Anterior tibialis EMG and airflow sensors have yet to be placed because of the infant's tactile defensiveness.

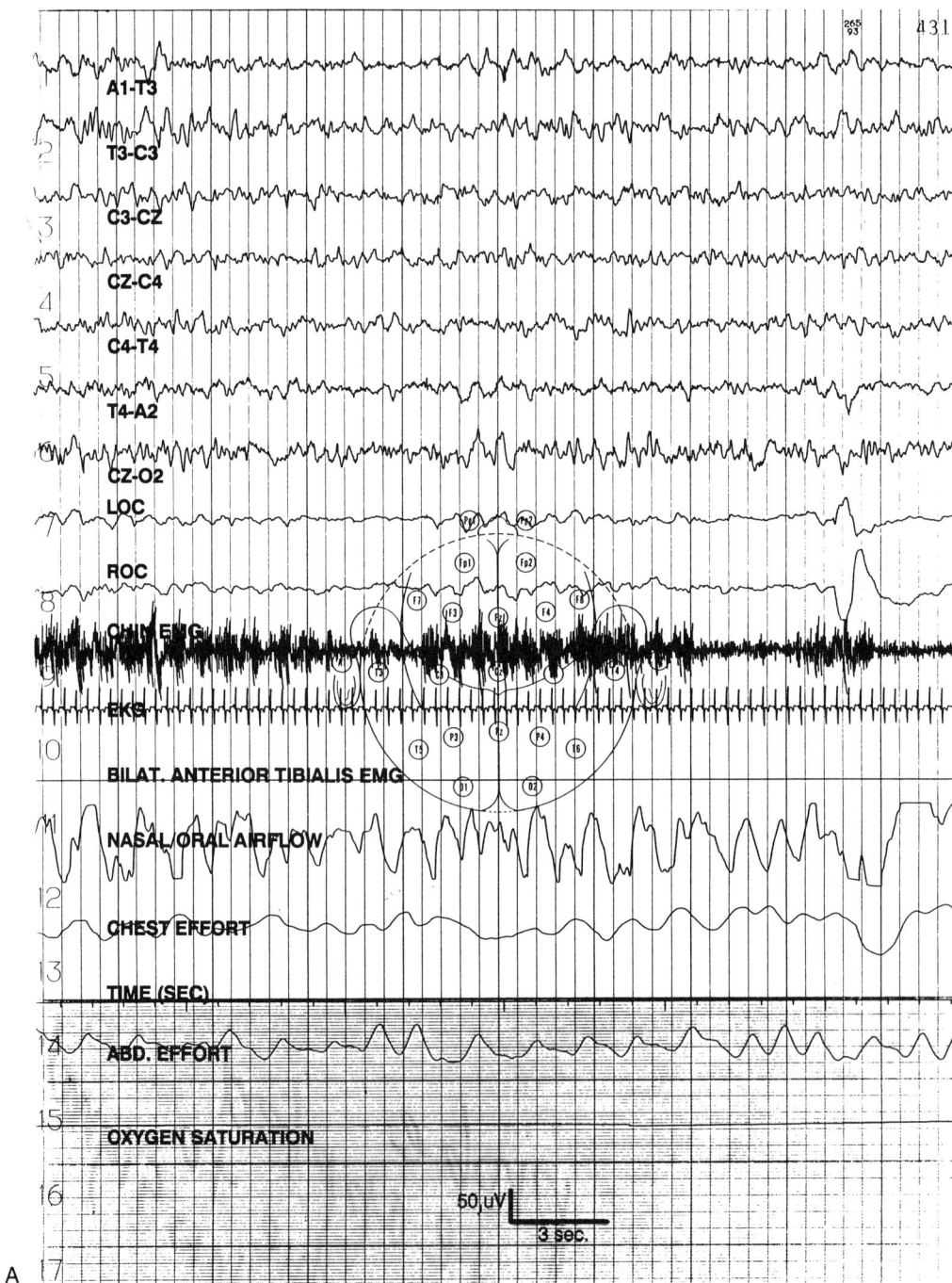

FIG. 10-7. A–B: Quiet wakefulness in a 5-month-old infant. There is a relatively low-voltage, mixed-frequency background rhythm interspersed with rhythmic 5- to 6-Hz activity characteristic of quiet wakefulness. Conjugate eye movements are present and the chin muscle tone is high (sucking artifact is present). Bilateral anterior tibialis EMG has not yet been placed. Nasal/oral airflow is being recorded and respirations are quite irregular.

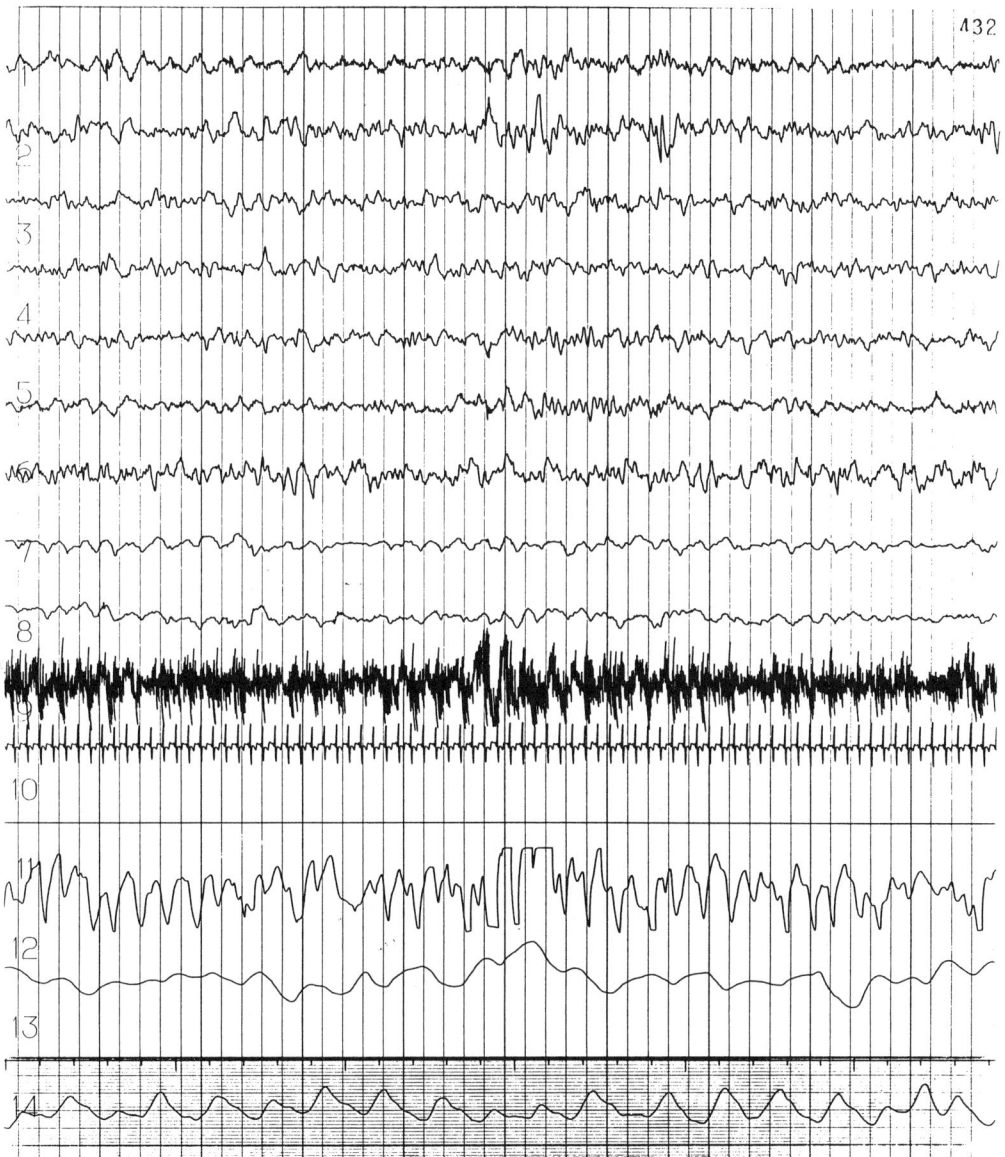

FIG. 10-7. *Continued.*

During wakefulness *EMG* activity is high and remains tonic. Movement artifact is frequent. Sucking artifact is commonly seen on chin muscle EMG and reveals periodicity during drowsiness and transitional states.

With the eyes open, *EOG* reveals conjugate eye movements. Occasional dysconjugate eye movements seen during the neonatal period become less frequent.

Heart rate ranges between 120 and 160 beats per minute. Heart rate typically increases during crying and/or vigorous activity. A sinus arrhythmia (respiratory variations) may be appreciated. *Respirations* are irregular and periods of tachypnea, respiratory pauses, and changes in respiratory effort are frequently seen. The normal waking respiratory rate during periods when the infant is quiet is 20 to 40 breaths per minute. *Oxygen saturation* remains stable (Figs. 10-6 and 10-7).

NREM Sleep

Differentiation of NREM-sleep states begins between 1 and 3 months of age. Between 4 and 6 weeks, sleep may be classified according to the predominant patterns. For example, some infants have a relatively immature pattern of state development and may be scored according to newborn criteria. Other infants reveal a more mature pattern and NREM-sleep states may be discernible. In these infants, state may be scored according to more mature criteria. Persistence of immature patterns after 6 weeks of age may denote delays in development that may not have yet been expressed clinically.

Transition from wake to sleep is generally rapid and smooth between 1 and 6 months of age. EEG reveals a gradual appearance of rhythmic, high-voltage 3- to 5-Hz waves with amplitudes of about 75 to 200 µV. They are widely distributed and continue for several minutes at the onset of sleep. As the infant matures, the transitional pattern begins to show occipital or widespread rhythmic asynchronous 4- to 5-Hz activity of moderate amplitude. Between 4 and 12 weeks of post-conceptional term, the infant will continue to transition from wakefulness into active sleep. Between 10 and 12 weeks of post-conceptional term, this transition begins to change to a more mature pattern of transition from wakefulness to sleep through NREM sleep and cycles every 40 to 50 minutes.

The tracé alternant pattern characteristic of quiet sleep in the neonate gradually changes after 1–3 weeks of age. By 4 weeks of age, the tracé alternant pattern is completely replaced by a high-voltage, slow-wave pattern of activity. At approximately 4 weeks of post-conceptional term, sleep spindles begin to appear and are generally well formed and established by 8 weeks of age. They begin to develop in the central regions during the first few weeks of life and become more widely distributed as development progresses. They tend to occur in bursts almost continuously throughout NREM sleep at the age of 2 to 6 months. Spindles are generally asymmetric and asynchronous in young infants. However, marked and persistent reduction in spindle activity over one hemisphere raises the question of unilateral depression of brain electrical activity. After 3 months of age, absence of spindles is probably abnormal.

Vertex sharp waves can be present during the neonatal period, but differ from more mature vertex waves by their lower amplitude. By 5–6 months, vertex sharp transients are generally well established and occur in bursts, especially during transitional sleep. Vertex waves are high-voltage (up to 250 µV) negative waves with a wide distribution about the vertex with a duration lasting less than 200 milliseconds.

By 6 months of age, a more mature pattern of NREM sleep is established. NREM sleep can be separated into at least 3 distinct states: stage 1 (transitional state), stage 2 (intermediate state), and slow-wave sleep. Slow wave sleep has been separated into two states dependent upon the percentage of slow-wave activity present (i.e., stage 3 is scored when each 30-second epoch consists of at least 20%, but less than 50% slow-wave activity; stage 4 is scored when each 30-second epoch consists of 50% or more slow waves). This separation is somewhat arbitrary since physiologic activity seems to be similar in both states.

Between 4 and 6 months of post-conceptional term the high-voltage, slow-wave activity of NREM sleep in infants begins to show a more mature, adult-like pattern with clear differentiation of stage 2 and slow-wave sleep. Descent through stages of sleep is quite rapid in young infants and the time from transition to slow-wave sleep may be only several minutes.

K-complexes are high-voltage slow waves that begin to appear after 4 to 6 months of age, are similar to vertex waves, but are much slower in frequency. There is an initial negative potential followed by a positive potential and return to the baseline. Often K-complexes are followed immediately by a sleep spindle. In contrast to vertex waves that appear during transitional stages of sleep, K-complexes occur during intermediate states. They may appear suddenly in response to a specific stimulus (e.g., auditory clicks, tactile stimulus) or may occur spontaneously.

NREM sleep during this period of development is also characterized by tonic muscle activity on chin muscle EMG. Movements are minimal and gross body movements generally signify a state change. EOG reveals no conjugate or saccadic eye movements and, often, the EOG is contaminated with frontal EEG artifact (Note: in our laboratories we tend to decrease EOG sensitivity in order to decrease EEG contamination. However, during slow-wave sleep and high-voltage activity, EEG contamination of the EOG is inevitable). Respiratory pattern is regular and monotonous. Heart rate is also regular and monotonous showing only minimal respiratory variation and normal sinus arrhythmia (Fig. 10-8A).

2-month-old—high-voltage slow-wave activity
(Fig. 8B)
2-month-old—high-voltage slow-wave activity
(Fig. 10-9A)
5-month-old—high-voltage slow-wave activity
(Fig. 10-9B)
5-month-old—high-voltage slow-wave activity
(Fig. 10-10A)
9-month-old—NREM-stage 2
(Fig. 10-10B)
9-month-old—NREM-slow-wave sleep

REM Sleep

Typically, REM sleep is distinguished from NREM sleep by the EEG pattern, EMG hypotonia, and the presence of saccadic, conjugate extraocular movements. Irregular breathing patterns are characteristic and muscle twitches, limb movements, and major body movements are common. However, these behavioral characteristics of REM sleep can also be seen in the presence of EEG patterns characteristic of NREM sleep; stability of respiration, absence of movements, and monotony of physiologic variation can also be seen in the presence of EEG that is characteristic of REM sleep. Furthermore, the EEG pattern of REM sleep in infants consists of activity in the 2- to 6-Hz frequency range that

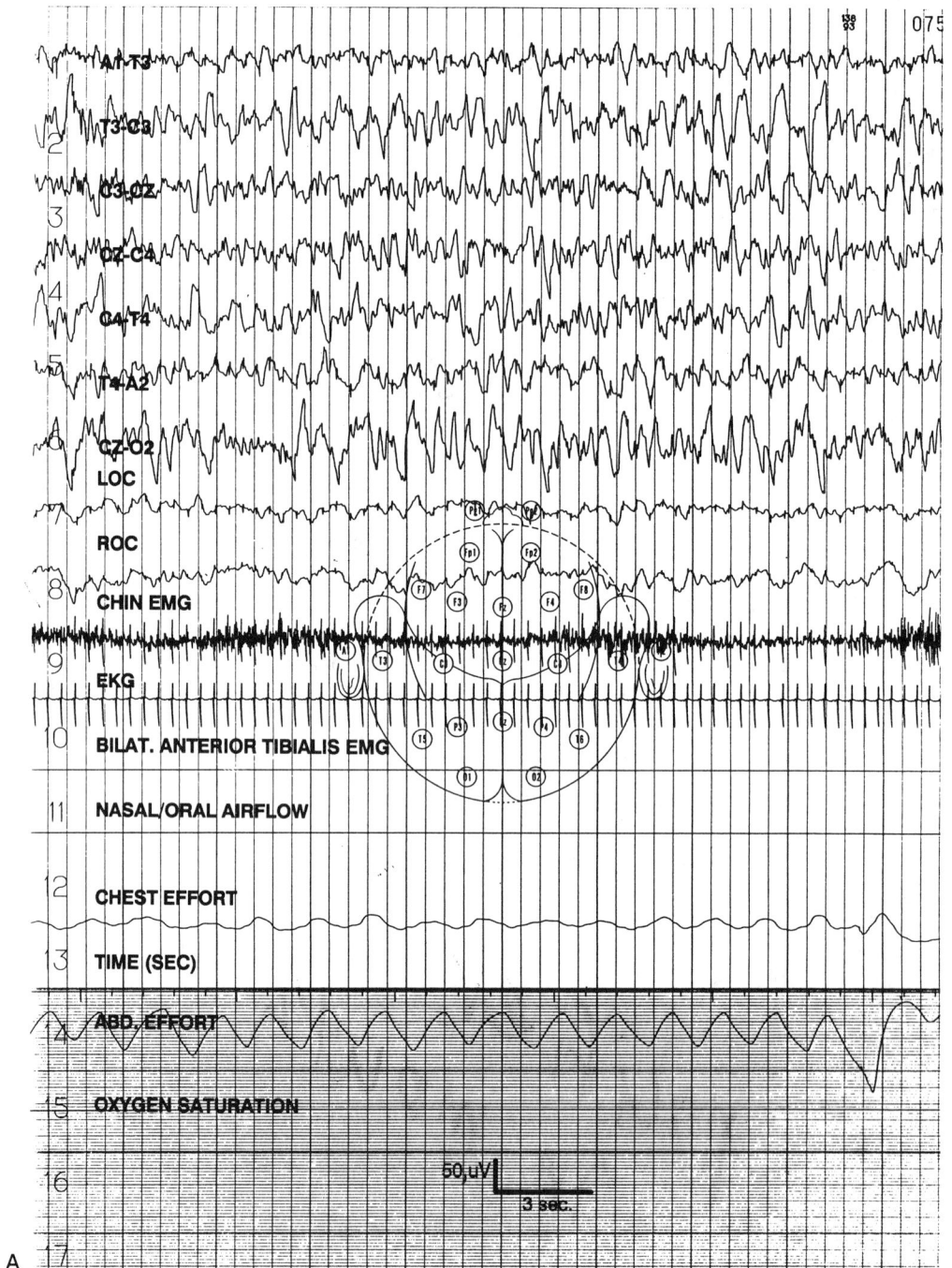

FIG. 10-8. A–B: Quiet sleep (NREM) in a 2-month-old infant. Continuous high-voltage slow waves are present; sleep spindles are absent; and K-complexes cannot be identified from the background rhythm. Eye movements are absent and the EOG reveals frontal EEG artifact. Chin muscle tone is somewhat decreased, although sucking artifact continues in this sleep state. A normal sinus arrhythmia may be seen in the EKG. Bilateral anterior tibialis EMG and nasal/oral airflow are not yet being measured (this is a good time for the technician to apply the remainder of the sensors). Respiratory effort is quite regular.

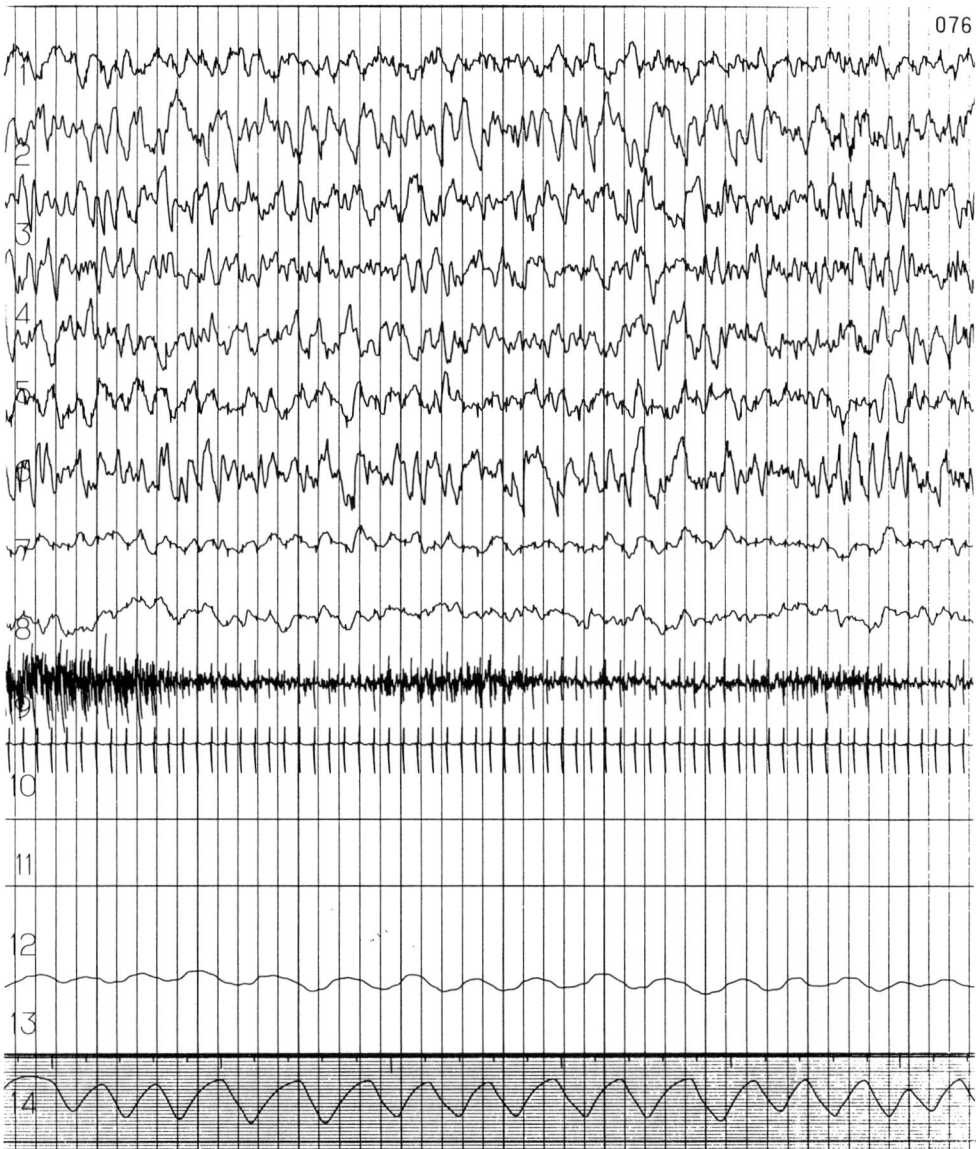

FIG. 10-8. *Continued.*

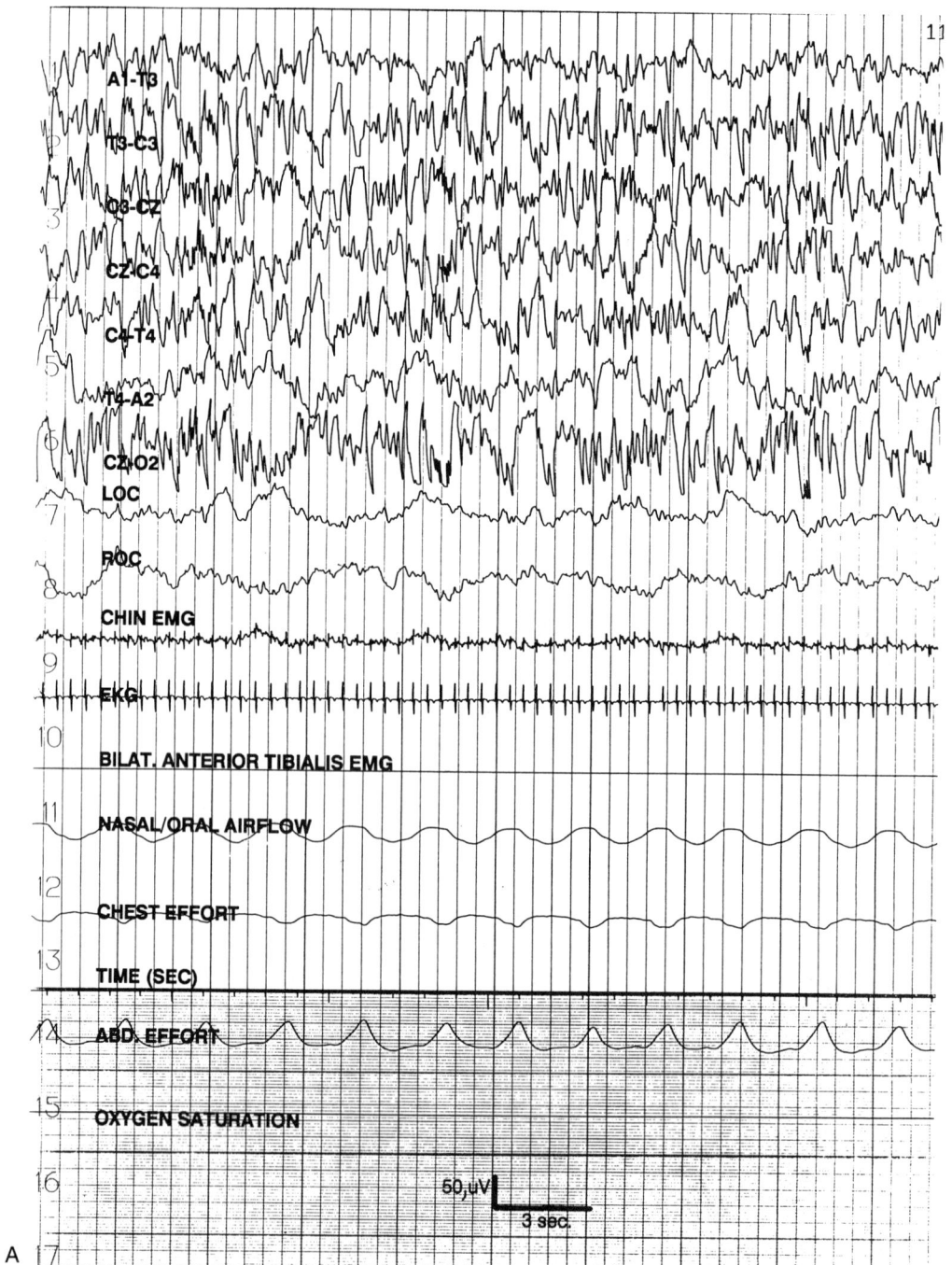

FIG. 10-9. A–B: NREM sleep in a 5-month-old infant. The EEG reveals relatively high-voltage activity with a background rhythm of about 5–6 Hz. Sleep spindles have appeared and K-complexes can be identified. Eye movements are absent and there is some sway artifact in the EOG from slight sweating. EMG tone is decreased from the waking state. EKG continues to show a normal regular sinus arrhythmia. Respirations are quite regular.

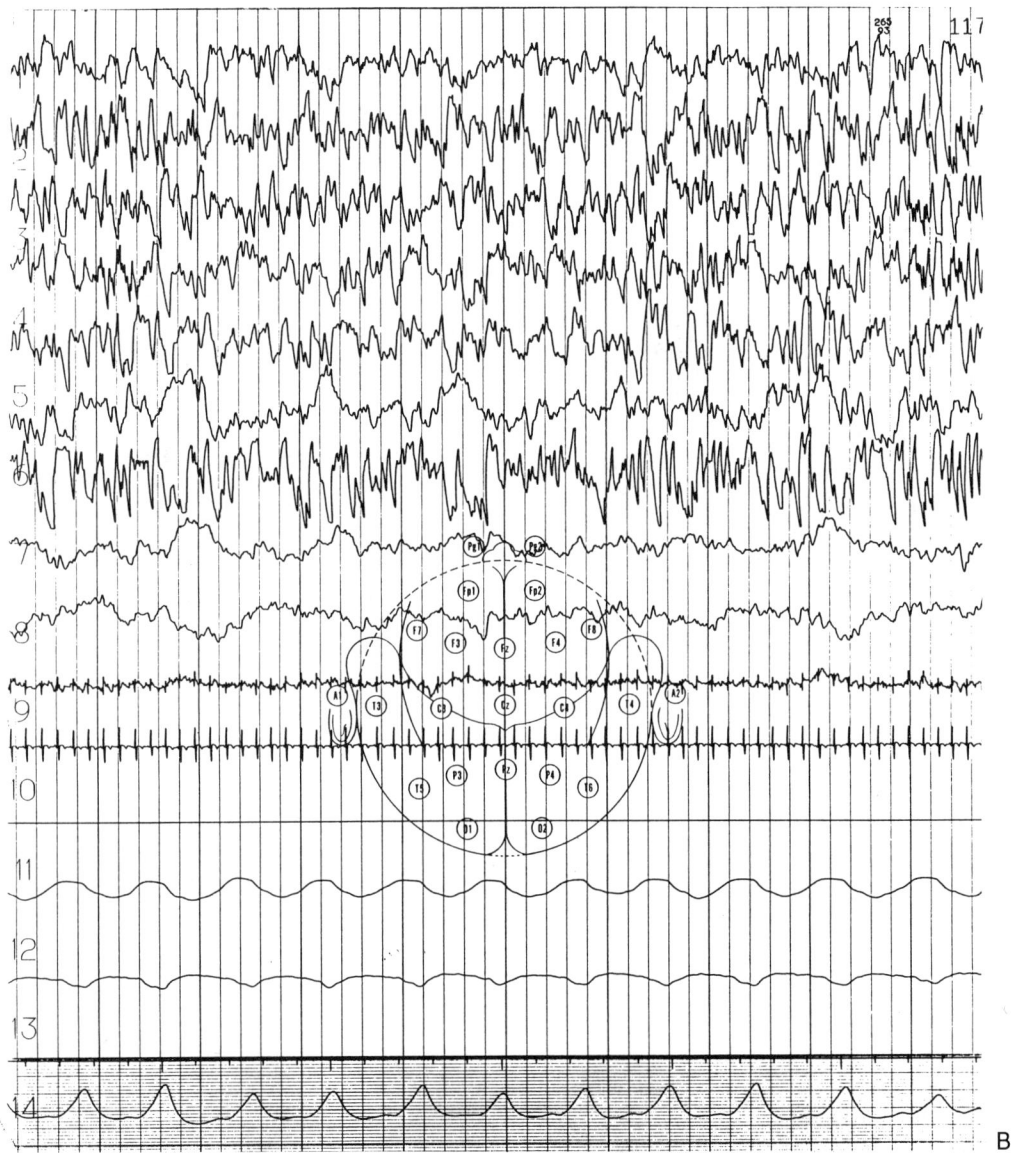

FIG. 10-9. *Continued.*

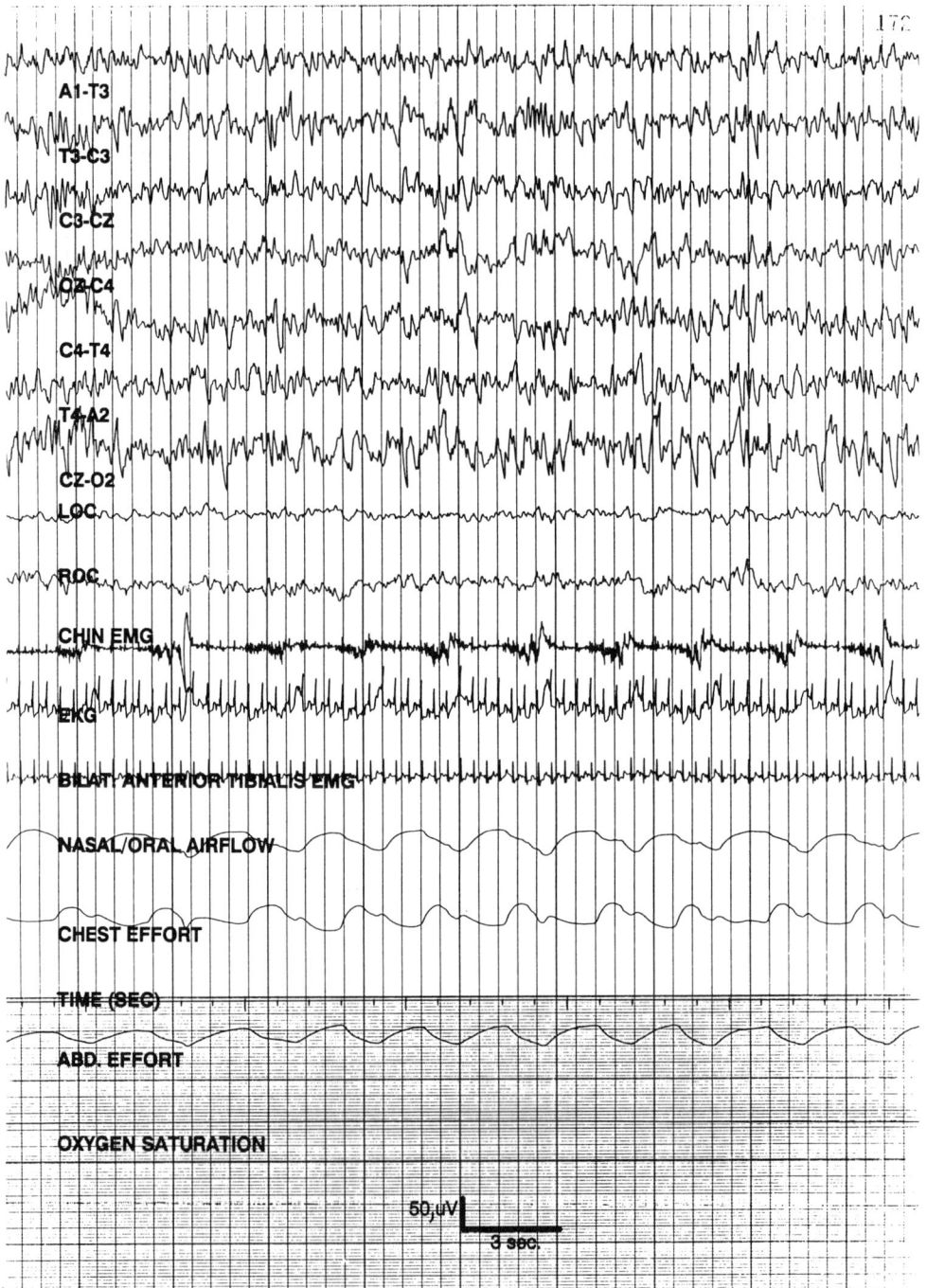

FIG. 10-10. A–B: NREM stage 2 in a 9-month-old infant. Voltage has decreased from earlier infancy and the EEG has assumed a more mature pattern. Sleep spindles are well formed and symmetric. K-complexes are clearly identified from background activity and appear to originate predominantly from the vertex. Background consists of relatively low-voltage, mixed-frequency activity ranging from 3–7 Hz. State differentiation is good. Eye movements are absent. Chin muscle tone is moderate and there is respiratory artifact present.

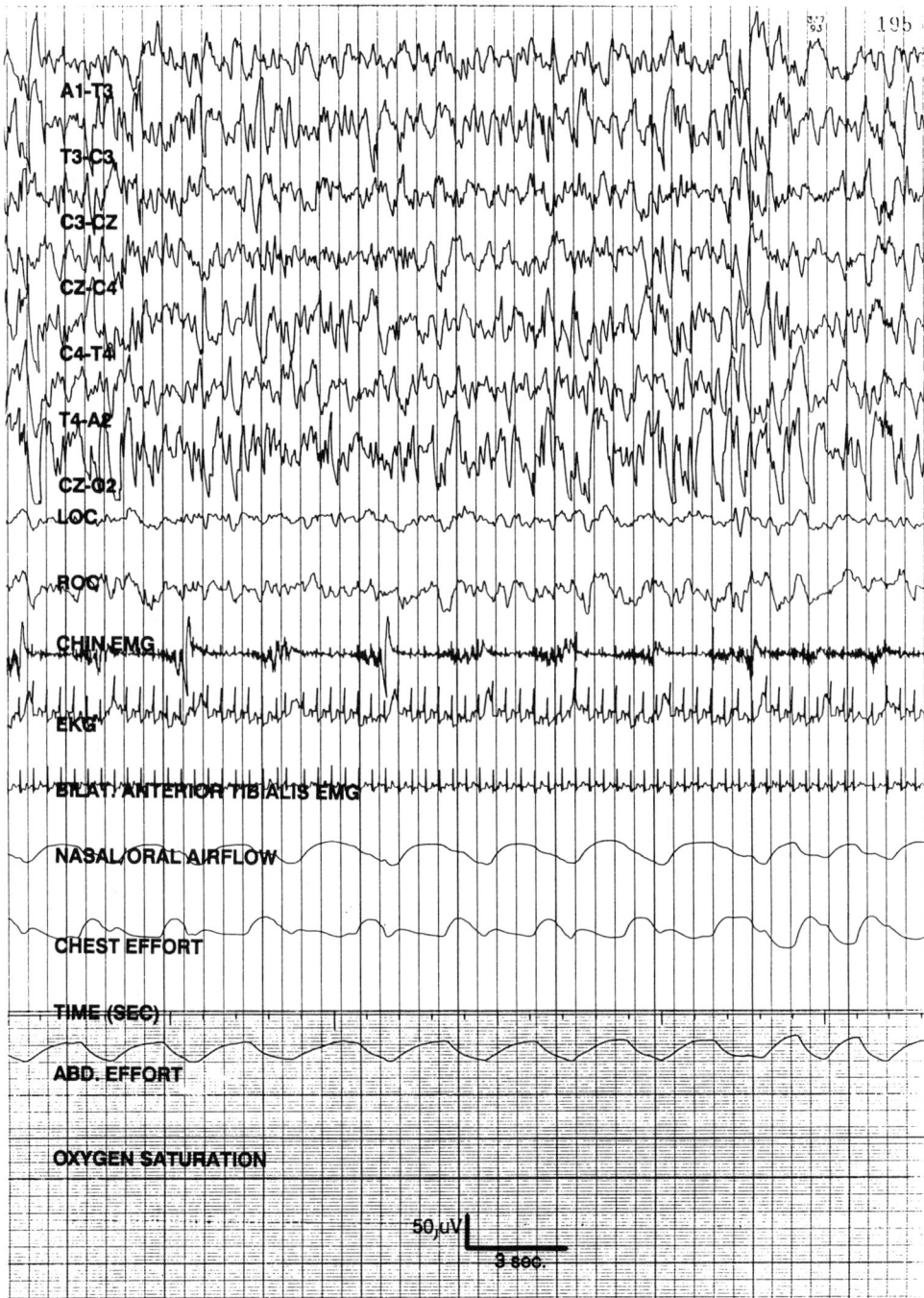

FIG. 10-10. *Continued.* NREM slow-wave sleep in a 9-month-old infant. State demarcation is good and high-voltage slow waves can clearly be identified from the background activity. Sleep spindles may still occur during slow-wave sleep. Eye movements are absent and frontal EEG artifact can be seen in the EOG. Chin EMG is tonic and respiratory artifact is still present. Respirations are quite regular. Anterior tibialis EMG has been applied and there is EKG artifact noted.

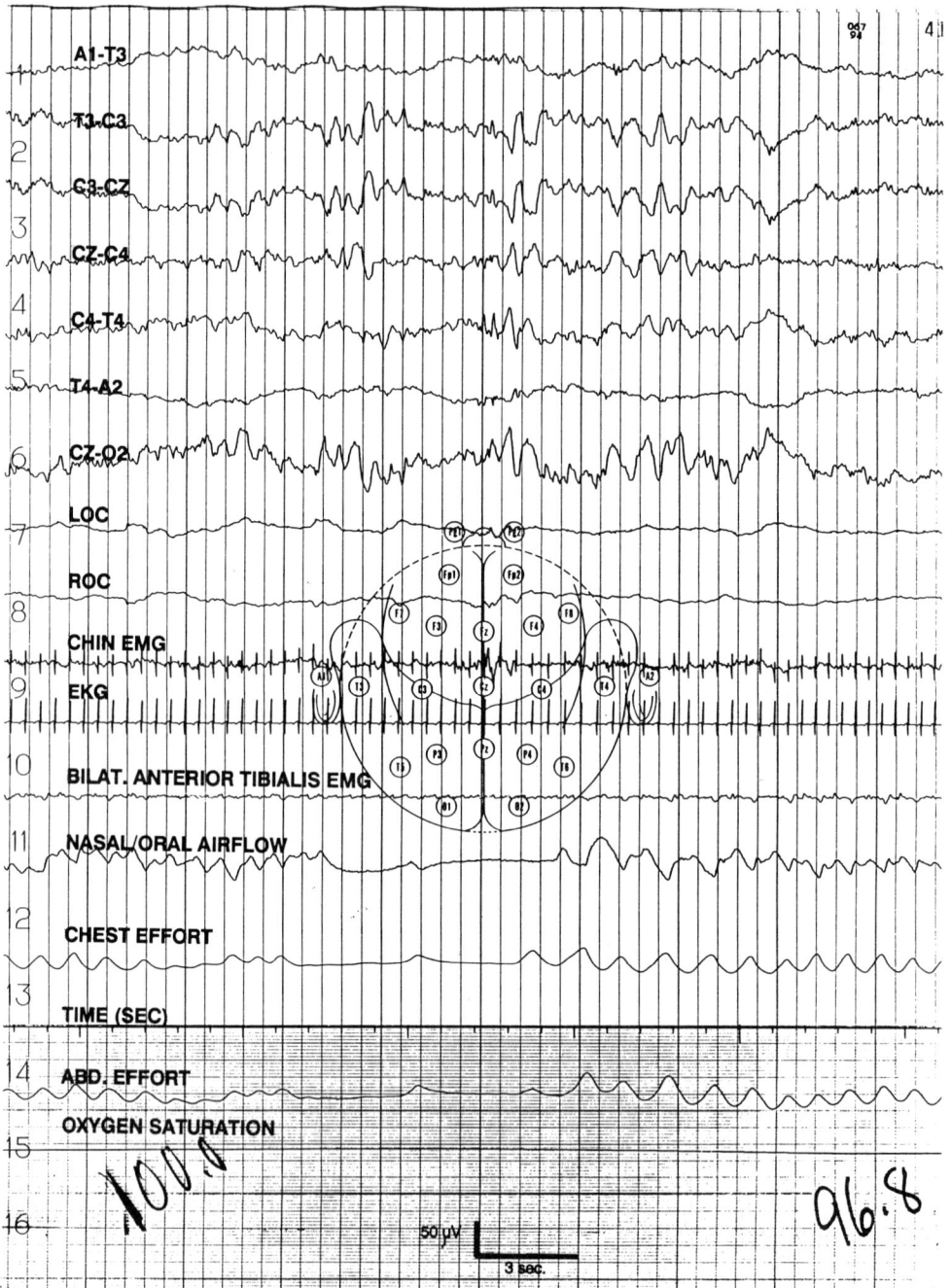

FIG. 10-11. A–B: Active/REM sleep in a 2-month-old infant. A relatively low-voltage, mixed-frequency background EEG rhythm is present. Conjugate eye movements are clearly noted in Fig. 10-11B. Chin muscle tone is considerably decreased. A sinus arrhythmia can be seen in

Continued.

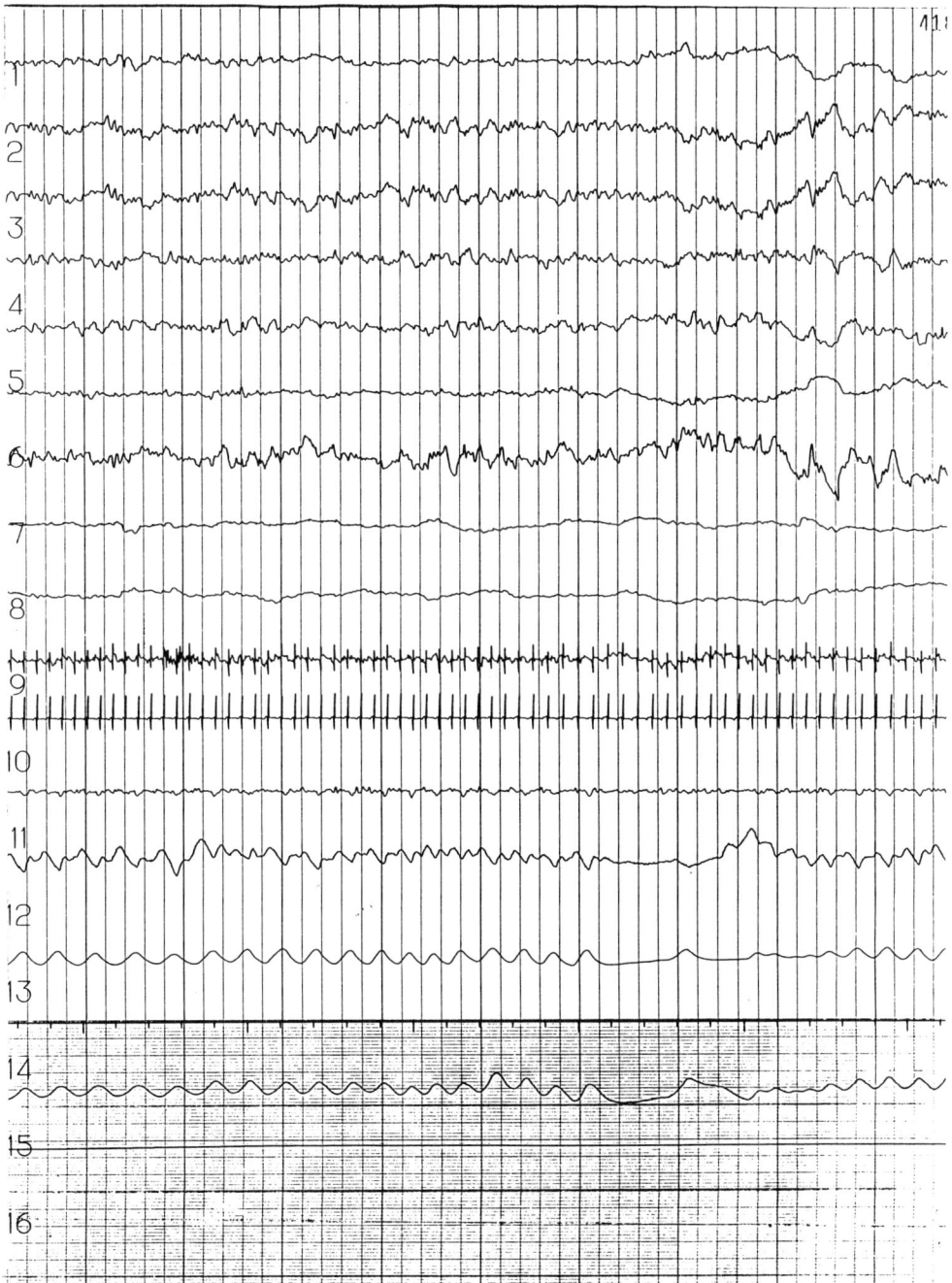

the chin EMG. Anterior tibialis EMG is also hypotonic. Significant respiratory instability is present with brief central pauses

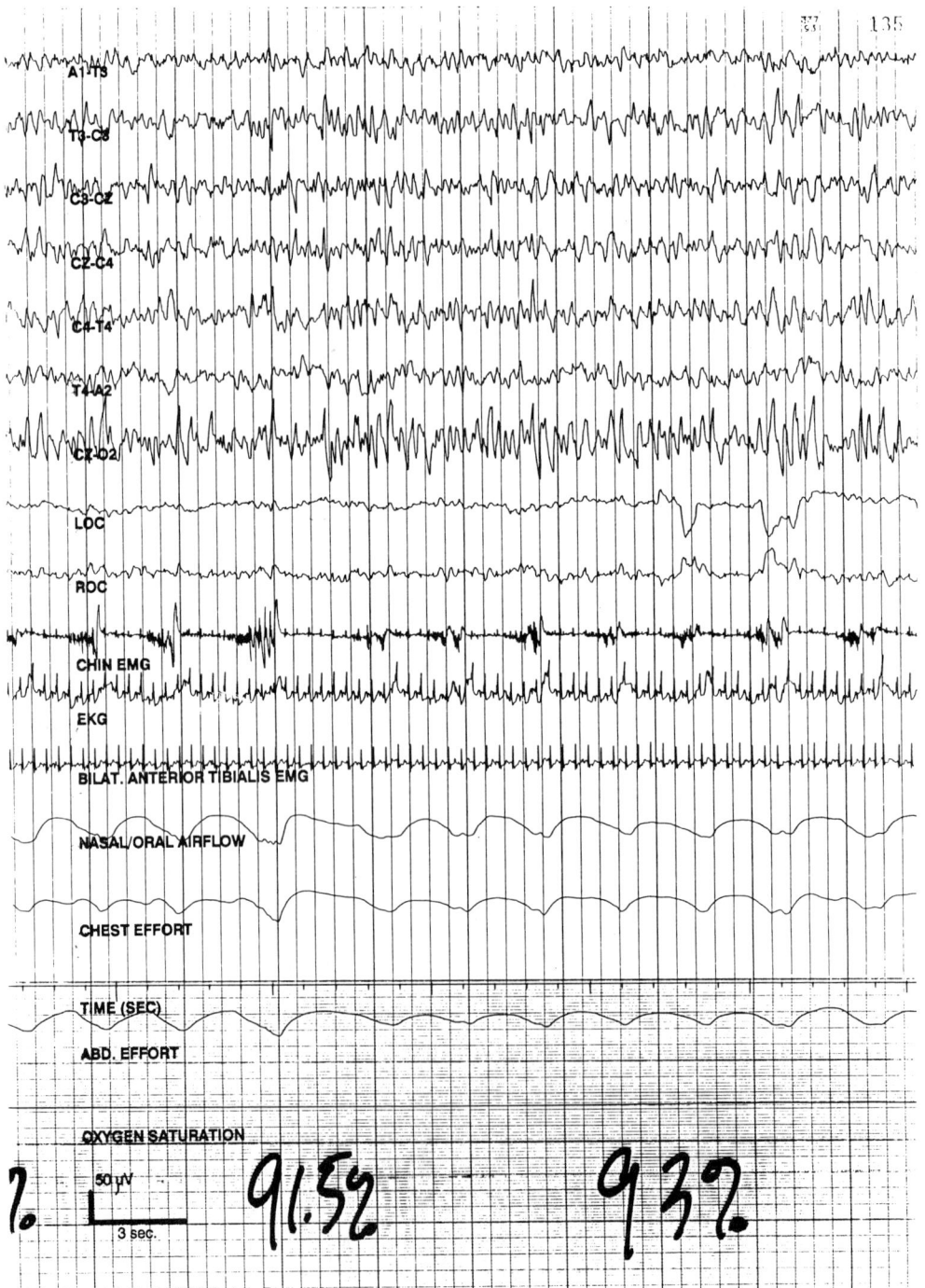

FIG. 10-12. A–B: Active/REM sleep in a 5-month-old infant. EEG activity is more mature and consists of moderate-voltage, 4- to 5-Hz activity. There are bursts of saw-tooth waves present. Clear saccadic eye movements can be seen. Chin muscle tone is decreased, but there is res-

Continued.

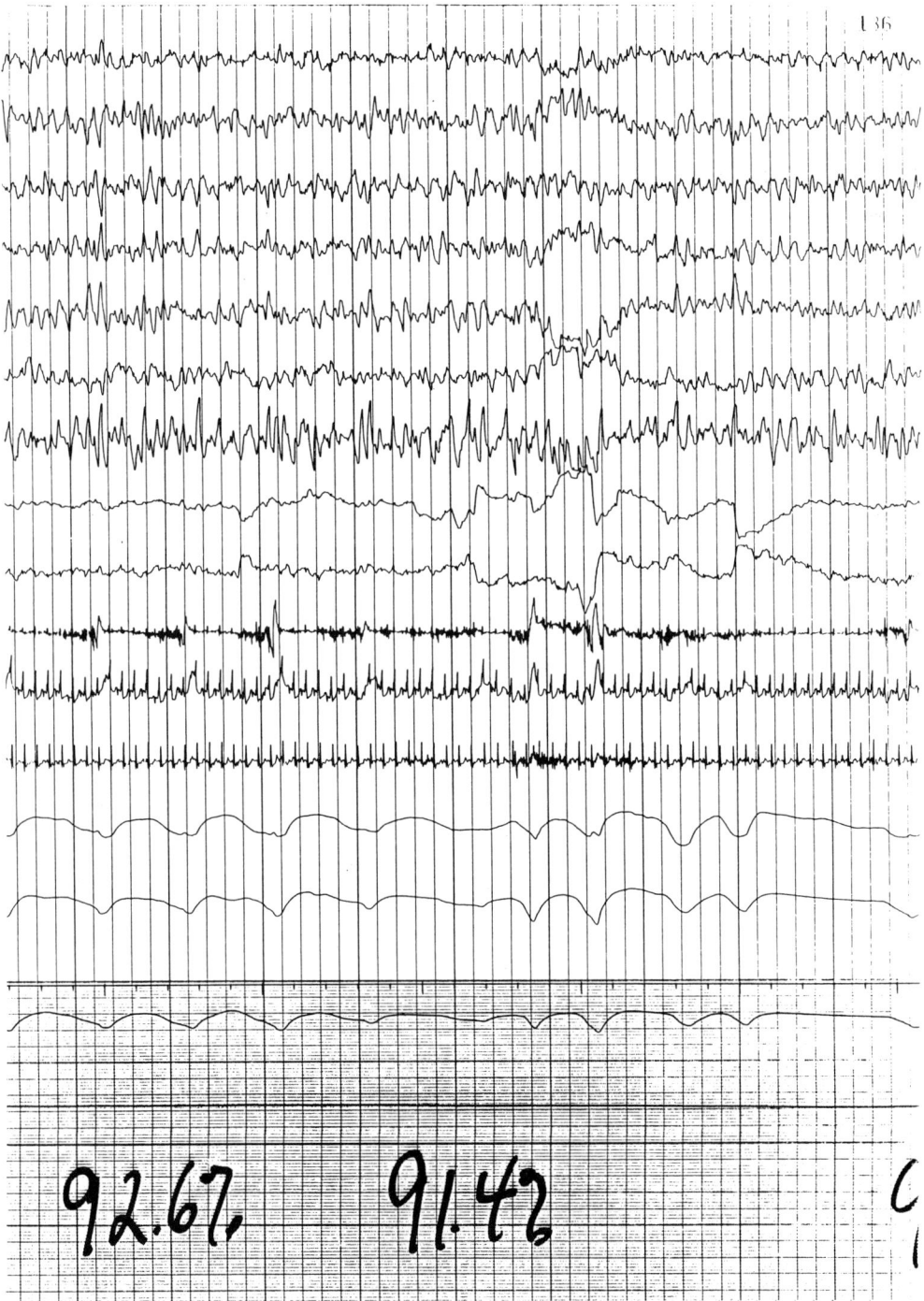

piratory artifact noted. Anterior tibialis EMG is hypotonic and there is significant EKG artifact. Sinus arrhythmia is present in the EKG and considerable respiratory instability is present.

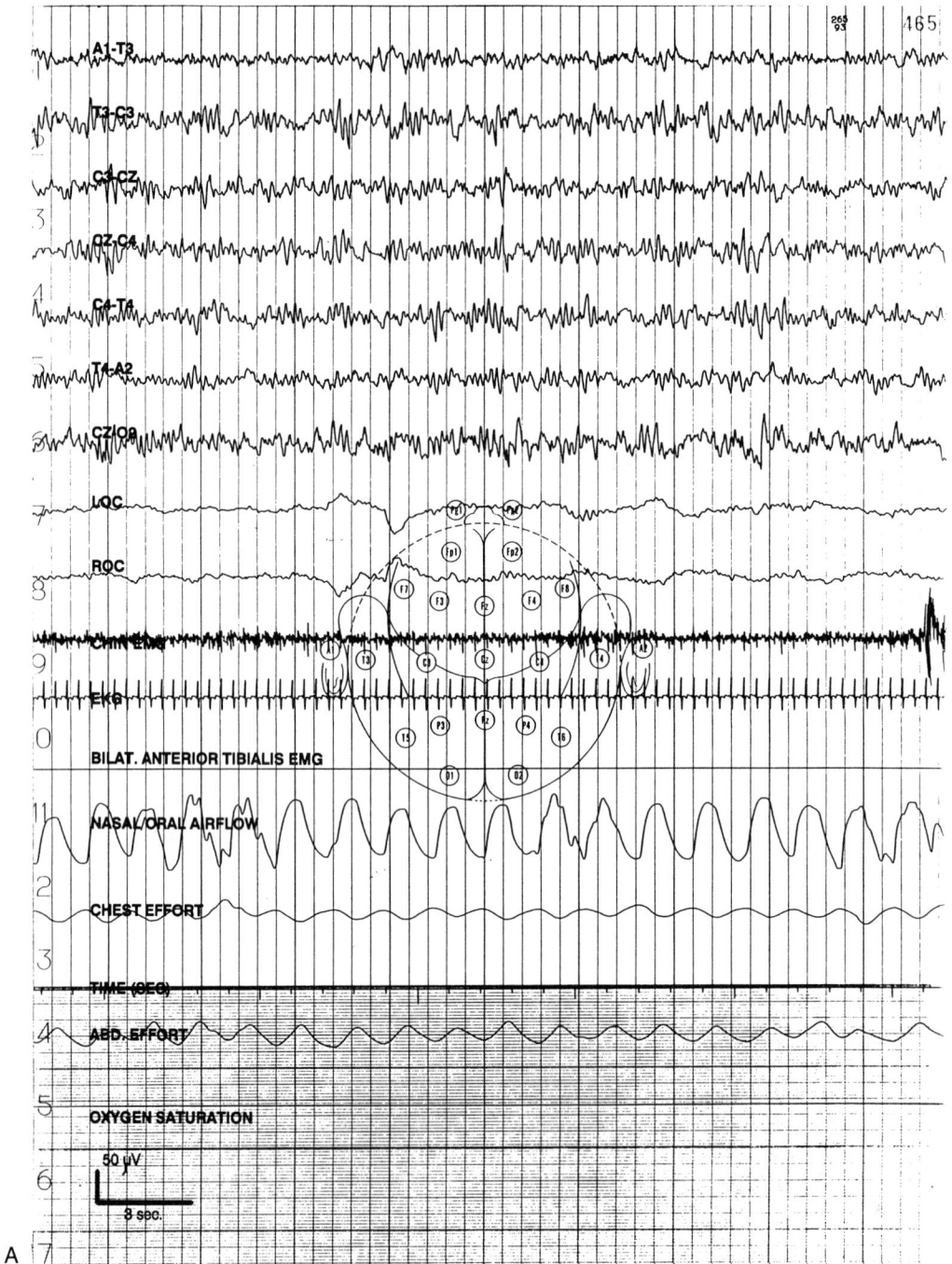

FIG. 10-13. A–B: REM sleep in a 9-month-old infant. EEG voltage has decreased somewhat from the 5-month-old pattern. Background frequency is similar at about 4–6 Hz. Eye movements are present on EOG and chin tone is decreased over NREM sleep level. Phasic twitch-

Continued.

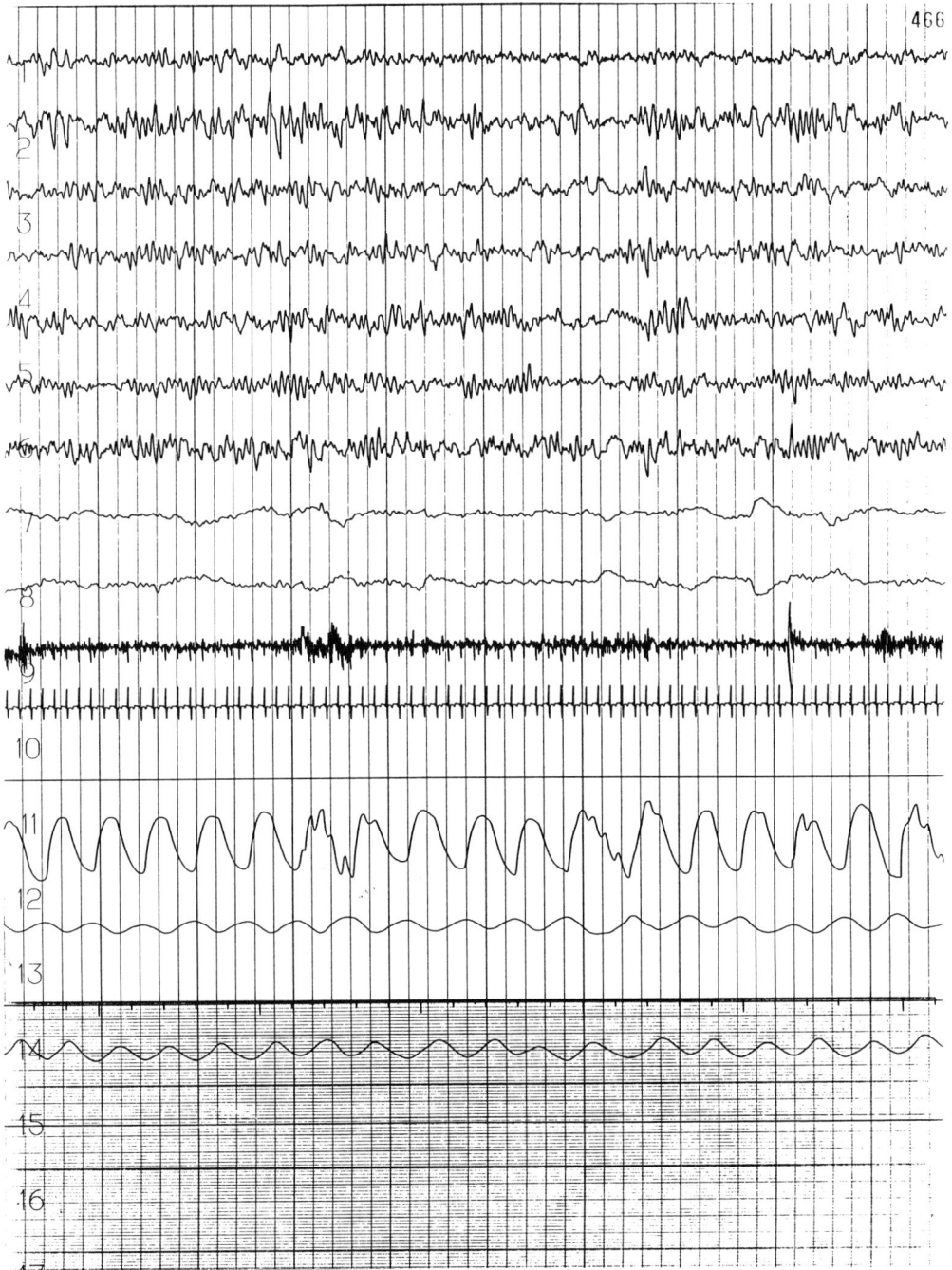

B

ing is also noted. EKG reveals a normal sinus arrhythmia. Respirations are somewhat stable during these two epochs.

gradually changes toward a pattern of relatively low-amplitude, mixed-frequency activity characteristic of adult REM EEG patterns. This indeterminant sleep (state dissociation/ status dissociatus) may hold special significance during infancy and during other stages of development (Figs. 10-11–10-13).

REFERENCES

1. National Institutes of Health Consensus Development Conference. *Infantile Apnea and Home Monitoring.* Bethesda, MD, US Department of Health and Human Services, Oct 1, 1987, NIH Pub No 87-2905.
2. Sheldon SH, Spire JP, Levy HB. *Pediatric Sleep Medicine.* Philadelphia: WB Saunders; 1992.
3. Sheldon SH, Onal E, Lilie J, Spire JP. Sleep-related post-inspiratory upper-airway obstruction in children. *Sleep Res* 1993;22:270.
4. Silverman A, Roy CC. *Pediatric Clinical Gastroenterology.* St Louis: CV Mosby; 1983:149–151.
5. Winter HS. Gastroesophageal reflux. In: Rudolph AM, Hoffman JIE, eds. *Pediatrics*, 18th ed. Norwalk, Connecticut: Appleton Lange; 1987:906–908.
6. Kahn A, Rebuffat E, Sottiaux M, Dufour D, Cadranel S, Reiterer F. Arousals induced by proximal esophageal reflux in infants. *Sleep* 1991;14:39–42.
7. Ferber R. *Solve Your Child's Sleep Problems.* New York: Simon & Schuster; 1985.

11

One Year to Five Years

By one year of age, sleep has achieved a relatively mature pattern. In contrast to the rapid changes that occur during early infancy, development over the next several years is slower and more consistent. Nocturnal sleep is fairly well consolidated into a single long period. Total sleep time and total sleep requirement gradually decreases. At the end of the first year of life, day-time sleep has generally consolidated into two diurnal naps (one morning nap and one afternoon nap). As the second year progresses, the naps gradually change in time and temporal relationship, coalescing into one afternoon nap by age 3. Naps are typically abandoned by 5 years. Circadian cycling has become fairly well established, state organization and differentiation are clear, and sleep-state cycles assume a mature, adult-like pattern. Sleep complaints generally surround symptoms of sleeplessness, especially difficulty in settling. However, because symptoms of sleeplessness are most commonly brought to the attention of the child health care professional, other sleep disorders and pathologies occur with equal (and perhaps greater) frequency. The sleepless child often comes to the attention of the health care professional because of the extreme disruption of the parents' sleep. Unfortunately, many other pathologic states exist that do not disturb the parents' sleep and may result in more significant morbidity during early childhood development (Table 11-1)

TABLE 11-1. *Indications for polysomnography*

Most common indications	Indicated under certain circumstances	Potential indications
Obstructive sleep apnea syndrome and UARS	Unexplained drop attacks	Hyperactivity/attention deficits
Follow-up apnea monitor alarms	Questionable syncope	Behavioral problems
Follow-up T/A for OSA	Unexplained weakness	Unexplained sleep-maintenance problems
Sleep-related seizures and uncontrolled seizure disorders	Frequent sleep terrors	Significantly restless sleep
Rhythmic movement disorders	Frequent sleepwalking	Periodic limb movement disorder
Paroxysmal nocturnal wanderings	Follow-up ALTE	Certain psychiatric syndromes
Unexplained CHF	Developmental delays	Nightmares with significant agitation
Hypotonia associated with neuromuscular conditions	Excessive day-time sleepiness	Injury associated with dream mentation
S/P cleft palate repair	Gastroesophageal reflux	Mental retardation syndromes
Mid-face cranial defects	Unexplained nocturnal limb pain	
	Periodic limb movements	

MOST COMMON INDICATIONS FOR POLYSOMNOGRAPHY

Obstructive Sleep Apnea Syndrom (OSAS)/
Upper-Airway Resistance Syndrome (UARS)

Obstructive sleep apnea syndrome (OSAS) and upper-airway resistance syndrome (UARS) are the most common indications for polysomnography (at the present time). The hallmark of OSAS/UARS is snoring (1). Loud snoring that can be heard in a room other than the youngster's bedroom is almost universally present in youngsters with this syndrome. The snoring is frequently associated with reports of pauses in snoring, snorts, gasping, and respiratory distress. Children who are chronic mouth breathers, have persistent nasal obstruction, and those children with hypertrophic tonsils and adenoids should have the benefit of polysomnography. Polysomnography can provide information regarding the severity of disease, and can also provide information regarding the likelihood of operative and/or post-operative complications. Polysomnography prior to tonsillectomy and adenoidectomy can also provide baseline information regarding the likelihood of persistence of obstructive respiratory disease after surgical intervention. Day-time symptoms include attention deficits, behavioral difficulties, hyperactivity alternating with hypersomnolence, developmental delays, failure to thrive, persistent systemic and/or pulmonary hypertension, and/or cor pulmonale. Youngsters with similar symptoms and chronic persistent otitis media may also be candidates for polysomnography to initially assess and follow the natural history of obstructive airway disease.

Follow-up Apnea Monitor Alarms

Probably the second most common clear indication for polysomnography is assessment of infants, toddlers, and young children who have experienced frequent cardiorespiratory monitor alarms. Comprehensive polysomnography can provide information regarding the presence or absence of significant cardiorespiratory disorders associated with frequent alarms. As important as the ability of polysomnography to provide information regarding the presence of disorders, it can also provide useful information regarding disorders that are *not* responsible for the frequent monitor alarms. After one year of age, the likelihood of SIDS is remarkably low and the need to continuous nocturnal monitoring controversial. Discontinuing monitoring is usually based on clinical findings. This assumes, however, that previous polysomnography did not reveal significant pathology that would be responsible for the apparent life-threatening event. Polysomnography can differentiate between obstructive and central apneas as well as apparently benign respiratory pauses associated with augmented breaths (post-sigh respiratory pause and sleep-related breath-holding spells/physiologic expiratory apneas) (2).

Follow-up Tonsillectomy/Adenoidectomy for Sleep-Disordered Breathing

Polysomnography is most likely indicated after surgery for hypertrophic tonsils and adenoids. Hypertrophic tonsils and adenoids are considered to be the etiology for upper-airway obstruction and is the most common cause of OSAS in children. This differs from the adult patient. However, in the presence of other facial deformities and especially if the respiratory distress index (RDI) is greater than 19 on the baseline study, residual apnea may be present after surgical intervention. Prior to surgical removal of the tonsils and adenoids, a baseline polysomnogram provides information regarding the likelihood of the individual youngster having complications of surgery and may estimate the risk of anesthesia. In addition, it can provide a baseline for the estimation of the likelihood of the presence of residual obstructive airway disease. After tonsillectomy and adenoidectomy, other interventions such as nasal CPAP may be required if residual airway obstruction is present. Therefore, it is recommended that polysomnography be conducted after surgery in patients whose RDI is greater than 19 on baseline study or in those patients presenting with residual symptomatology after surgical intervention.

Sleep-Related Seizures and Uncontrolled Seizure Disorders

Paroxysmal disorders are common indications for polysomnography. Seizures may occur diurnally, nocturnally, or both. Seizures during sleep alone are not uncommon. If there is suspicion of a seizure disorder and routine EEG has not been able to identify the presence of seizure activity, nocturnal (sleep-related) polysomnography can provide more information. A circadian rhythm of seizure activity seems to exist and seizure foci may become more active during early morning hours near the nadir of the body temperature. Another indication for polysomnography in patients with seizure disorders includes poor medication control. Patients who seem to be under good control during the day but have poor diurnal functioning may require nocturnal polysomnography to determine the adequacy of anticonvulsant therapy during sleep.

Rhythmic Movement Disorders

Stereotypic behavior confined to the sleep period is often an indication for polysomnography. If these behaviors are frequent and/or severe, polysomnography should be conducted to rule out the presence of another paroxysmal disorder. This is more likely indicated when the rhythmic movements are stereotypic, confined to a single side of the body, or occur solely during sleep. Those conditions where rhythmic movement disorders are associated with sleep-wake transitions are less likely to require polysomnography.

Paroxysmal Nocturnal Wanderings

Paroxysmal nocturnal wanderings are often difficult to differentiate clinically from quiet or agitated sleepwalking. They tend to occur during NREM sleep and are often associated with significant EEG abnormalities and often respond well to anticonvulsant therapy. Behaviors are commonly stereotypic and often consist of automatisms ranging from crawling to posturing to running through the house. They can appear at any time during sleep. Semi-purposeful and violent behaviors are also common characteristics in some of these patients.

Unexplained Congestive Heart Failure

Upper-airway obstruction may underlie or contribute to significant congestive heart failure. Cor pulmonale can occur in the presence of severe upper-airway obstruction. In the presence of sleep-disordered breathing, congestive heart failure can be significantly improved by application of nasal CPAP. Intrathoracic pressure changes that occur during the course of nasal CPAP treatment results in changes in preload and afterload permitting more efficient cardiac output.

Hypotonia Associated with Neuromuscular Conditions

The presence of hypotonia associated with neuromuscular conditions affects all muscle groups. Because skeletal muscles of the upper airway are also affected, signs and symptoms of sleep-related airway obstruction may occur. All nocturnal symptoms that would typically lead to consideration of polysomnography need not be present. Polysomnography is most likely indicated in the presence of both diurnal and nocturnal symptomatology. Difficulty handling secretions as well as swallowing difficulties indicate dysfunction of pharyngeal muscular activity. Functional abnormalities of both the afferent and efferent neurologic control of the pharyngeal musculature as well as primary muscle dysfunction can result in sleep-related and state-related obstructive-breathing patterns.

Status Post Cleft Palate Repair

After the creation of a pharyngeal flap during the course of cleft palate repair, severe upper-airway obstruction can occur. This is typically dependent upon the lumen and patency of the pharyngeal airway after the surgery. Severe obstructive sleep-disordered breathing can occur and can result in significant cardiorespiratory compromise. If fragmentation of sleep, restless sleep, and diurnal symptoms, which suggest the presence of sleep-disordered breathing, are present, polysomnography is indicated to evaluate the degree of upper-airway obstruction present after repair.

Mid-Face Cranial Defects

Mid-face cranial defects (e.g., Crouzon's disease, choanal stenosis) may result in upper-airway obstruction and resultant cardiorespiratory abnormalities. Symptoms can range from high UARS to frank severe OSAS.

Prader Willi Syndrome

Patients with Prader Willi syndrome frequently have associated obstructive sleep apnea (3). Although not universal, the frequency is high enough so that patients with Prader Willi syndrome should be evaluated in the sleep laboratory. The sleep-related breathing disorder appears to respond well to nasal CPAP.

POLYSOMNOGRAPHY INDICATED UNDER CERTAIN CIRCUMSTANCES

Unexplained Drop Attacks

In unexplained drop attacks with a normal neurologic examination and normal EEG, polysomnography might be considered to assist in the differential diagnosis. Polysomnography may be particularly helpful in patients who completely lose muscle tone but maintain consciousness during the spell. The family history is very important to rule out cataplexy (narcolepsy syndrome). Cataplectic attacks can appear fairly similar to syncopal episodes and/or drop attacks and a sleep laboratory evaluation may be quite helpful during the course of evaluation.

Unexplained Syncope

In patients with unexplained syncope, sleep laboratory evaluation may assist in the differentiation of a variety of causes of symptoms that appear similar clinically. Often attempts at traditional management of syncopal attacks in children should be attempted prior to sleep laboratory evaluation. However, because symptoms of cataplexy may appear quite similar to syncope, sleep center evaluation may be quite helpful in sorting out the variety of causes.

Unexplained Episodic Weakness

Patients with unexplained episodic weakness, especially when associated with a normal neurologic evaluation, can be studied in the sleep laboratory. If the family history is positive for excessive day-time sleepiness, sleep attacks, or narcolepsy syndrome, sleep laboratory evaluation is further indicated. Although exact percentages are unknown, some childhood narcoleptic patients will present with cataplexy as the only symptoms. Therefore, consideration of this diagnosis is important with any patient who experiences unexplained loss of muscle tone or weakness.

Frequent Sleep Terrors

Patients with sleep terrors that occur more than 3 times per week or episodes that are associated with significant displacement from the bed should undergo polysomnography. Certain paroxysmal disorders (e.g., temporal lobe seizures) may present with similar symptoms during early childhood and polysomnography can assist in evaluation of these patients. In addition to the ability of comprehensive polysomnography to rule out seizures as a possible cause, it can provide useful information regarding the underlying cause for the partial arousal (if one is present) and provide insight into the possibility of precipitating events.

Frequent Sleepwalking with Agitation

Like sleep terrors, somnambulism is considered a partial arousal parasomnia. Frequent sleepwalking (more than 3 times per week) associated with agitation may be associated with considerable risk of injury. If associated automatisms and/or stereotypic behaviors are present, seizure disorder might be considered. If agitation and body movements occurs in the presence of clear dream mentation, REM motor parasomnia may also be considered and differentiation requires sleep laboratory evaluation.

Developmental Delays

Polysomnography can be especially helpful in evaluation of developmental delays, especially if it is associated with failure to thrive or other sleep-related symptoms (e.g., loud snoring, restless sleep, periodic limb movements). Baseline information regarding state development can be obtained and polysomnography can assist in differentiating environmental and behavioral causes from physiologic/biologic causes.

Follow-up Apparent Life-Threatening Events

Apparent life-threatening events (ALTEs) occurring in infancy may be initially evaluated and longitudinally followed polysomnographically. If the youngster is greater than 1 year old at the time of the ALTE, sleep laboratory evaluation can assist in providing diagnostic information. Polysomnography can rule out a variety of sleep-related causes. Polysomnography can provide significant information regarding the absence of significant sleep-related pathologic causes for the ALTE, but should not be used to determine whether or not to monitor patients at home.

Excessive Day-Time Sleepiness

Excessive day-time sleepiness is a clear indication for sleep laboratory evaluation and polysomnography. However, in the 1- to 5-year-old age group it is often quite difficult to determine what is "excessive." Unless the excessive sleepiness is profound and the youngster is in the preschool period of development, determination is almost impossible. Normative data in this age group is scant making interpretation of diurnal symptoms quite difficult. Additionally, diurnal symptoms of intermediate degrees of sleepiness are quite different from profound sleepiness in youngsters and excessive day-time sleepiness in adults. Young children are more often hyperactive, may experience hyperactivity alternating with somnolence, behavior problems, attention span problems, learning difficulties, and other seemingly unrelated symptoms. Nocturnal polysomnography can be done, however, to rule out nocturnal sleep-related pathology that could contribute to excessive sleepiness during the day.

Gastroesophageal Reflux

Nocturnal respiratory symptoms secondary to sleep-related gastroesophageal reflux is uncommon in this age group. Gastroesophageal reflux is normally present in most children under one year of age (4). Cardioesophageal sphincter tone has become generally well developed by 12 months and significant reflux is uncommon. When persistent, it can be severe, resulting in significant failure to thrive, and typically presenting with diurnal symptoms as well as nocturnal symptoms. Nocturnal symptoms generally include frequent arousal, abdominal or substernal chest pain, wheezing, choking, coughing, gagging, and gasping. Neurologic abnormalities may also be present especially if there are persistent pulmonary findings, since neurologic abnormalities may affect pharyngeal reflexes that protect the airway.

A small "H" type tracheo-esophageal fistula without esophageal atresia can be missed early in infancy and childhood. It may present later in childhood with frequent pneumonias, unexplained periodic wheezing, or unexplained nocturnal laryngospasm or sleep-related respiratory abnormalities similar to that seen with esophageal reflux into the pharynx.

When GER is suspected as being a cause of nocturnal symptoms, we generally schedule two consecutive nights of polysomnography. The first night is a baseline night without the presence of an esophageal pH probe. This can provide significant information regarding the presence of sleep-related symptoms or identify other sleep-related pathology that may be the cause of the nocturnal symptoms without the confounding variable of an indwelling foreign body in the pharynx. If the cause for the nocturnal symptoms can be identified on the first night of polysomnography, the second night need not be conducted. If the baseline night does not provide sufficient information, the second night is performed with an indwelling esophageal pH probe. Polysomnography is time coordinated with the pH study and the presence of sleep-related symptoms compared with the presence or absence of GER. Interestingly, GER can be present, but not be the cause of the sleep-related abnormality. Therefore, time coordination of the pH study and polysomnogram is essential. It is ideal to patch the pH signal into the polygraph, if possible. If not, clock synchronization is mandatory in order to interpret the study.

Unexplained Nocturnal Limb Pain and Periodic Limb Movements

Nocturnal limb pain is fairly common in youngsters close to 5 years of age. It tends to be more common in slightly older children, but youngsters in this age group can present with nocturnal wakings and complaints of limb pain. Comprehensive work-ups generally cannot explain the reason for the pains. If the pains are frequent and result in significant sleep-maintenance insomnia, polysomnography is probably indicated. Periodic limb movement disorder can occur in young children and other parasomnias might explain the nocturnal symptoms.

POTENTIAL INDICATIONS FOR POLYSOMNOGRAPHY

Hyperactivity/Attention Deficits

Excessive day-time sleepiness (EDS) and increased sleep pressure have been recently suggested as underlying causes for the attention deficit hyperactivity complex (5). In older youngsters it is more easily identified. Because of the absence of normative data in children between the ages 1 and 5 years, diagnosis in the sleep laboratory is extremely difficult and variable. Youngsters with attention span problems and hyperactivity tend to have moderate degrees of sleepiness and a hypoarousal state can be identified (6). They do not fulfill standard established criteria for EDS established for adults, adolescents, and older children. Sleep laboratory evaluation might be considered if there is hyperactivity alternating with excessive sleepiness and the youngster is falling asleep at other inappropriate times (e.g., during meals, parties). It also might be considered in youngsters who are hyperactive but show significant improvement in activity, attention span, and performance on a variety of activities after a nap. This improvement might be brief in nature, but is definitely identifiable. Because of the absence of normative data for this age group, evaluation and assessment of data is quite difficult, but initial evaluation during this period of time provides a baseline for further study.

Unexplained Behavioral Problems

Unexplained behavior problems or behavior problems that do not appear to be based on any environmental factors may or may not have associated sleep-related symptoms. If there are symptoms referable to the youngster's sleep time, these may contribute to or underlie the problem. History is important in evaluating these patients and will provide the information required to determine whether polysomnography can provide insight into the etiology.

Unexplained Sleep-Maintenance Problems

In children with sleep-maintenance problems, the history is most important in evaluating the possible causes. Initially, behavioral and/or environmental approaches should be made. If there is no response to initial interventions and compliance appears to be appropriate, further evaluation may be necessary. If there are sleep-maintenance difficulties that do not appear to be associated with sleep-onset difficulties, the likelihood of there being sleep-related abnormalities underlying the nocturnal wakings increases and consideration for polysomnography would be greater.

Significantly Restless Sleep

Significantly restless sleep associated with falls from bed, excessive day-time sleepiness, hyperactivity, or behavioral problems may be indications for sleep laboratory evaluation. High UARS, periodic limb movement disorder, or other physiologic abnormalities that disrupt the continuity of sleep can underlie or contribute to restless sleep and diurnal symptoms.

Periodic Limb Movement Disorder

Periodic limb movement disorder occurs in youngsters and can result in nocturnal symptoms of restless sleep and diurnal symptoms of excessive day-time sleepiness. Historic information may reveal restless sleep, frequent movements and arousals, frequent nocturnal wakings, limb discomfort, diurnal hyperactivity, attention span problems, learning difficulties, and behavior problems. The family history may be positive for periodic limb movements of sleep or excessive day-time sleepiness.

Certain Psychiatric Syndromes

A number of sleep-related disorders can be interpreted as psychiatric syndromes in early childhood. Narcolepsy syndrome, OSAS, periodic limb movement disorder, agitated sleep waking, and sleep-related seizure disorders have all been associated in initial diagnosis as psychiatric syndromes ranging from schizophrenia and childhood autism to attention deficit-hyperactivity disorder.

Nightmares with Significant Agitation

Parents often will state that their child is having "nightmares" when a variety of nocturnal symptoms are present. A complaint of nightmares is common whenever the youngster screams, cries, or presents with agitated symptoms during their sleep. At times there is significant dream mentation and nightmares can easily be diagnosed on historic grounds alone. Episodes can occur any time of night, but tend to cluster during early morning hours. There is full awakening, report of clear dream mentation, and the waking episode tends to be prolonged (30 minutes or more). Agitation may be present, but tends to be rather mild. The youngsters are most often easily comforted by parents. In comparison, sleep terrors tend to occur early in the sleep-period time (during slow-wave sleep). It is heralded by a piercing scream, intense autonomic discharge (diaphoresis, pupillary dilatation, tachycardia, and tachypnea), intense agitation, and the youngster tends to become worse upon parental intervention, often fighting and pushing away from the caretaker. They are typically short lived (lasting only a few minutes), the youngster rapidly returns to sleep, and there is amnesia for the event. At times sleep terrors can be frequent (occurring several times per night), prolonged (lasting for hours), and can be associated with displacement from the bed. When there is severe agitation and displacement from the bed, injury is common and the injuries are potentially fatal. Children have been reported to jump out of windows, run through plate glass doors, out of the house and into the middle of busy streets. When symptoms are frequent and there is significant displacement from the bed, polysomnography is indicated. Medication management may be required. It is also important to differentiate these episodes from other treatable causes, e.g., sleep-related seizures, episodic nocturnal wanderings. It is also important to be able to determine whether there are any other sleep-related precipitating causes, e.g., obstructive sleep apnea, periodic limb movements. In addition, REM-sleep motor disorder has been reported in children (7) and polysomnography can provide needed information regarding the state of sleep out of which the episodes occur. Treatment may also be guided by polysomnographic findings.

Mental Retardation Syndromes

Some mental retardation syndromes may be associated with significant sleep-related abnormalities. Similar criteria are required for referral for comprehensive sleep evaluation and polysomnography. However, some sleep difficulties in these youngsters may be primary and related to underlying central nervous system (CNS) pathology, or may be related to environmental and/or behavioral factors. When environmental and behavioral factors are involved, children with mental retardation are as likely as other children to have sleep-related pathology. Under certain circumstances, when control of diurnal symptoms is poor or when nocturnal symptoms are significantly disruptive, quality of life for the patient and family may be improved when attention is paid to the sleep-related symptoms. Polysomnography may provide information regarding the presence of associated sleep-related pathology (e.g., apnea, seizures), physiologic basis for the problems, level of maturation of the CNS, and functional status by state organizational relationships.

TECHNICAL CONSIDERATIONS AND TECHNIQUES

Preparation

Children between the ages of 1 and 5 years of age can be the most difficult patients to study in the sleep laboratory. It is a time of development in which there are fears (both environmental fears and fear of strangers), tactile defensiveness, noncompliance, and resistance to interventions. In order to obtain a reliable sleep study in the laboratory that can approximate the youngster's habitual sleep, the environment (as well as personnel) must appear safe and the youngster must feel relatively secure. Parents are required to remain with their child during the entire course of the study. They are encouraged to visit the laboratory prior to the scheduled date of the study so that the laboratory will not be a strange environment on the night of the investigation. The child should be allowed to play with the sensors and, at times, should be allowed to take certain sensors home to become more familiar with the equipment. Dolls and manikins can be used. The child can apply the sensors to the doll or manikin and can manipulate the environment in order to achieve the greatest degree of security and comfort. Other techniques to gain the youngster's confidence in personnel can be utilized.

Parents are encouraged to arrive at the laboratory at 2000. This generally provides the youngster time to adapt to the sleeping environment, undergo set-up, and prepare for bed at a time similar to that at home. Set-up is done in a room distant from the sleeping room. The sleeping/monitoring room should appear safe for the child and devoid of as much technical equipment as possible. It should be furnished and adorned in a developmentally appropriate manner. We, therefore, keep all set-up equipment, electronic monitoring equipment, resuscitation equipment, and medical paraphernalia in the set-up room. If repair of electrodes is required during the course of the study, equipment is brought to the child's room on a small cart when needed and returned to the set-up room after use. Hospital beds and hospital cribs are not used in our laboratory. Traditional junior beds and home style cribs provide for a more home-like environment and make the child feel more comfortable in the laboratory.

During set-up, it is advisable to enlist the assistance of the parent in holding and gently restraining the youngster. The parent's lap is typically an ideal location for set-up. The youngster will feel most comfortable and safe on the parent's lap and the parent can provide assistance (as well as a second pair of hands) in skin preparation and electrode placement. Occasionally, in younger children, swaddling in a sheet may be required. Restraint is not always advisable since it may result in over-stimulation of the youngster and provide for spurious polysomnographic results. It is also associated with struggling and sweating under the sheet, making electrode placement and signal quality poor.

The parent's lap and technician's lap makes for an excellent preparation table. With the parent and technician sitting and facing each other, knees can be positioned to touch each other and a sheet or other protective covering draped over the technician's and parent's lap. The youngster is positioned supine on the two laps with the child's head in the technician's lap and feet and hands toward the parent. The parent can restrain the youngster's feet under her arms and can also hold the child's hands during the procedure. This frees the technician's hands to control the child's head, prepare the electrode site, and secure the electrodes with minimal difficulty. EEG electrodes may be best applied with the parent holding the youngster on her shoulder (Figs. 11-1 and 11-2). It is still advisable In younger children during this developmental period, to wrap the child's head with Kerlix in order to assure equal pressure on the electrodes and to protect them from displacement during the course of the study. Head wrapping can also be easily accomplished with the youngster laying supine in both the parent's and technician's lap. Arm board and arm restraints are not advisable in this age group since they have the potential for disrupting the study.

Often it is difficult, if not impossible to completely set-up a young toddler during the set-up period prior to the study. Young toddlers exhibit extreme tactile defensiveness, especially from strangers. Parents can help apply some of the sensing devices, but these youngsters will often be resistant even to the parents' attempts. Instead of forcing and restraining the youngster for the set-up procedure, it is more appropriate to attach those

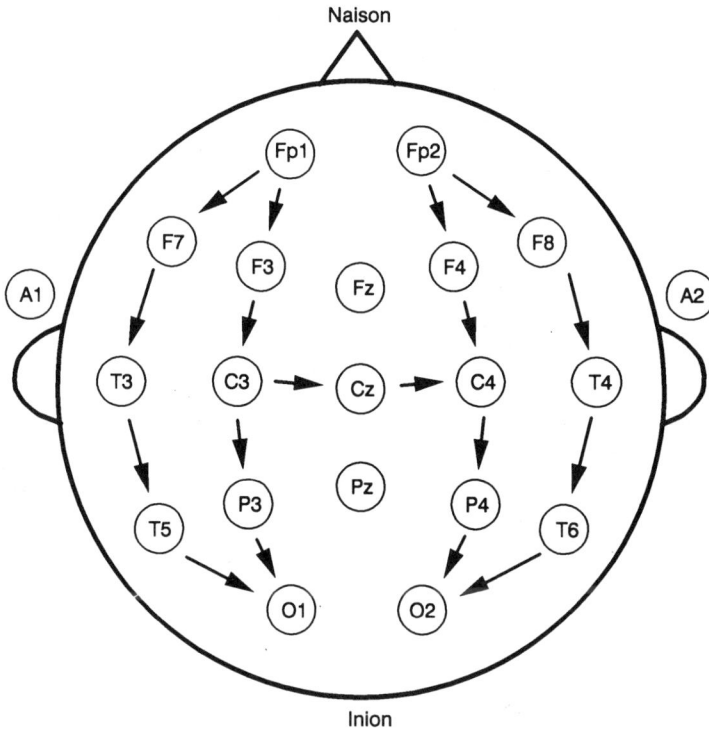

FIG. 11-1. Parasagittal montage. The two coronal bipolar channels are utilized to identify vertex activity.

electrodes that can be attached, document the difficulties, and develop a plan for placement after the youngster is asleep. The arousal threshold is typically very high in children in this age group. Once the child has achieved slow-wave sleep, the technician and parent can usually apply the remaining electrodes and sensing devices. The ability to better apply electrodes and sensors shortly after sleep onset with minimal interference provides for much better signal quality, acceptance of the procedure, and interpretable and reproducible data.

Length of Study

The study should be conducted as close as possible to the youngster's habitual sleep period. Attempts should be made to obtain at least 400 minutes of sleep. On the first night in the laboratory, it may not be possible. In younger toddlers, nocturnal wakings may be prolonged and because of frequent movements and the need for occasional technician intervention to repair recording electrodes, total sleep time may be less than 400 minutes. It is important to record several sleep cycles and it is equally important to obtain sleep cycles during the early morning hours in order to record events that exhibit their peak frequency or severity during this time period. Although sleep progression and architecture is developing a more mature, adult-like pattern, in younger toddlers (closer to 1 year of age) slow-wave sleep can be evenly distributed throughout the sleep period and

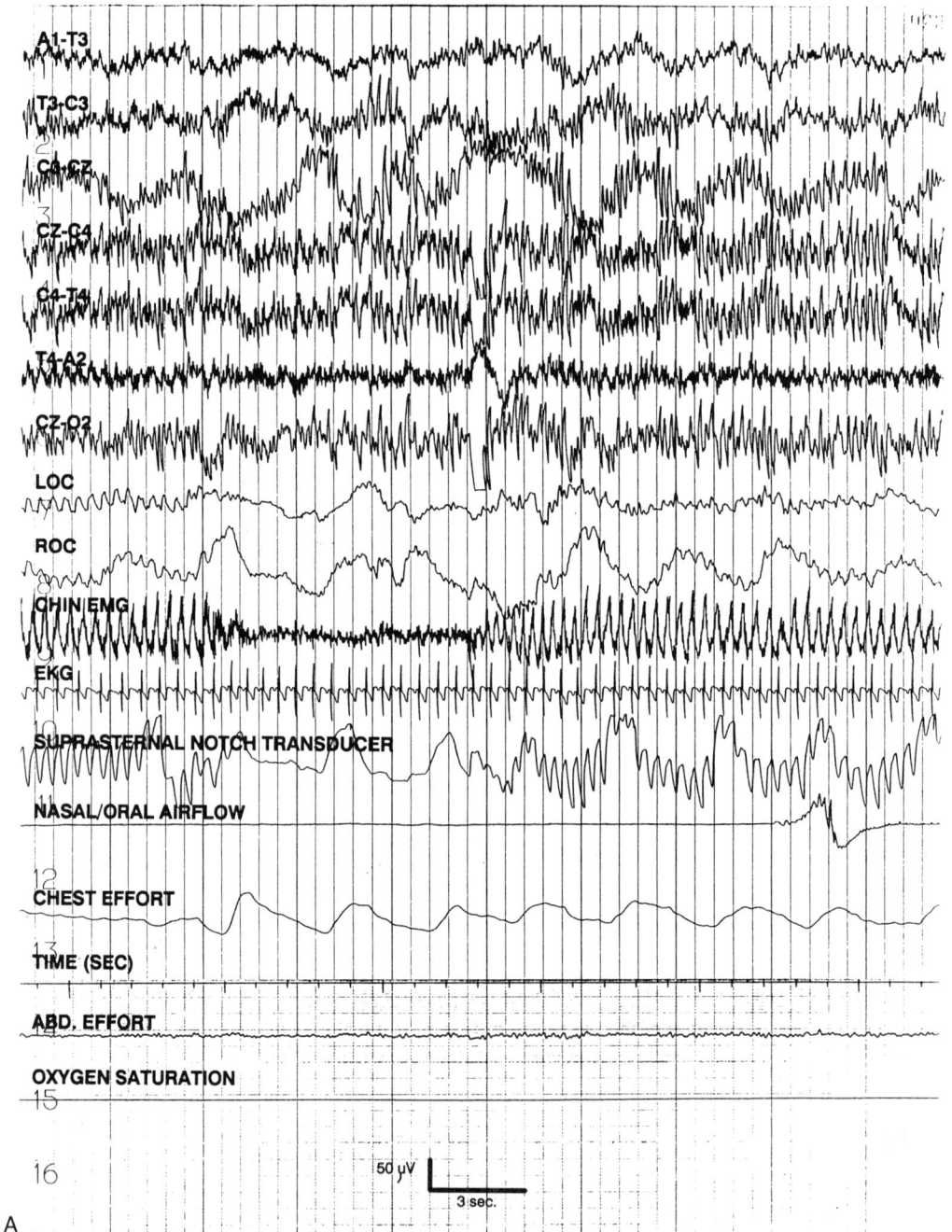

FIG. 11-2. A–B: Quiet wake in a 14-month-old toddler. EEG reveals moderate-voltage activity at about 5–7 Hz. Some conjugate eye movements are present, but these are difficult to discern due to the presence of sweat artifact. The patient is sucking on a bottle and this artifact can be identified in the chin muscle EMG. Swallowing artifact can be seen in the suprasternal notch transducer. EKG rhythm is rather stable and minimal respiratory variation is present. Nasal/oral thermistor has not yet been placed. Respiration, however, is variable and the variations are associated with sucking and swallowing.

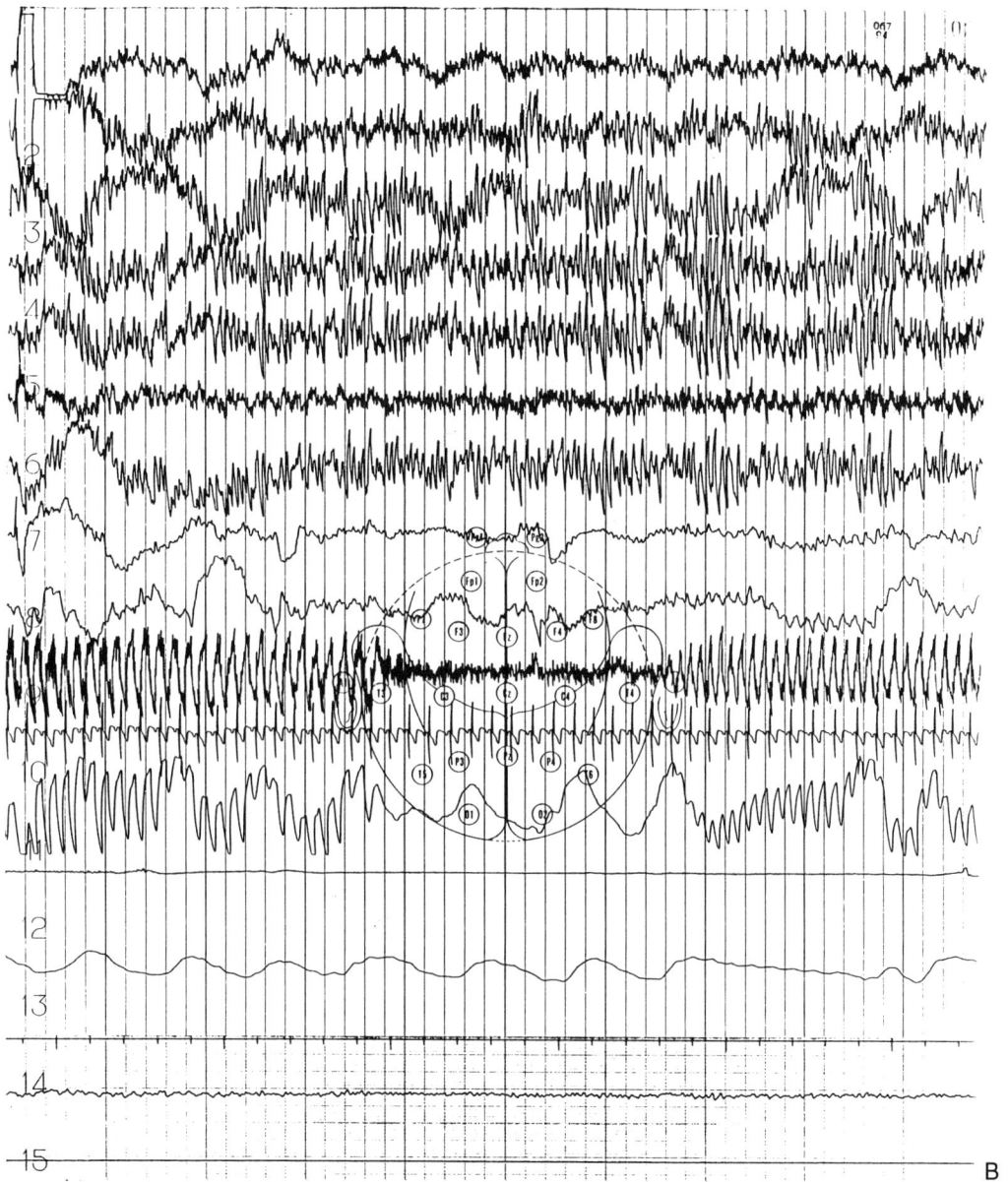

FIG. 11-2. *Continued.*

cycle with REM-sleep episodes that are rather equal in length. Despite these differences in sleep-stage progression, some pathologies of sleep still reveal circadian differences in severity and absence of early morning recordings (e.g., recordings between 0400 and 0700) may miss the frequency and severity of the pathophysiologic process.

Recommended Equipment

Standard polysomnographic equipment is recommended. It may be advisable to have developmentally appropriate toys and games to amuse the youngsters during set-up and during adaptation periods in the laboratory. Additional recording equipment should be determined by the indication for the study. For example, esophageal pH probes and recording equipment may be required in the evaluation of patients with GER; an esophageal manometer may be required to determine exact changes in intrathoracic pressures when high UARS is suspected; $TcPCO_2$ monitors may be required when assessing for central and/or alveolar hypoventilation syndrome; home apnea monitors for assessment of frequent alarms; laryngeal microphones can be utilized when specific vocalizations or respiratory sounds require recording; and nasal CPAP and bilevel CPAP equipment available for those youngsters undergoing titration. Supplemental oxygen must be available in all sleep laboratories and centers.

Technical Considerations

EEG

A bipolar transcoronal montage is the standard EEG recording in our laboratories. Not only does this montage provide for accurate identification of sleep transitions and state determination, it affords the ability to screen for abnormal hemispheric activity, and asymmetries. The montage can be easily modified during the course of the study (when appropriate electrodes are placed at the beginning of the study) into a more diagnostic array. It also provides a much better estimate of the maturity of the EEG, waking and sleeping background rhythms, and can clearly differentiate active, normal, vertex, sharp-wave activity from abnormal electrical activity. When studying children for REM and/or NREM parasomnias or when there is a high index of suspicion of a sleep-related seizure disorder, a parasagittal bipolar montage is generally recommended. This montage can yield a greater appreciation of temporal lobe activity and can identify temporal lobe abnormalities more clearly than the transcoronal montage. In many instances, standard-single and double-channel polysomnographic montage (C3-A2, C4-A1, O2-A1, etc.) have completely missed abnormal electrical activity (some suspected and some unsuspected). Therefore, we only reserve the standard polysomnogram montage for conducting multiple sleep latency tests, after a complete night when a transcoronal or parasagittal montage has been assessed as normal (Fig. 11-1).

Other Physiologic Parameters

Other physiologic parameters should be determined by the needs of the study. We generally utilize the bilaterally linked anterior tibialis EMG channel for all studies on children over 1 year of age. At times, arm movements may also be required. In this situation, we will also record bilaterally brachioradialis EMG. EOG, chin EMG, EKG, respiratory channels, and video/audio are also recorded for all studies. Esophageal pH, intraesophageal pressure, suprasternal notch retraction, are optional. Rarely, additional EOG electrodes are required when the direction of eye movements is in question. This has generally only been required for research and investigational purposes. Often it is important to determine the patency of tracheostomy and/or whether the tracheostomy can be discontinued. When these studies are performed, an addition airflow channel from the tracheostomy site is added. Adequacy of flow through the tracheostomy, patency of the tracheostomy, and the patency of the upper airway when the tracheostomy is capped can be clearly identified polysomnographically.

Machine Calibrations

Standard machine calibrations should be conducted well before the beginning of the study. It is sometimes advisable to conduct machine calibrations prior to the patient arriving at the sleep disorders laboratory. This provides the technician time to make any adjustments or repairs to the recording equipment prior to patient set-up and delays in the beginning of the recording can be easily avoided. Pen alignment must be checked. If there is misalignment of pens, simultaneous electrophysiologic activity may be missed and it will be difficult to interpret this activity and differentiation of artifact (e.g., seizure spikes from occasional EKG artifact). High-frequency filters function and settings, low-frequency filters (time constants) function and setting, and line filter (60 Hz) should be calibrated with 20, 50, and 100 μV square pulses. Paper speeds should be verified. Pulse oximeter should be calibrated and the scale recorded on the tracing. Capnograph should also be calibrated with known concentrations of CO_2.

Patient Calibrations

In this age group, children often fall to sleep during set-up. In addition, they are frequently not at a developmental level where standard patient calibrations can be conducted. It is advisable prior to the time of lights-out to check the impedance of all recording electrodes. Impedance should be below 5,000 ohms in order to provide the most reliable signal and to significantly eliminate artifact. If the electrode test reveals leads that are greater than 5,000 ohms, they should be reapplied prior to the onset of the study, preventing iatrogenic disruption of the study to replace the electrode after the study has begun. In young patients who cannot comply with patient calibration instructions, technician observations and recording of observations on the recording are essential to further assessment of electrophysiologic parameters. The technician should record whether the patient is awake and moving, crying, eating, sucking, or quiet, with eyes open or closed, asleep, squirming, and all other behavioral observations needed in order to adequately evaluate the youngster's state. Parents feeding the youngster, patting the child, lying with the child, and diaper changes should be recorded. Older preschool children can generally respond to patient calibration instructions. Standard instructions include: keep eyes open, keep eyes closed; look left, right, up, down; blink 5 times; flex right leg then left leg; grit teeth, and hold breath.

It is important for the technician to identify the direction of airflow and respiratory effort of the chest and abdomen (i.e., the direction of inspiration and exhalation on all respiratory recording channels. Polarity of effort channels should be in phase when the chest and abdominal efforts are in phase. Paradoxical breathing can then be easily identified. It is generally advisable to also adjust the polarity of the EKG recording channel so that positive deflections are upward (EKG convention is opposite from standard EEG convention which requires negative potentials deflecting the pen upward). P waves, QRS complexes, and T waves will then generally result in upward deflection of the pen in lead 2.

Initial Polygraph Parameters

Initial polygraph parameters should be standard (see pages 110–111). At the beginning of the study, during the first slow-wave sleep period, pen blocking is common since wave-form amplitude is very high. Adjustments to the gain can be made at this time. Gain should be adjusted for maximum pen deflection during slow-wave sleep without blocking. Once adjusted, it should not be changed for the remainder of the study, unless very poor quality signal is being recorded that requires an increase in gain in order to accurately interpret the tracing. These changes must be clearly documented on the record and recorded so that the changes can be easily identified.

EVALUATION AND SCORING OF POLYSOMNOGRAMS OF CHILDREN ONE TO FIVE YEARS OF AGE

Behavioral Observations

Behavioral observations prior to and during the course of polysomnography are again essential in determination of state and assisting in identification of movements and artifact from electrophysiologic events. The technician's recordings of observations during the course of polysomnography can be the most important aspect of the recording.

Wake

During the early portion of this developmental period, wakefulness is sometimes difficult to differentiate from transitional sleep in some infants. Behavioral observations and documentation on the record is essential for accurate interpretation. Often the youngster may be crying and moving about. Movement artifact obscures much of the record.

EEG

When quiet, occipital rhythms of relatively high voltage (50–150 μV) may be present at 1 year of age. The amplitude decreases as the youngster matures, but remains quite high in comparison to the adolescent and adult record. At about 1 year of age, the occipital rhythm consists of 6- to 8-Hz activity of approximately 50–75 μV, which is clearly attenuated with a decrease in amplitude and change to mixed frequency by eye opening. This activity slowly progresses more anteriorly to the parieto-central regions as the youngster ages. Resting wakefulness is closer to the adult pattern when compared to earlier in infancy. Waking EEG can provide significant information regarding structural abnormalities and metabolic defects whereas sleeping EEG provides for activation and identification of epileptiform activity.

Between the ages of 1 and 5 years, resting wakefulness consists of an admixture of alpha and theta activity, which is of higher voltage than that of older children and adults. As the youngster matures, alpha rhythm becomes more clearly formed and consists of a sinusoidal pattern of waves at a frequency of about 8–13 Hz. It is most prominent over the posterior regions of the head, but may extend more anteriorly to the central regions as the youngster ages. It is most prominent during relaxed wakefulness when the eyes are closed and is attenuated by eye opening, focusing attention, and cognitive efforts. The frequency of alpha activity slowly increases with age and becomes quite stable in a given individual. By the end of the 5th year, it reaches a frequency of about 9 to 11 Hz and remains fairly constant throughout adolescence and adulthood. However, at 5 years of age, alpha rhythm may still be undergoing maturation.

Delta activity during wakefulness decreases in prominence with age. Theta activity is more prominent during wakefulness up to about 4 years of age. At 5 years of age, the percentage of alpha and theta activity occurring during wakefulness is about equal. Beta activity can occur in young children and is most often associated with medication effect. When it occurs spontaneously, it can be normal unless there is persistent asymmetry.

EOG

Conjugate eye movements, saccadic eye movements, and blink artifact are common. High-voltage activity may yield frontal EEG artifact if gains are set too high. If there is significant crying and/or activity, sweat artifact may be rather prominent.

EMG

Chin muscle EMG is tonic and may reveal a variety of movement artifacts including, but not limited to: sucking, swallowing, chewing, crying.

EKG

Lead 2 EKG reveals a sinus rhythm. Sinus tachycardia may be present and there can be considerable respiratory variability present, especially during periods of crying. Normal waking heart rates at rest may range from 90 beats per minute to 150 beats per minute at 1 year of age (mean 119 beats per minute) to 65 beats per minute to 130 beats per minute at 5 years of age (mean 100 beats per minute) (8).

Respiration

Respiratory effort is variable and inconsistent during active wakefulness. During quiet wake respirations may be more regular, yet some variability remains. There may be respiratory pauses due to breath holding during movements and/or crying. Airflow may cease during periods of feeding and swallowing. Airflow may also be quite variable during times of non-nutritive sucking. Oxygen saturation in the presence of normal pulmonary and cardiac function generally remains about 95% (depending upon the oximeter used) and artifactual decrease in SpO_2 is common with movements due to poor pulse signals (Figs. 11-3–11-4).

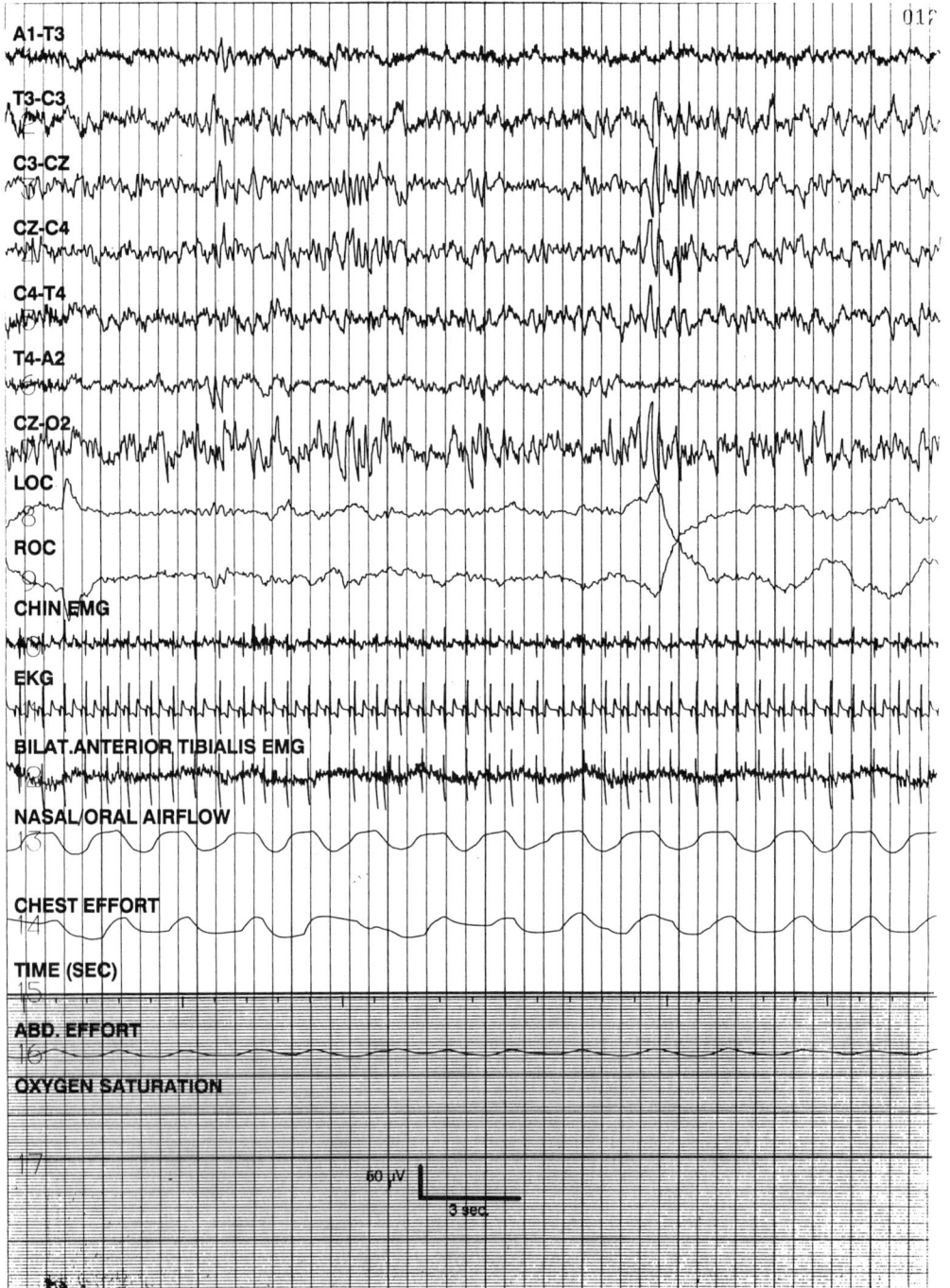

FIG. 11-3. A–B: Quiet wake in a 3-year-old youngster with transition into sleep by epoch (**B**). Waking rhythm consists of moderate-voltage activity of about 6–7 Hz in frequency. Conjugate eye movements are present. Chin muscle tone is somewhat decreased and EKG reveals a normal sinus arrhythmia. Anterior tibialis EMG is tonic, and there are no leg movements or

Continued.

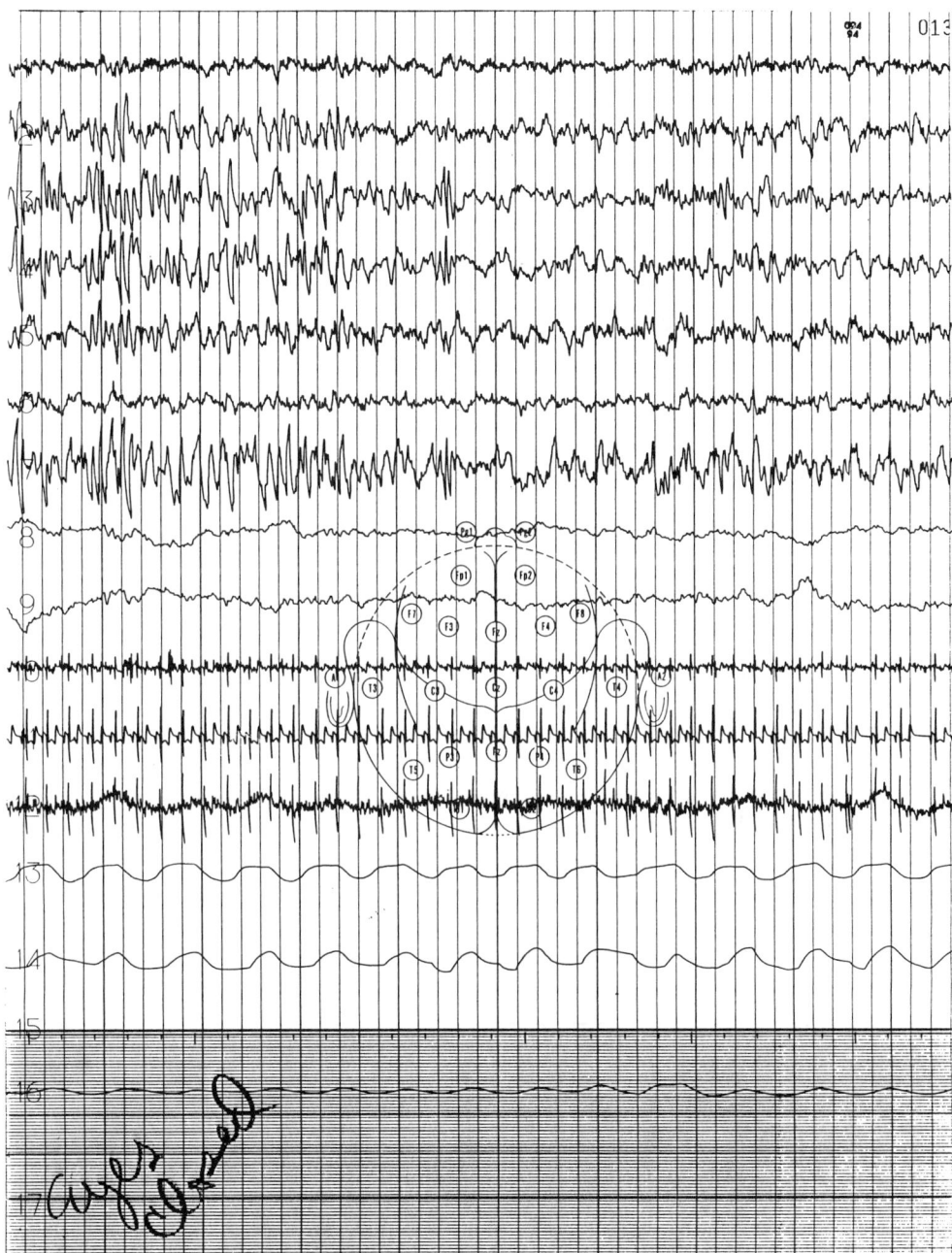

B

phasic activity to be seen. Respiration is regular. As the transition to sleep occurs, the EEG background voltage increases slightly and decreases in frequency. Bursts of hypersynchronous theta activity (hypnogogic hypersynchrony) can be identified. Conjugate eye movements disappear and are replaced with slow, rolling eye movements. Chin and anterior tibialis tone remains present. Respirations remain regular. The technician's note that the eyes are closed is quite helpful in determining the transition to sleep in this patient.

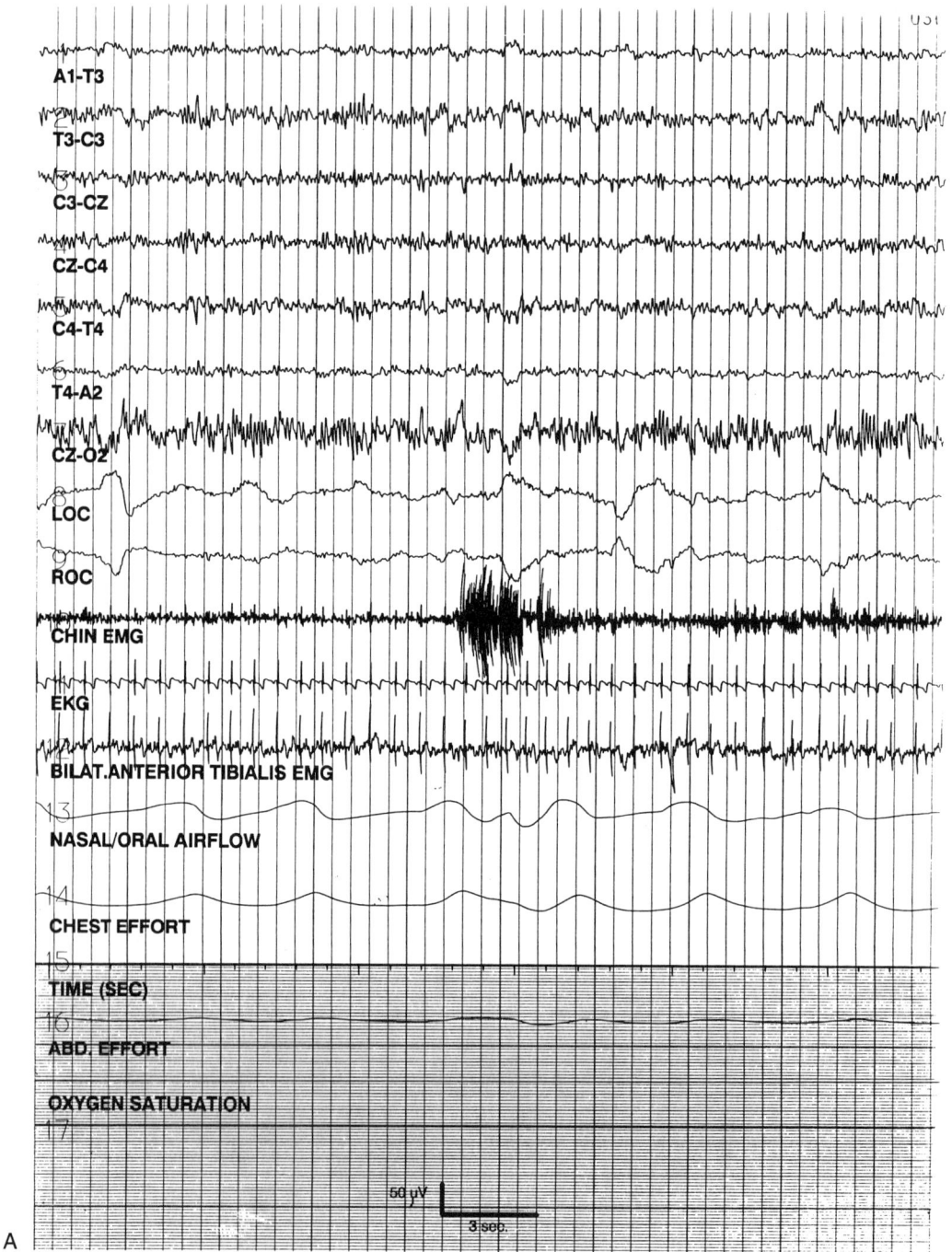

FIG. 11-4. A–B: Quiet wake in a 5-year-old youngster. The EEG pattern has become quite mature. Background voltage has decreased and there is well-formed alpha activity, seen especially well in the posterior region of the head. Conjugate eye movements are present and chin tone is high. Chin movements can also be seen. Normal respiratory variation in heart rate is present on EKG.

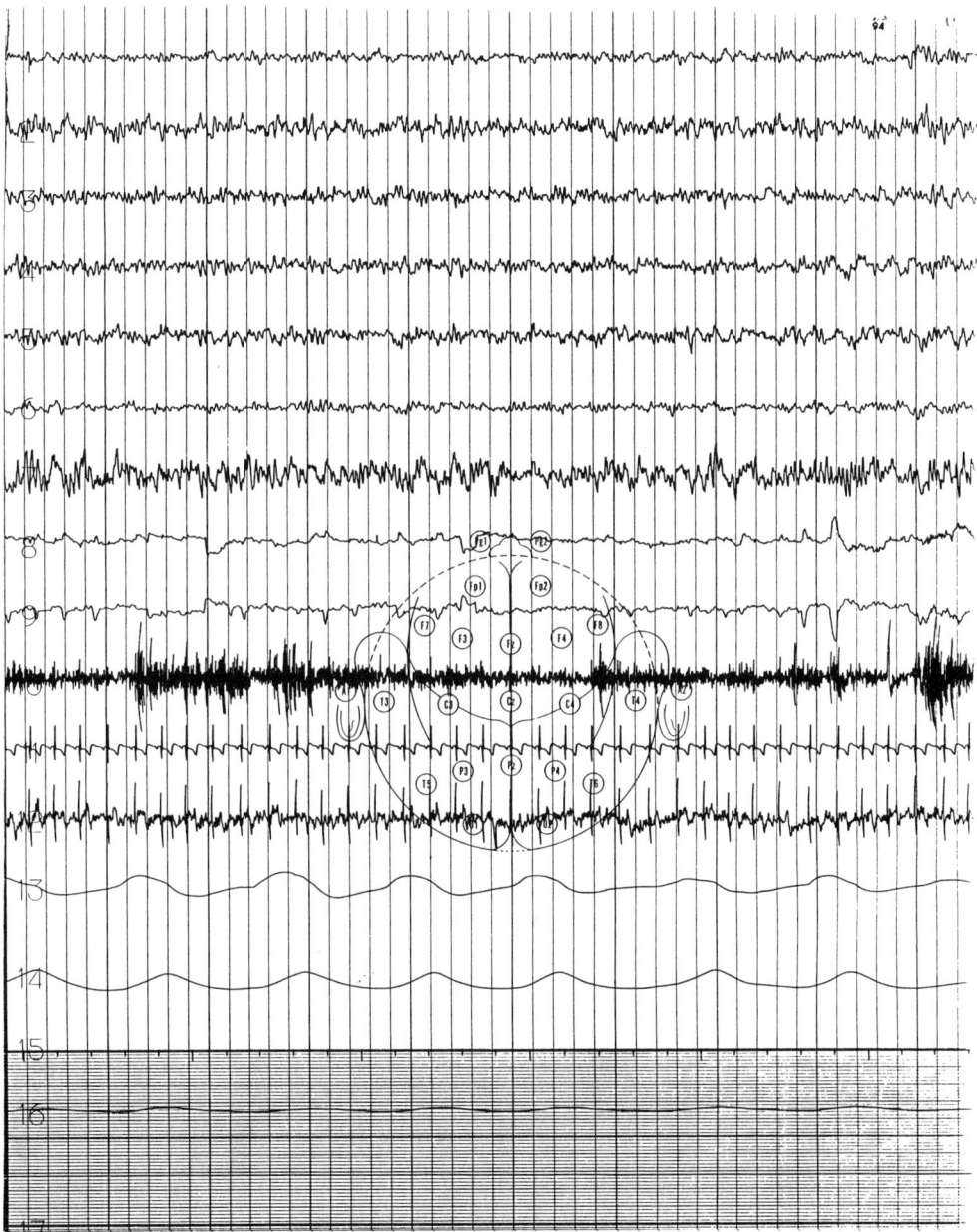

FIG. 11-4. *Continued.*

Transitional Sleep

Transitional sleep (or stage 1 sleep) in youngsters in this developmental period is variable. In younger toddlers, the transition can be quite rapid with electrophysiologic evidence of sleep onset occurring within one minute or less. In older children there is generally a slightly longer (1–5 minutes) period of drowsiness and micro-sleep episodes that herald transition into sleep. This period of drowsiness gradually transitions into stage 2 sleep, or micro-sleep periods become more frequent and coalesce into an identifiable sleep pattern.

EEG

During drowsiness in this developmental period, two EEG patterns may be present. Bilateral synchronous or hypersynchronous high-amplitude wave forms appear in the 3- to 5-Hz frequency. This typically is present during the middle portion of the first year of life and can continue until 4–5 years of age. In addition, rhythmic 6-Hz activity of medium amplitude begins to appear, especially in the frontal region by the time the youngster reaches 5 years of age. Hypersynchronous activity in the theta range is very frequent in the 1- to 5-year-old age group and is often termed *hypnogogic hypersynchrony*. The clinical significance of this hypersynchronous theta activity is questionable. It is typically present during lighter stages of sleep. However, in youngsters with partial arousal slow-wave sleep parasomnias (such as sleep terrors and somnambulism) can reveal intense hypersynchronous theta activity during all stages of NREM sleep and reveal a pattern of theta-delta activity during slow-wave sleep (Fig. 11-5). The clinical and pathophysiologic significance of this finding has yet to be elucidated.

EOG

EOG reveals a disappearance of conjugate eye movements. Saccadic eye movements are replaced with slow and rolling eye movements more characteristic of adult stage 1 sleep. Because of occasional state discordance during transitional sleep, a rare conjugate eye movement may be seen in the presence of an EEG pattern clearly associated with transitional sleep. Rhythmic 6-Hz activity of medium amplitude appears bilaterally in the frontal region during this transition phase and may appear as frontal EEG artifact in the EOG.

EMG

EMG remains tonic or may reveal a moderate fall in chin muscle tone. Non-nutritive sucking artifact frequently persists into drowsiness and transitional sleep (Fig. 11-6).

EKG

EKG is relatively stable during this transition phase. Beat-to-beat variability occurs and identification of respiratory variability (normal sinus arrhythmia) can be identified.

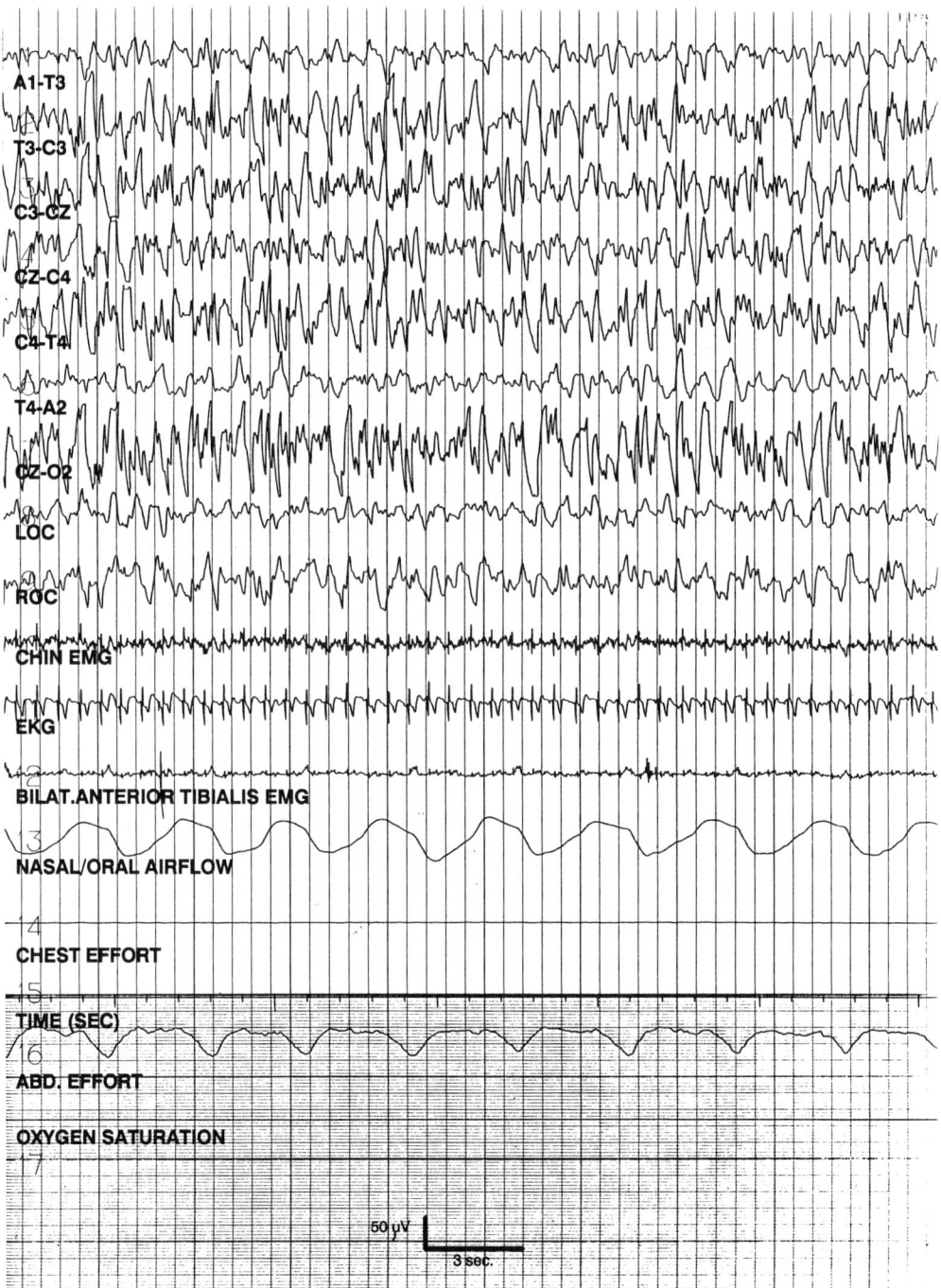

FIG. 11-5. Theta intrusion. At times EEG theta activity is so ubiquitous in youngsters that it may pervade all stages of NREM sleep. Note the moderate-voltage 4- to 6-Hz activity superimposed upon high-voltage 0.5- to 1.0-Hz waves. Although the clinical significance of this finding is unknown, it is most likely a normal phenomenon.

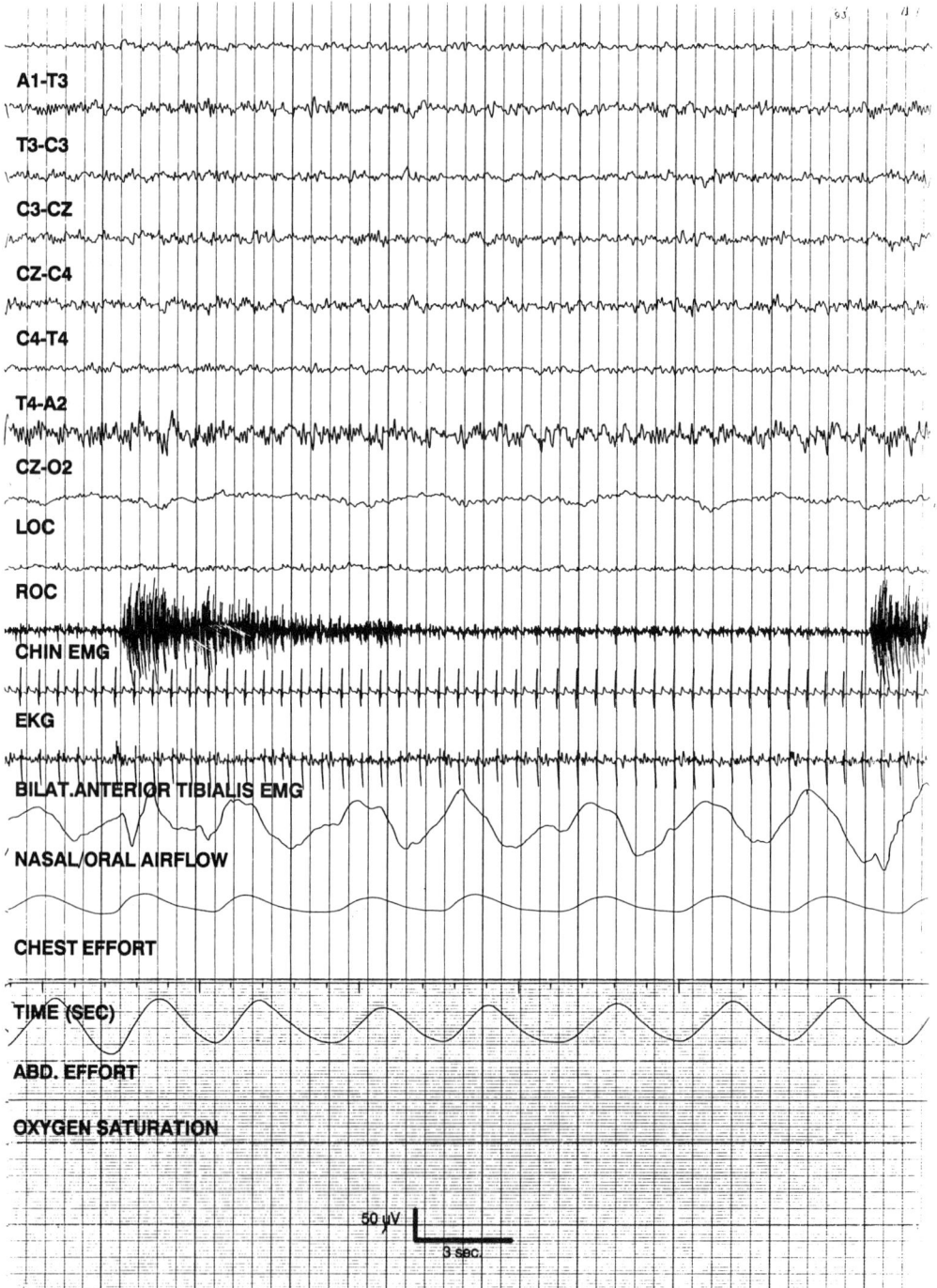

FIG. 11-6. Sucking artifact. The patient is sucking on a pacifier resulting in waxing and waning of chin muscle EMG tone.

Respiration

Respiration becomes regular and stable, in contrast to the high respiratory variability associated with wakefulness. Transitional hypopneas are not uncommon and are typically of little consequence as long as they are not associated with significant oxygen desaturation, are prolonged, or are associated with EKG changes or arousal. Oxygen saturation remains stable and generally above 95%. Small changes in PaO_2 generally occurs. If the position of the hemoglobin-oxygen saturation curve remains normal, there is a limited fall in SaO_2 since the PaO_2 is generally on the shallow portion of the curve.

NREM Sleep

Between the ages of 1 and 5 years, NREM sleep shows patterns of maturation and there is apparent emergence of new patterns. NREM sleep can more clearly be differentiated into an adult-like pattern of 4 states (assuming stage 1 is the transitional stage discussed above and separating slow-wave sleep into stage 3 and stage 4). Separation of slow-wave sleep into two distinct stages for scoring purposes is easier in adults than in children. Descent into deeper stages of sleep during early childhood occurs very rapidly (young children tend to plummet into slow-wave sleep) and separation of slow-wave sleep into two distinct physiologic states is probably unnecessary and artificial. In addition to changes in sleep structure, state percentages tend to assume a more adult character. Sleep cycles tend to lengthen from about 50 to 60 minutes at 1 year of age to the adult level of 80–90 minutes by age 5 years. REM-sleep percentage gradually decreases as a percent of the sleep-period time from about 30% at 1 year of age to the adult level of about 20% to 25% at 5 years of age. Arousal thresholds are generally very high during this stage of development and are probably the highest of any time during the life cycle.

EEG

EEG reveals a well-formed background rhythm during NREM sleep that consists of moderate-voltage, mixed-frequency activity. Sleep spindles are generally well formed, mature, synchronous, and symmetric in appearance. The absence of well formed and symmetric sleep spindles after one year of age is abnormal. Spindles often occur immediately after the appearance of a K-complex. Frequent bursts of vertex sharp waves lasting 3 to 12 seconds (or more) appear during stage 1 sleep and during the transition into deeper stage 2. Positive sharp transients of sleep (POSTs) begin to appear during transitional sleep. Descent into slow-wave sleep is generally rapid. High-voltage slow waves (generally greater than 250 µV) appear and rapidly occupy more than 50% of each 30-second sleep epoch. Sleep spindles can be present during slow-wave sleep. Hypersynchronous theta activity can also occur but seems to be more prevalent in youngsters who are prone to partial arousal NREM-sleep parasomnias. The first slow-wave sleep cycle lasts for a considerable uninterrupted period in youngsters in this developmental age period. It ends with a major body movement with ascent to a lighter stage of NREM sleep. Frequent body movements in slow-wave sleep *without* state change can be seen in youngsters with partial arousal NREM motor disorders.

EOG

EOG reveals absence of conjugate eye movements. Because of the high amplitude of slow waves during NREM sleep in children between 1 and 5 years, frequent frontal EEG artifact is noted, even when the gain of the eye channels are turned down to rather low levels. The eye channels need not be adjusted at this time to eliminate the frontal EEG artifact. If the gain is turned down too low, eye movements during REM sleep would be obscured.

EMG

EMG remains tonic during NREM sleep. Rare phasic activity may be present, however, the clinical significance of this phasic activity is unknown. Occasionally bruxism may be noted. Rhythmic movements of the mandible may be associated with teeth grinding or may be isolated teeth clenching, not associated with the characteristic sound of bruxism. Jaw thrusting may also occur during NREM sleep. Characteristic rhythmic EMG and muscle artifact appears (Fig. 11-7).

EKG

EKG remains stable during NREM sleep, especially during slow-wave sleep. Beat-to-beat variability may be identifiable and respiratory variation may occur.

Respiration

Respiration is also remarkably stable during slow-wave sleep. Breath-to-breath variability is minimal and respiratory effort is monotonous. Slow-wave sleep also tends to offer protection from abnormal occlusive upper-airway events. Even in the presence of significant OSAS, respiration may appear remarkably normal during this state. Oxygen saturation also remains stable, although normal NREM decrease in respiratory efforts and mild hypoventilation, which normally occurs during NREM sleep, results in a minimal fall in the baseline oxygen saturation (Figs. 11-8–11-13).

REM Sleep

EEG

Similar to NREM sleep, REM sleep assumes a more mature pattern during this stage of development. Background EEG rhythm consists of moderate-amplitude, mixed-frequency activity. Notched theta activity in the 5- to 7-Hz frequency range occur in long bursts. Sometimes this activity is almost continuous. Sleep spindles may be present, especially during the first and second REM sleep period. Mixed states are fairly common during this time. Scoring of REM state should be based on the preponderant activity of a combination of physiologic variables that are being continuously measured.

It should be remembered that scoring of state is somewhat artificial in that there are a variety of neuronal networks that become activated during various states and state transitions, thereby resulting in changes in the variety of physiologic parameters measured

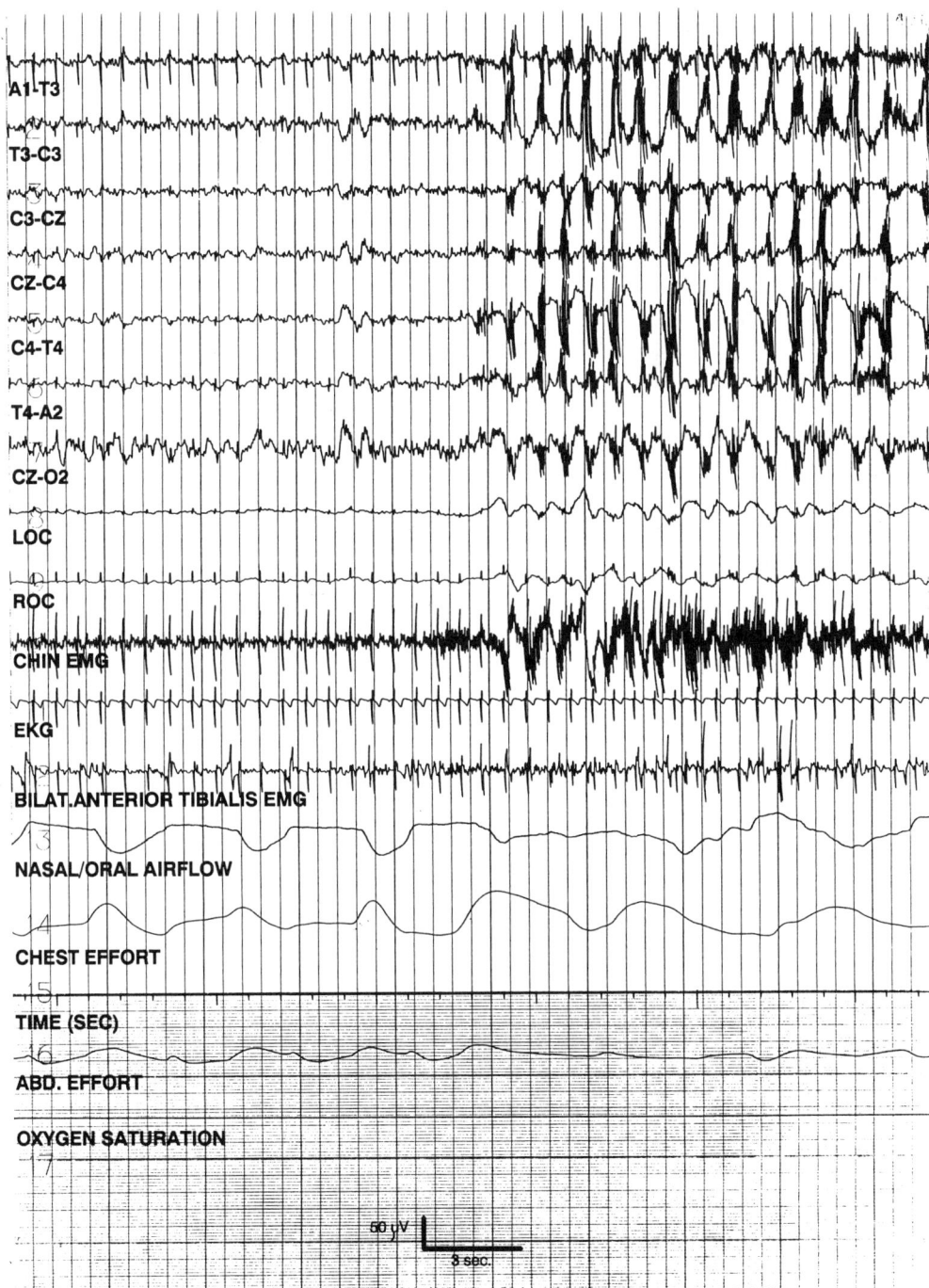

FIG. 11-7. Bruxism. Note the rhythmic chin muscle movements. Rhythmic muscle artifact is also present in the EEG (secondary to rhythmic temporalis muscle movements).

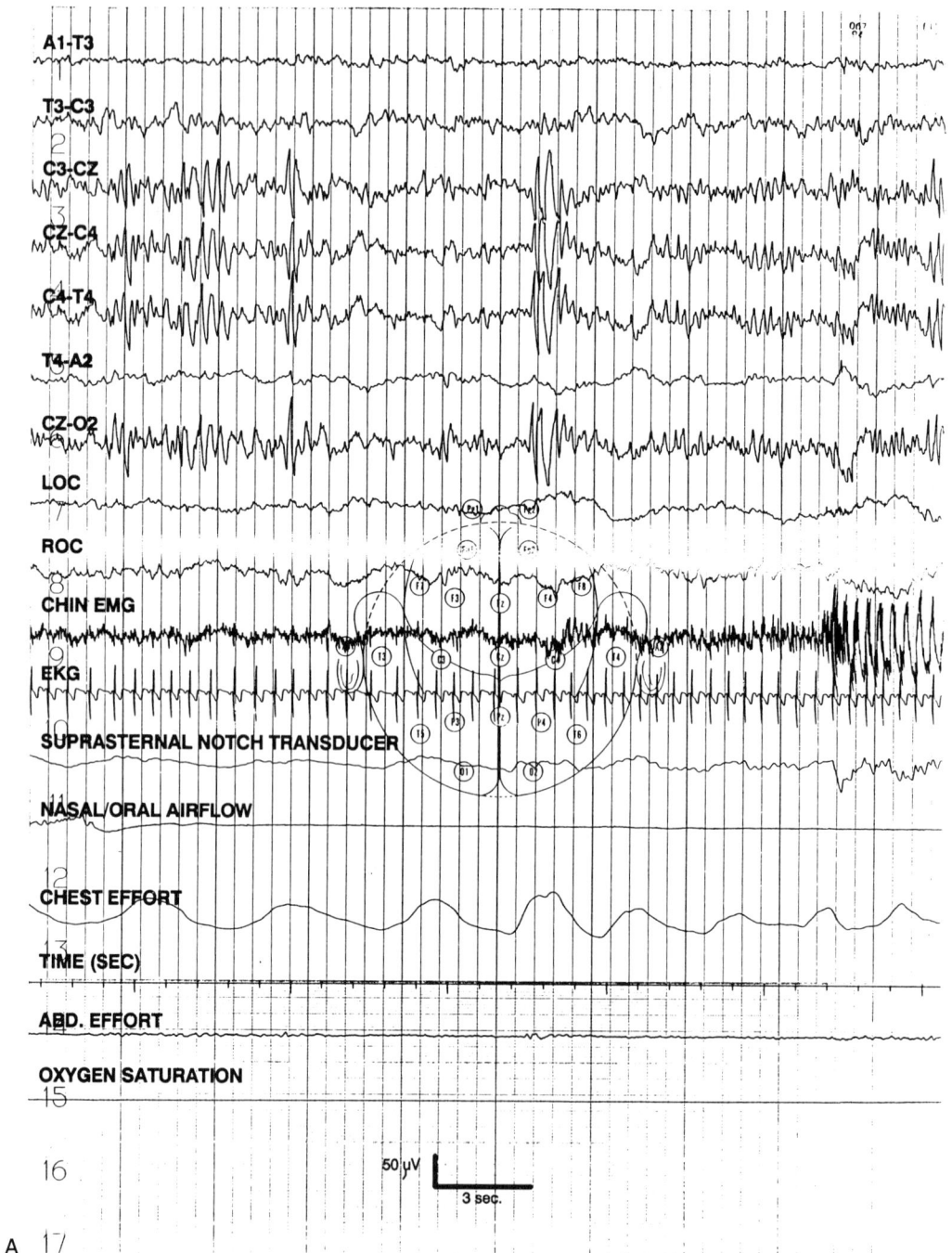

FIG. 11-8. A–B: NREM stage 2 in a 14-month-old toddler. A mixed-frequency, relatively low-voltage background EEG rhythm is present. K-complexes and vertex activity can be noted. Eye movements are absent and chin tone is moderate. Sucking movements can persist into NREM sleep and suck artifact can be seen in the chin EMG. Respiratory variation in heart rate can be seen. Signal is poor from the nasal/oral thermistor due to occlusion from a pacifier.

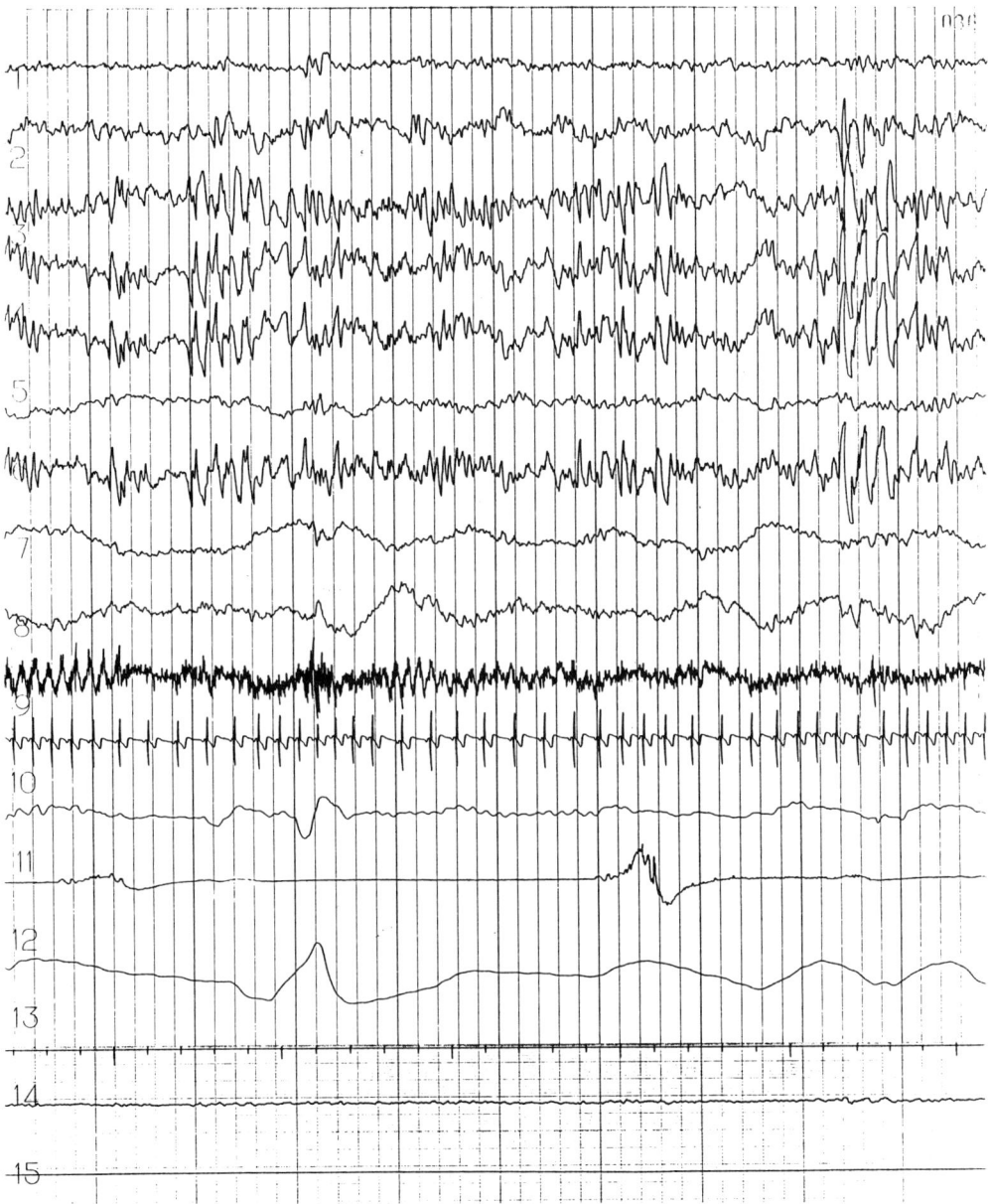

FIG. 11-8. *Continued.*

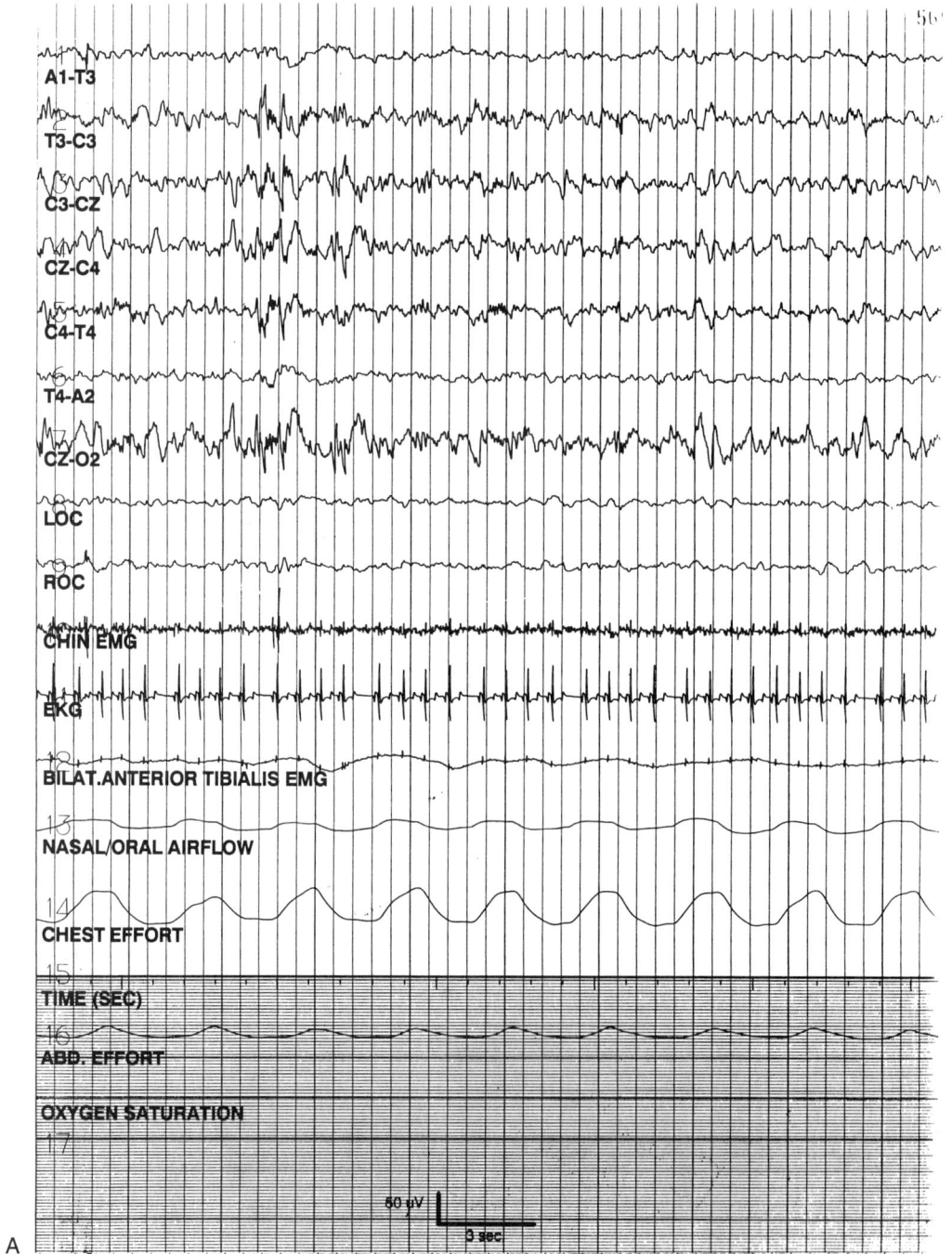

FIG. 11-9. A–B: NREM stage 2 in a 3-year-old youngster. A more mature pattern is present. Note the well formed and symmetric sleep spindles of about 8–10 Hz. Eye movements are absent, chin EMG is tonic, and a normal sinus arrhythmia is present in the EKG. Respirations are quite regular.

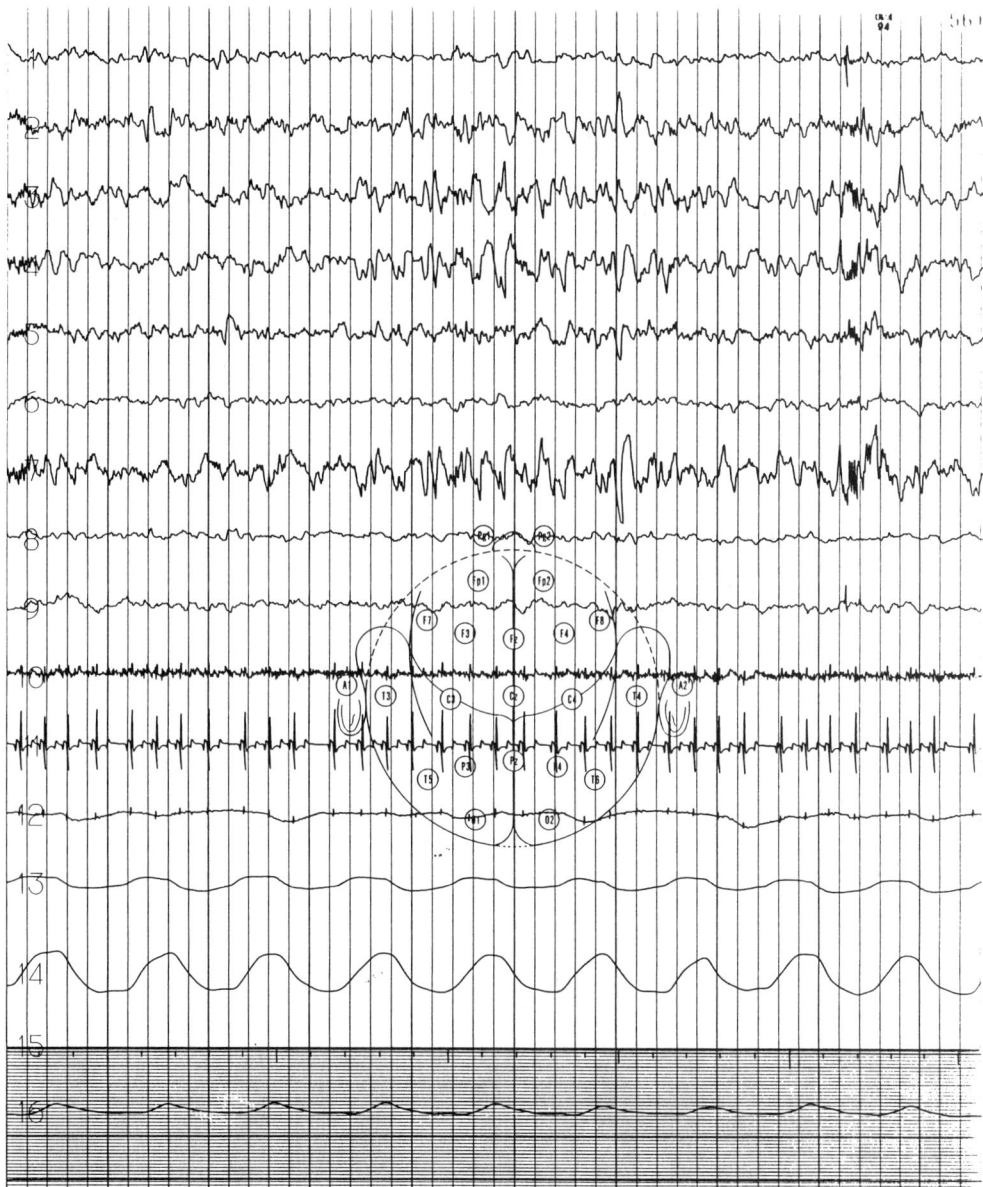

FIG. 11-9. *Continued.*

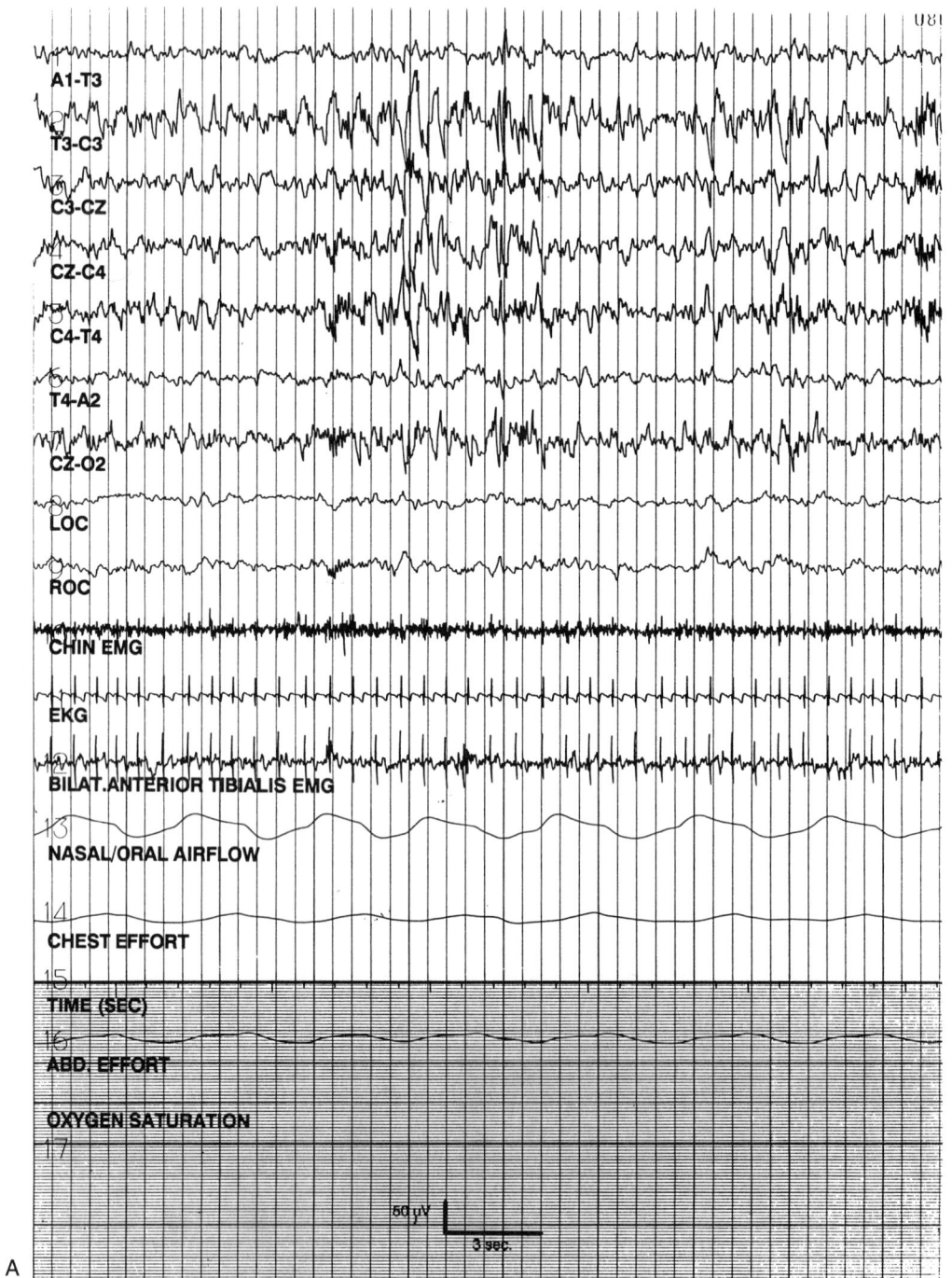

FIG. 11-10. A–B: NREM stage 2 in a 5-year-old youngster. The EEG pattern is now quite mature. Note the well-formed sleep spindles (which are occasionally quite long), K-complexes, and vertex activity. Again, chin EMG is tonic and there are no eye movements present. Anterior tibialis EMG reveals some EKG artifact and some phasic activity. Respiration is regular.

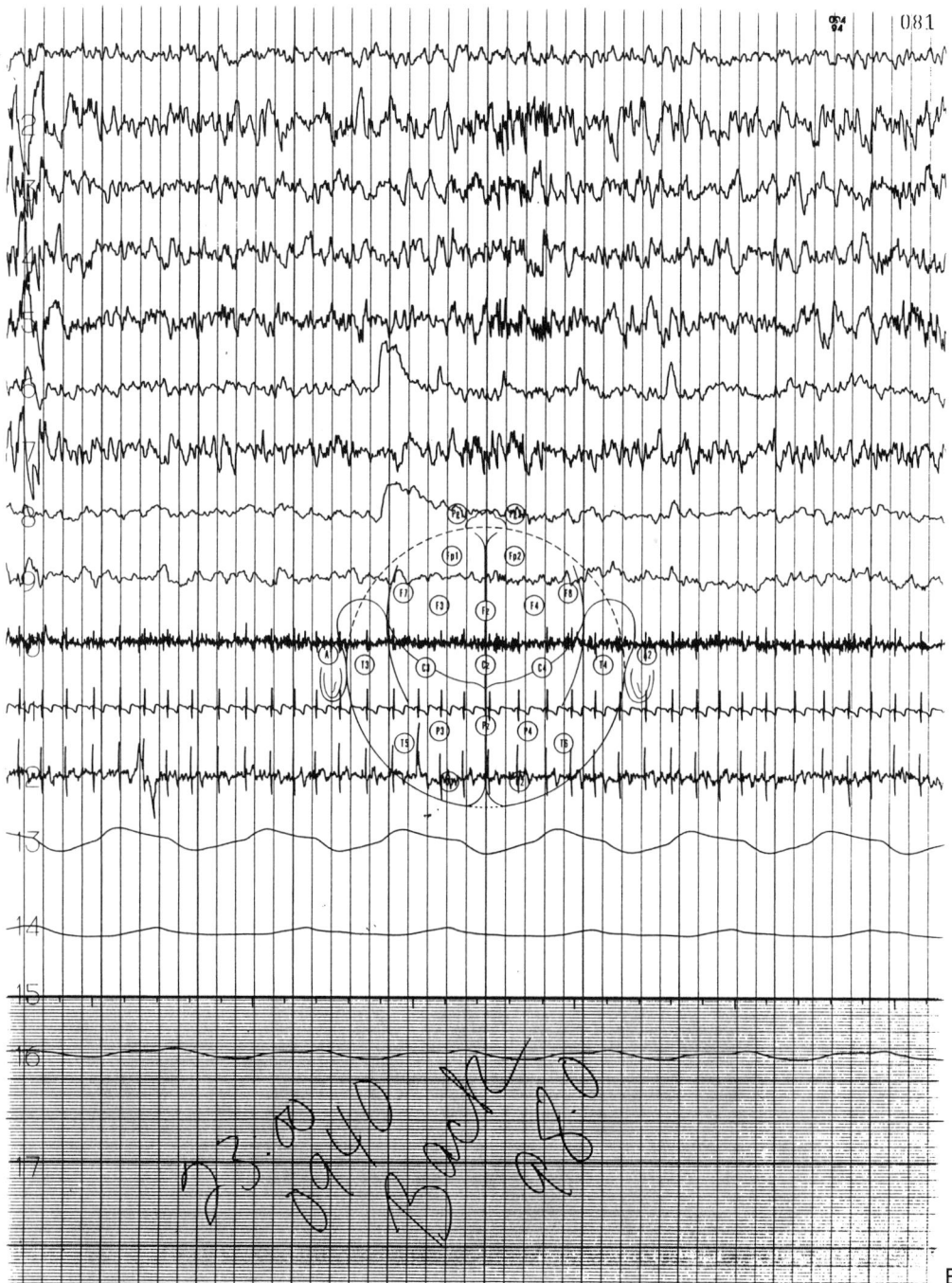

FIG. 11-10. *Continued.*

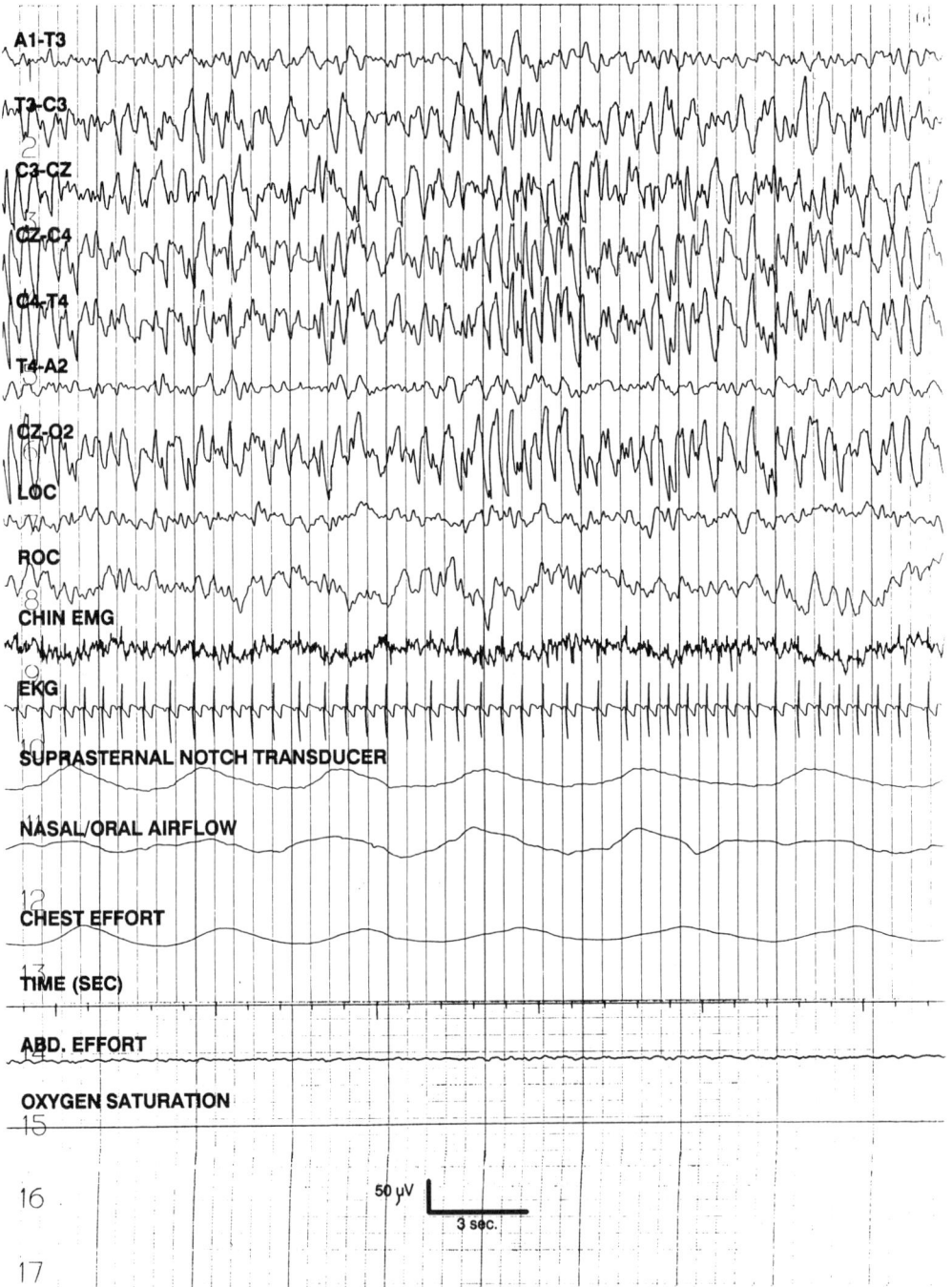

FIG. 11-11. A–B: NREM slow-wave sleep in a 14-month-old toddler. State demarcation is clear and the vast majority of the 30-second epoch consists of high-voltage activity at about 1–2 Hz. Frontal EEG artifact is present in the EOG.

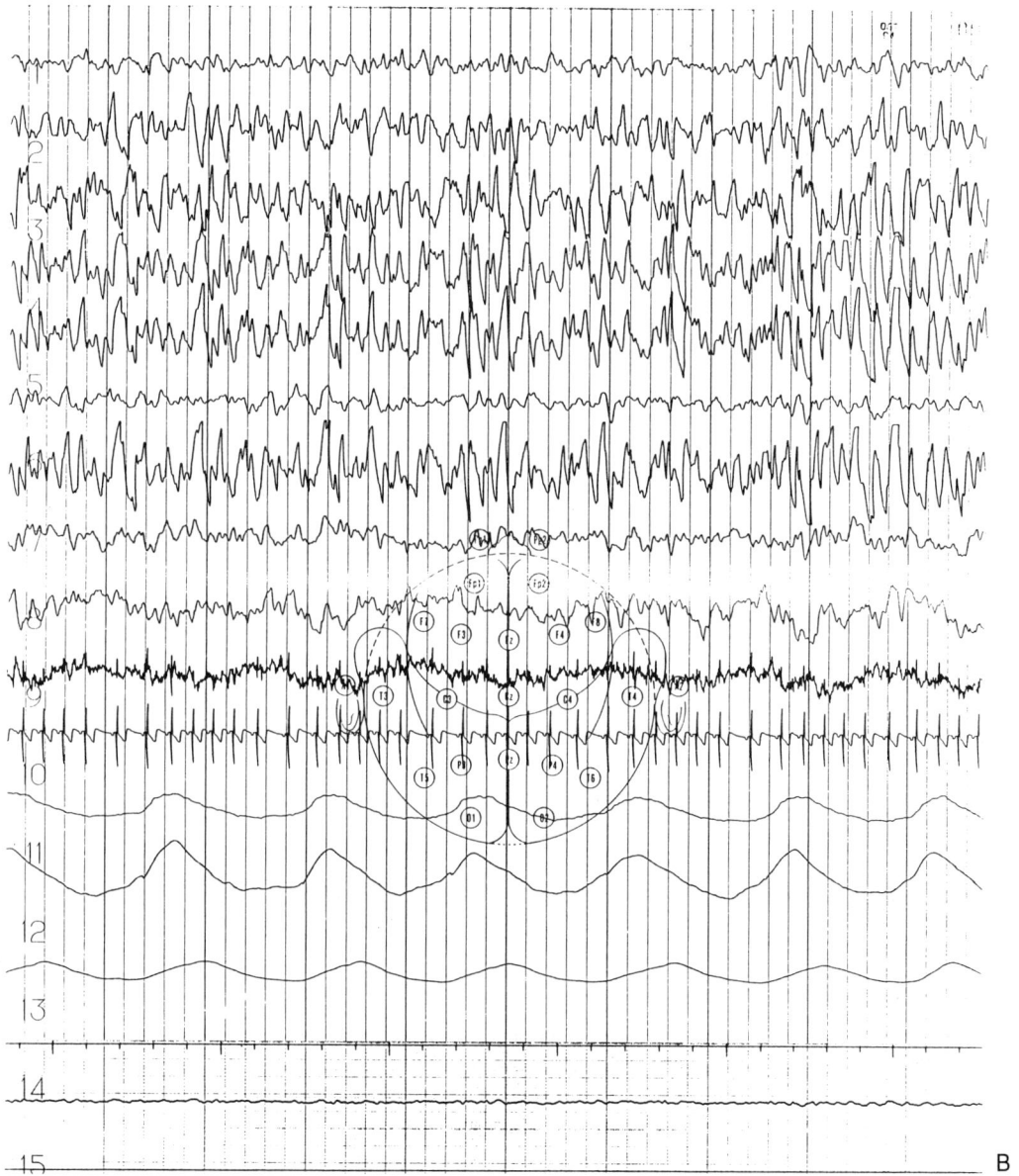

FIG. 11-11. *Continued.*

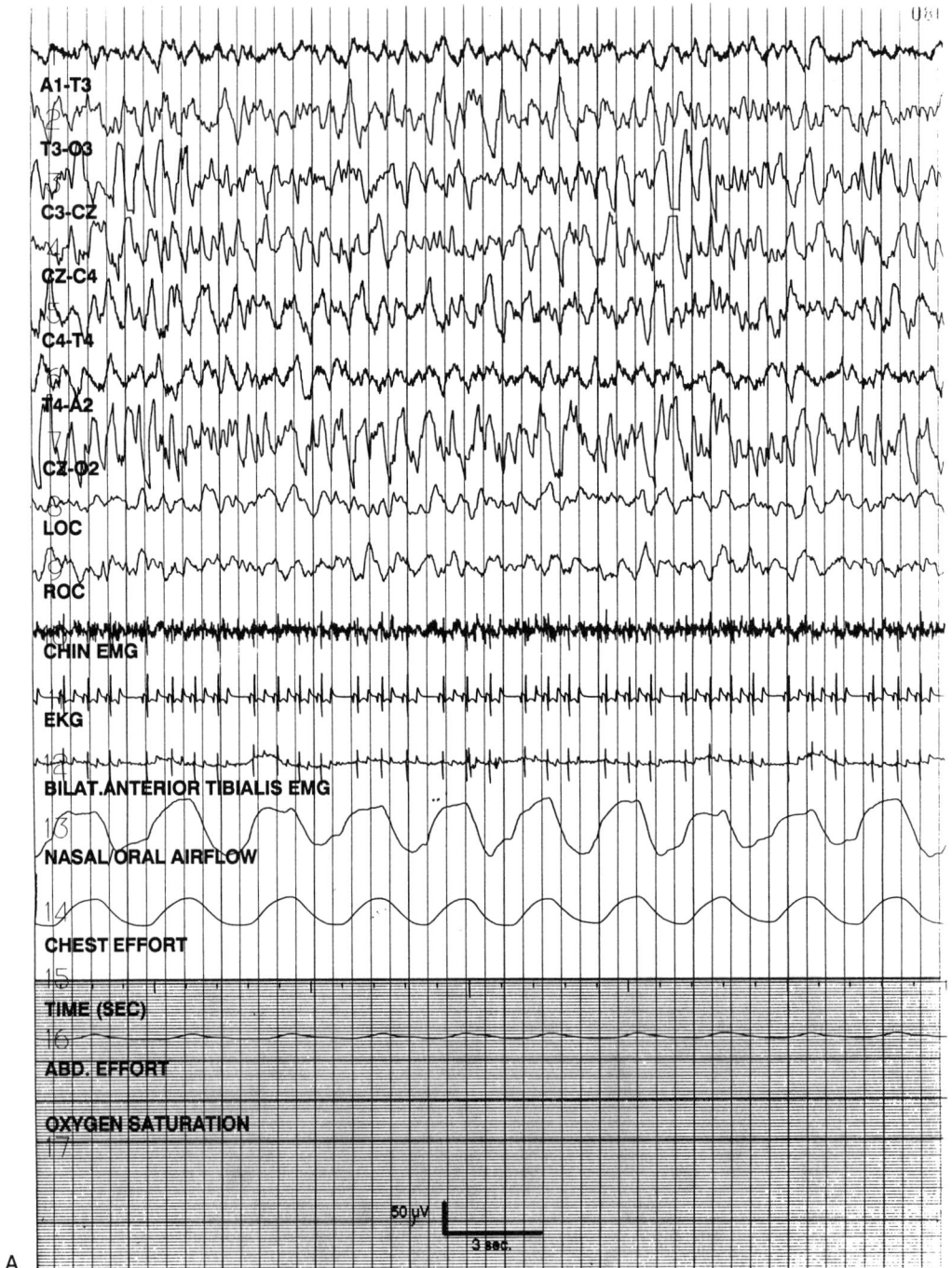

FIG. 11-12. A–B: NREM slow-wave sleep in a 3-year-old youngster. State demarcation is quite clear. High-voltage activity at about 0.5–1 Hz is present throughout the epochs.

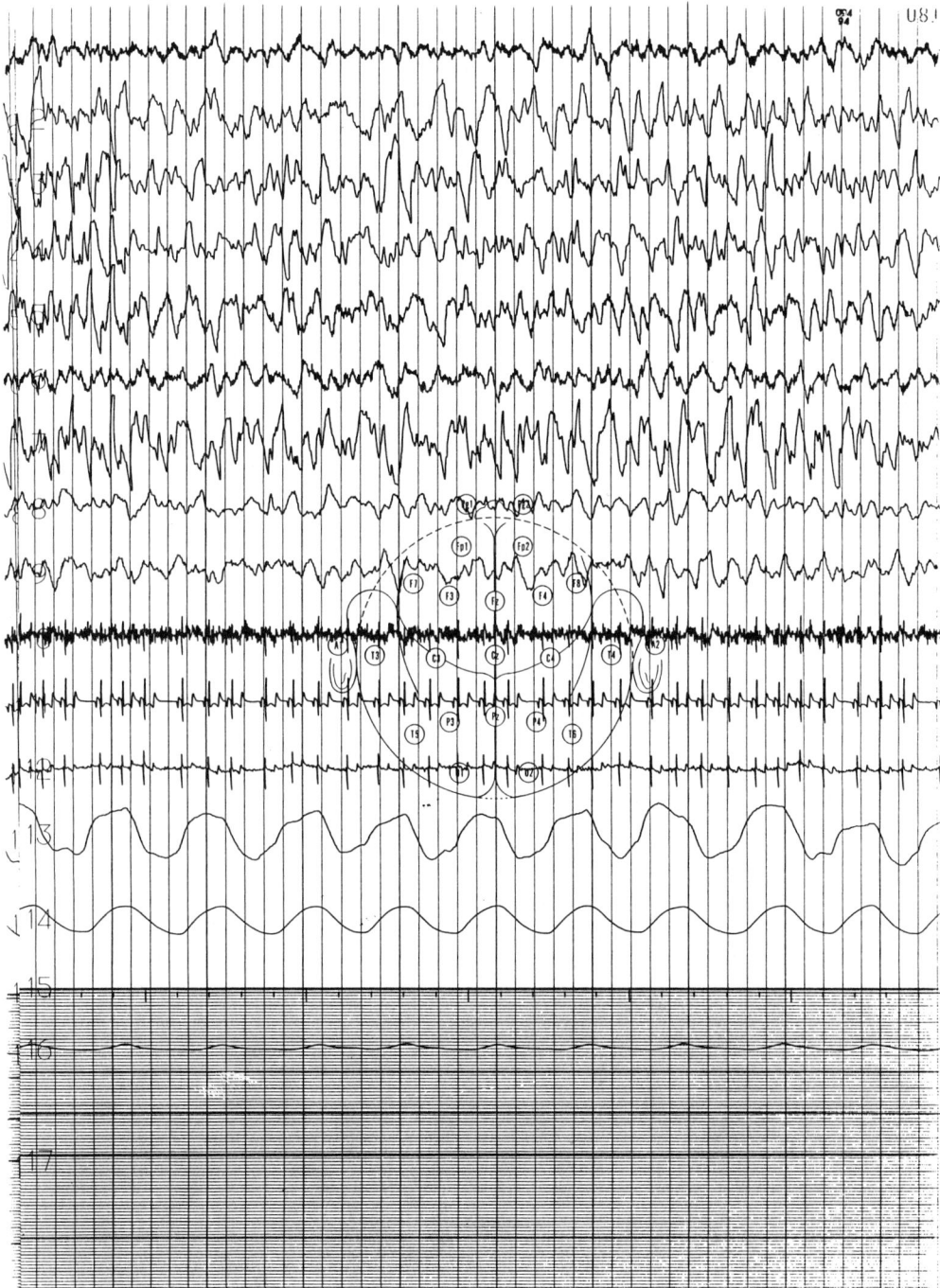

FIG. 11-12. *Continued.*

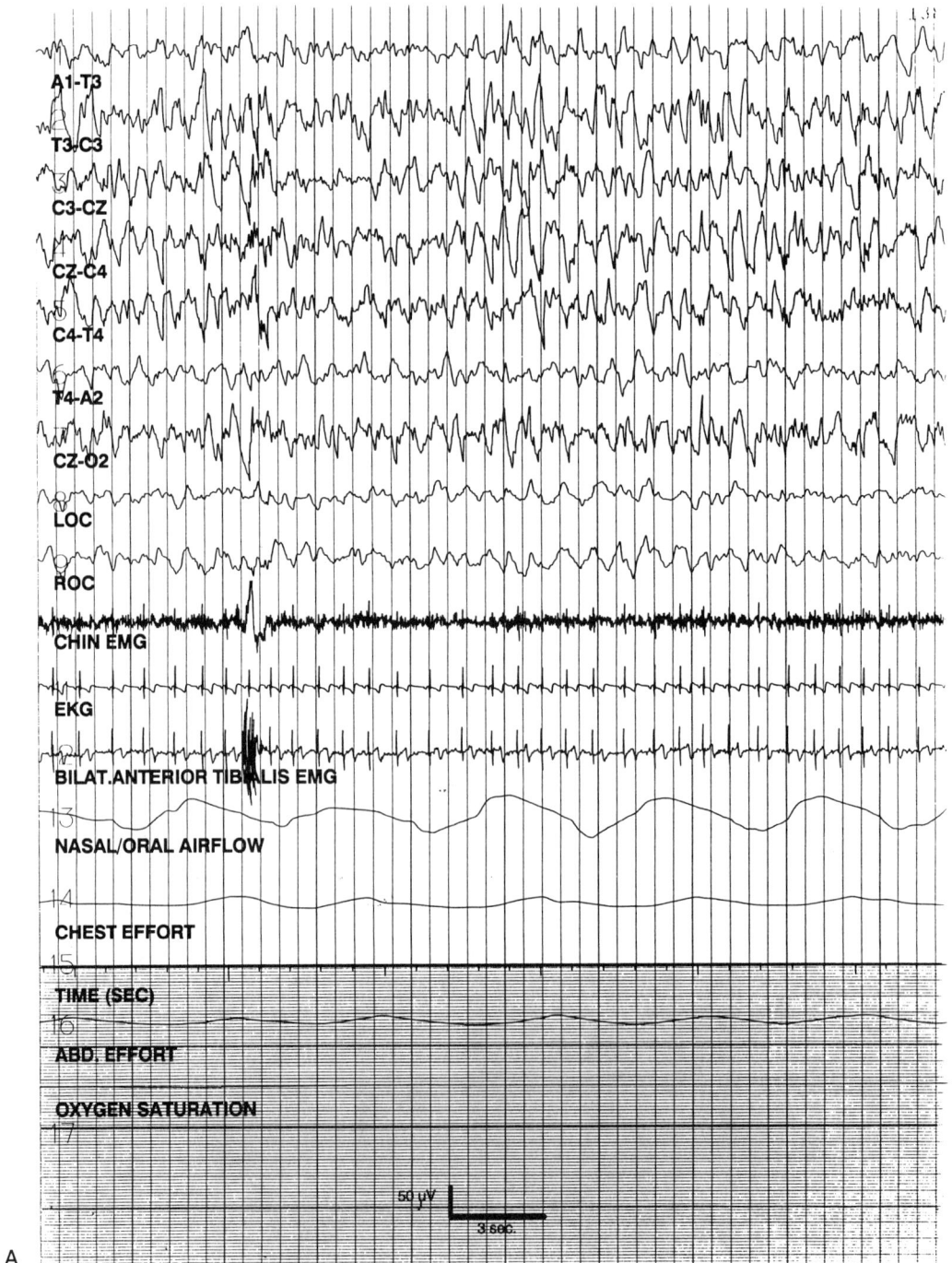

FIG. 11-13. A–B: NREM slow-wave sleep in a 5-year-old youngster. This pattern is very mature. Along with the high-voltage slow waves, sleep spindles may occur. A phasic twitch in the anterior tibialis EMG can be seen. A normal sinus arrhythmia is present in the EKG.

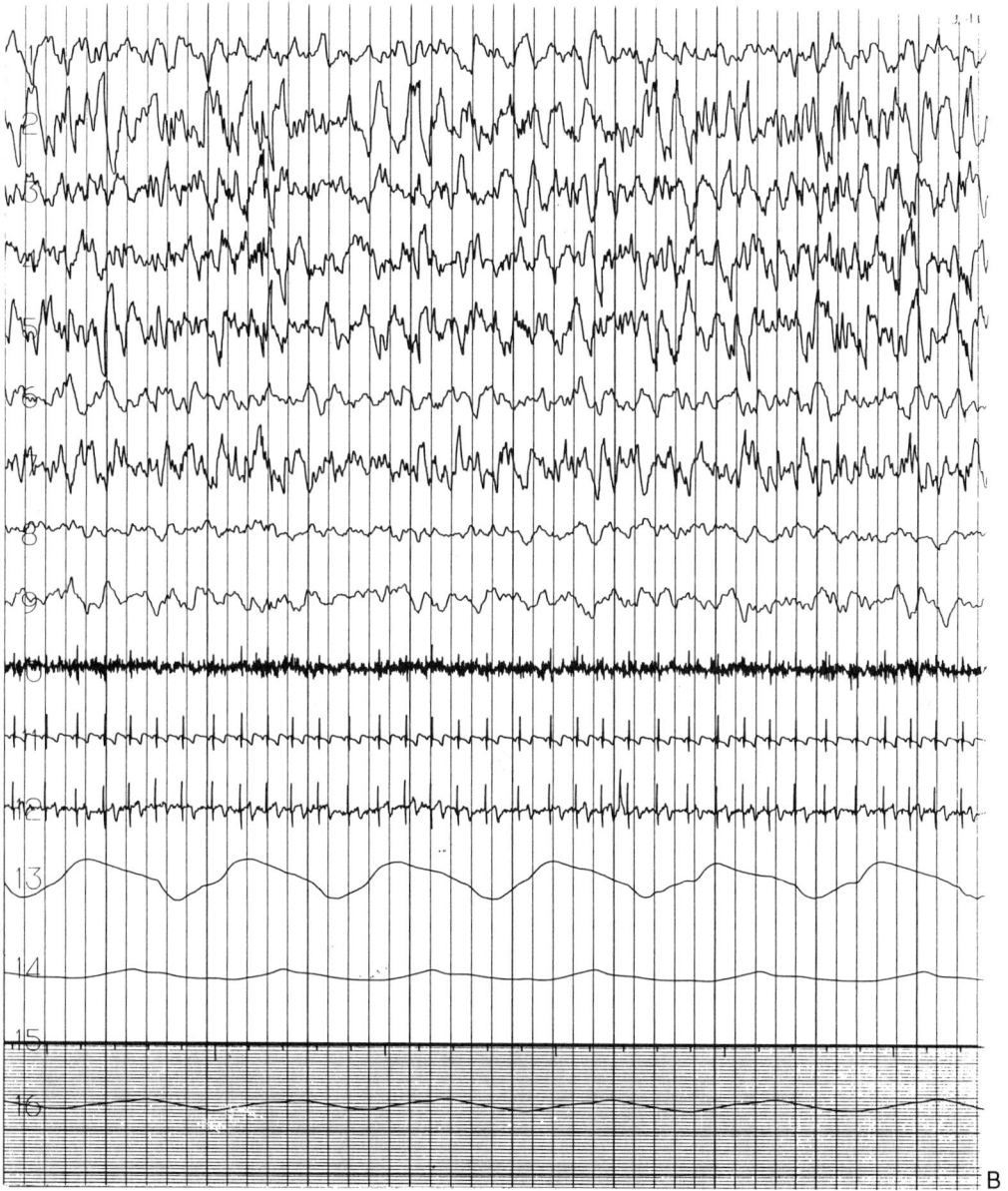

FIG. 11-13. *Continued.*

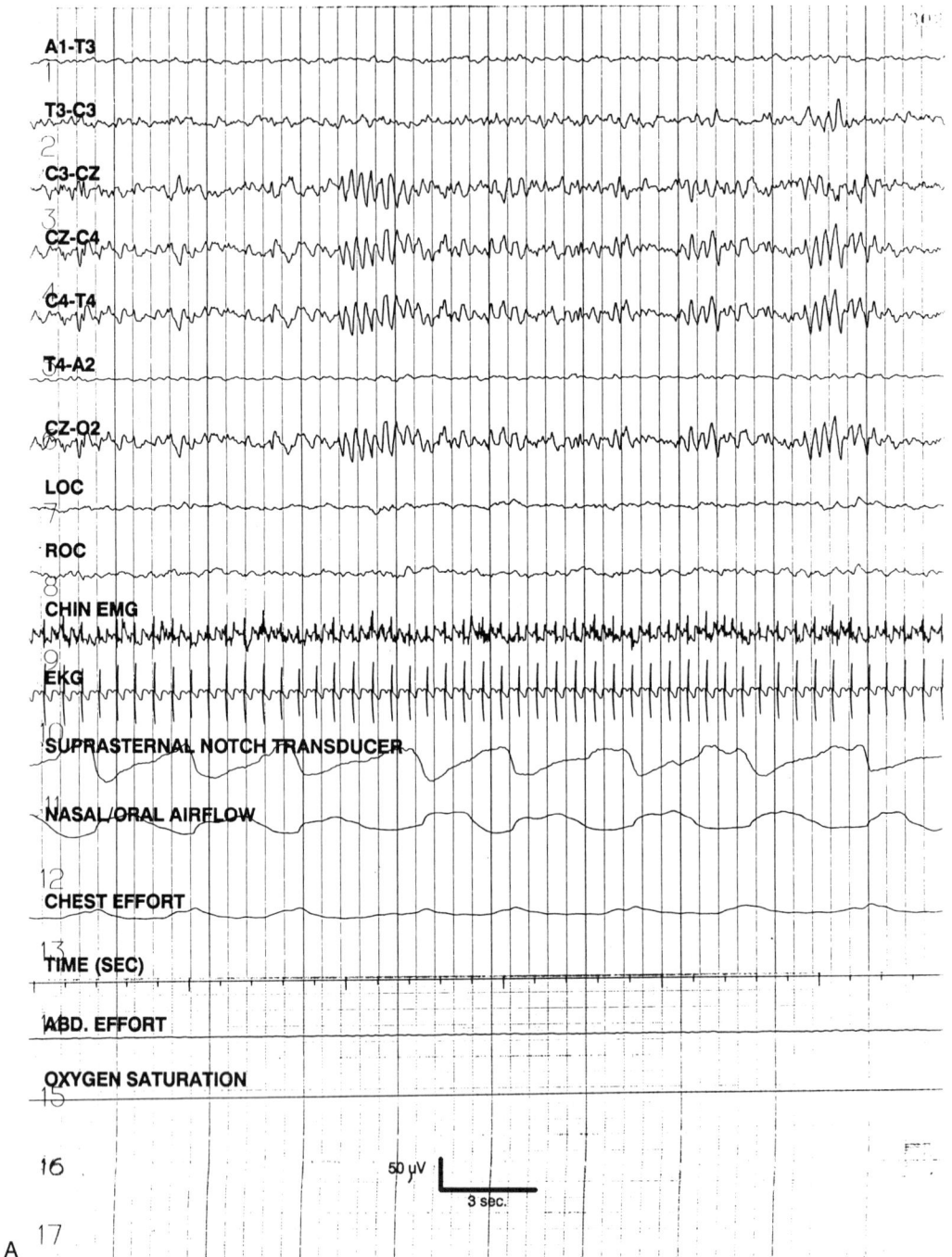

FIG. 11-14. A–B: This is the first REM episode of the sleep period for this 14-month-old toddler. EEG background rhythm is relatively low in voltage and shows a mixed-frequency pattern. Clear saw-tooth waves are present. Chin tone is considerably decreased from NREM stages. However, eye movements are sparse and respiration is rather regular. This is common during the first sleep cycle on the first night in the laboratory. It may be scored as stage 1 and is similar to an indeterminate, mixed state.

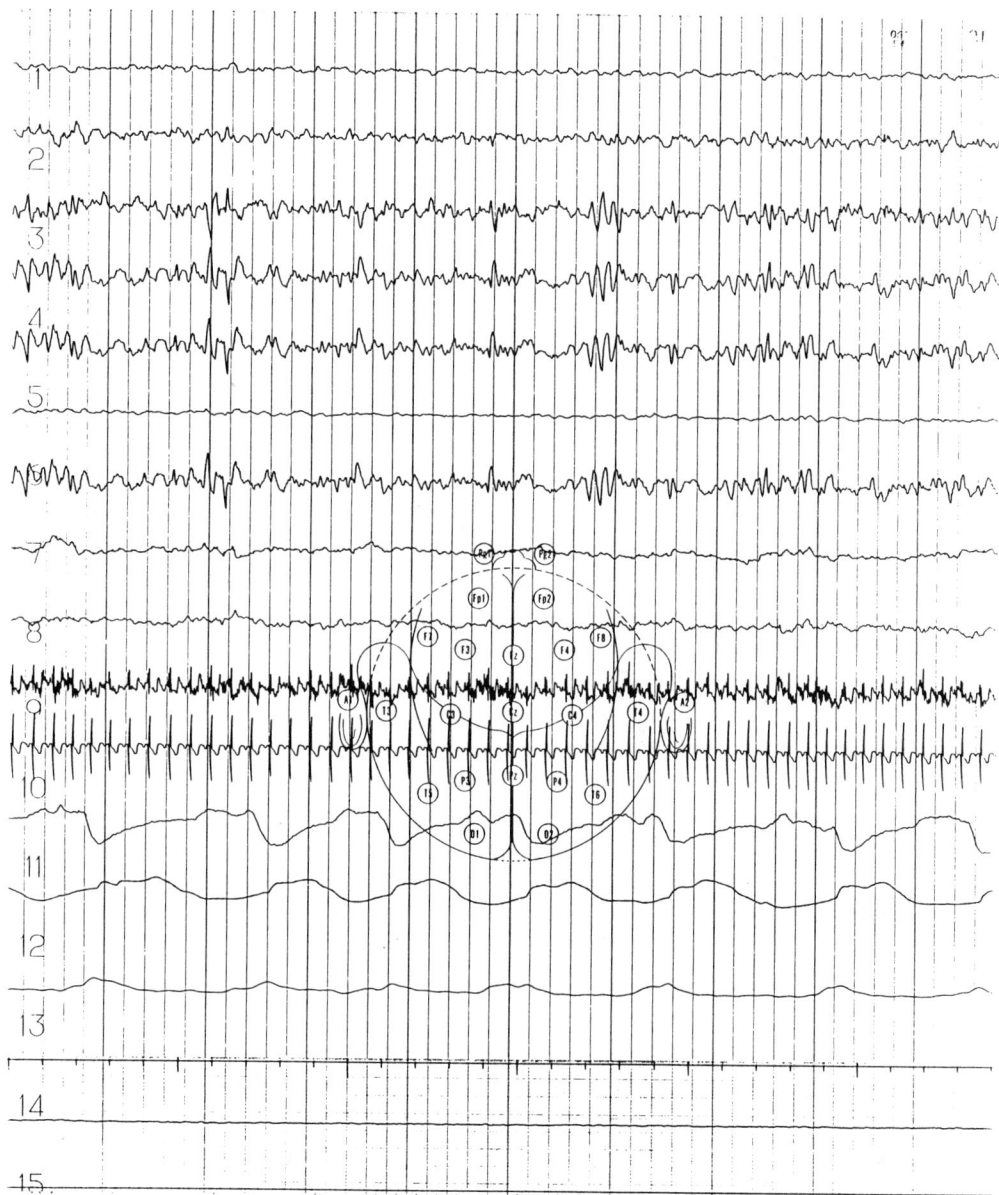

FIG. 11-14. *Continued.*

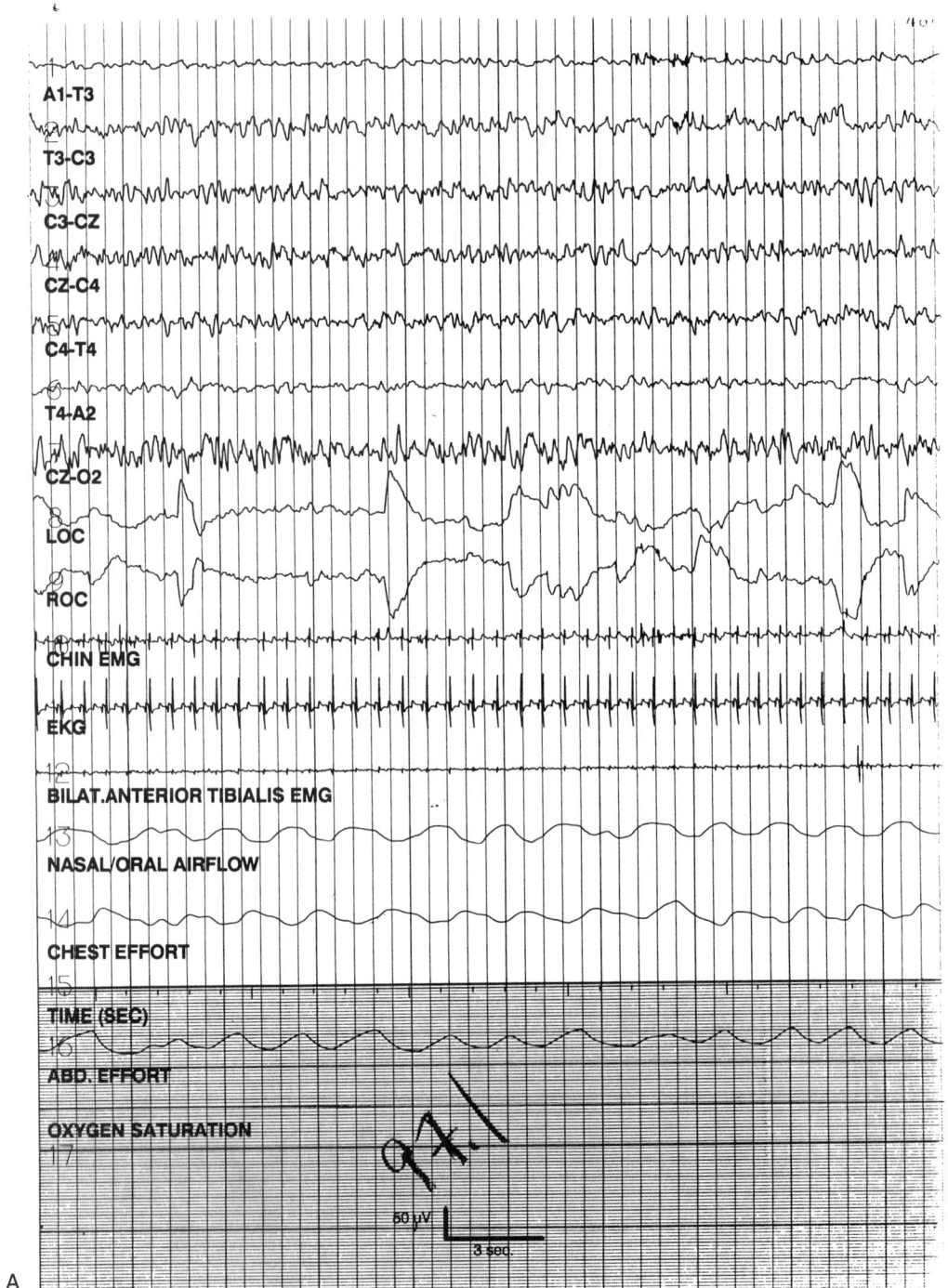

FIG. 11-15. A–B: Unequivocal REM in a 3-year-old youngster. The EEG rhythm is clearly different from NREM states and reveals a mature pattern. Bursts of saw-tooth waves are present. Dense rapid eye movements are seen and the chin muscle tone is very low. Phasic twitches are also present. Phasic twitches can also be identified in the anterior tibialis EMG. Cardiorespiratory instability is also present.

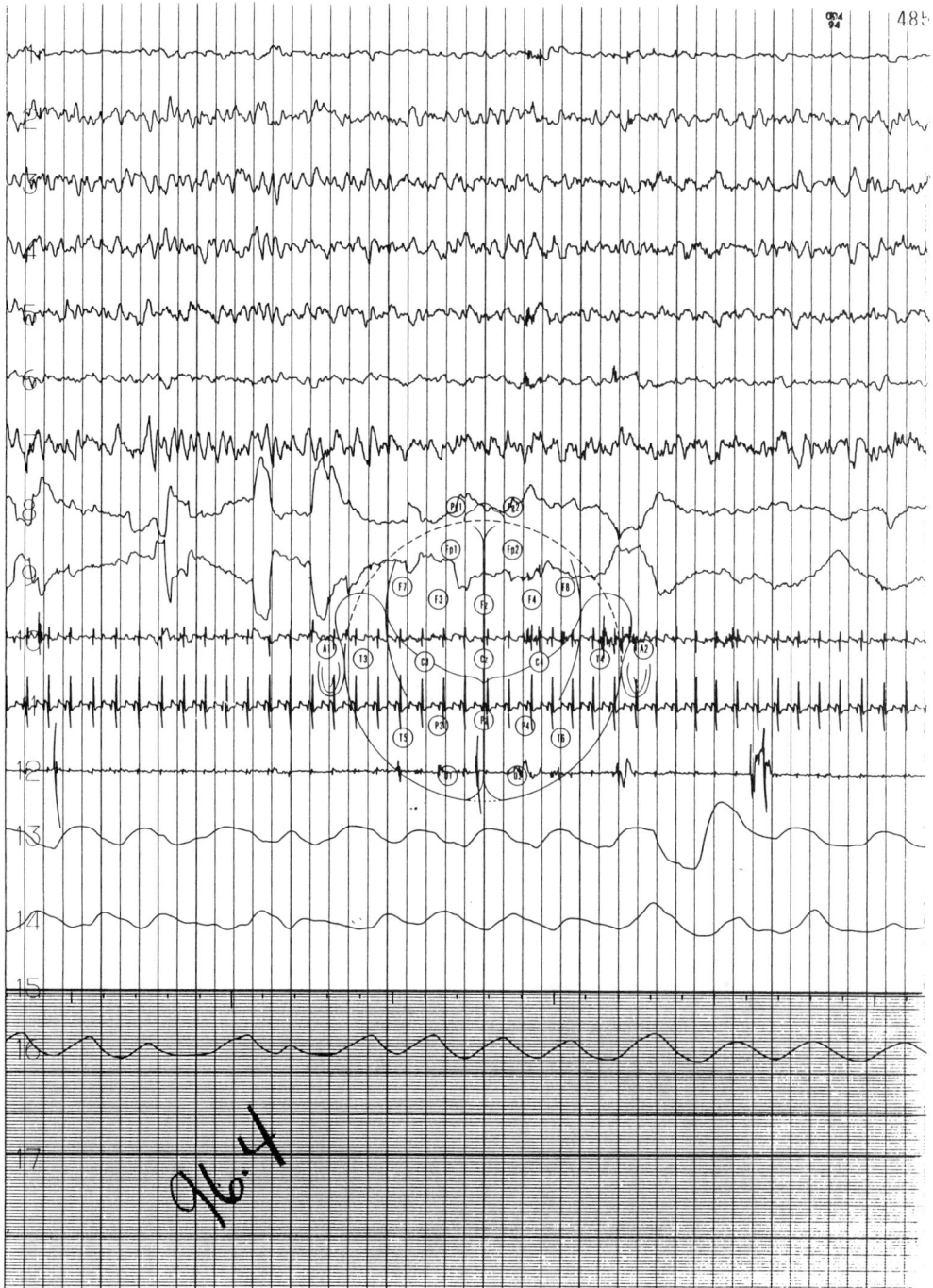

FIG. 11-15. *Continued.*

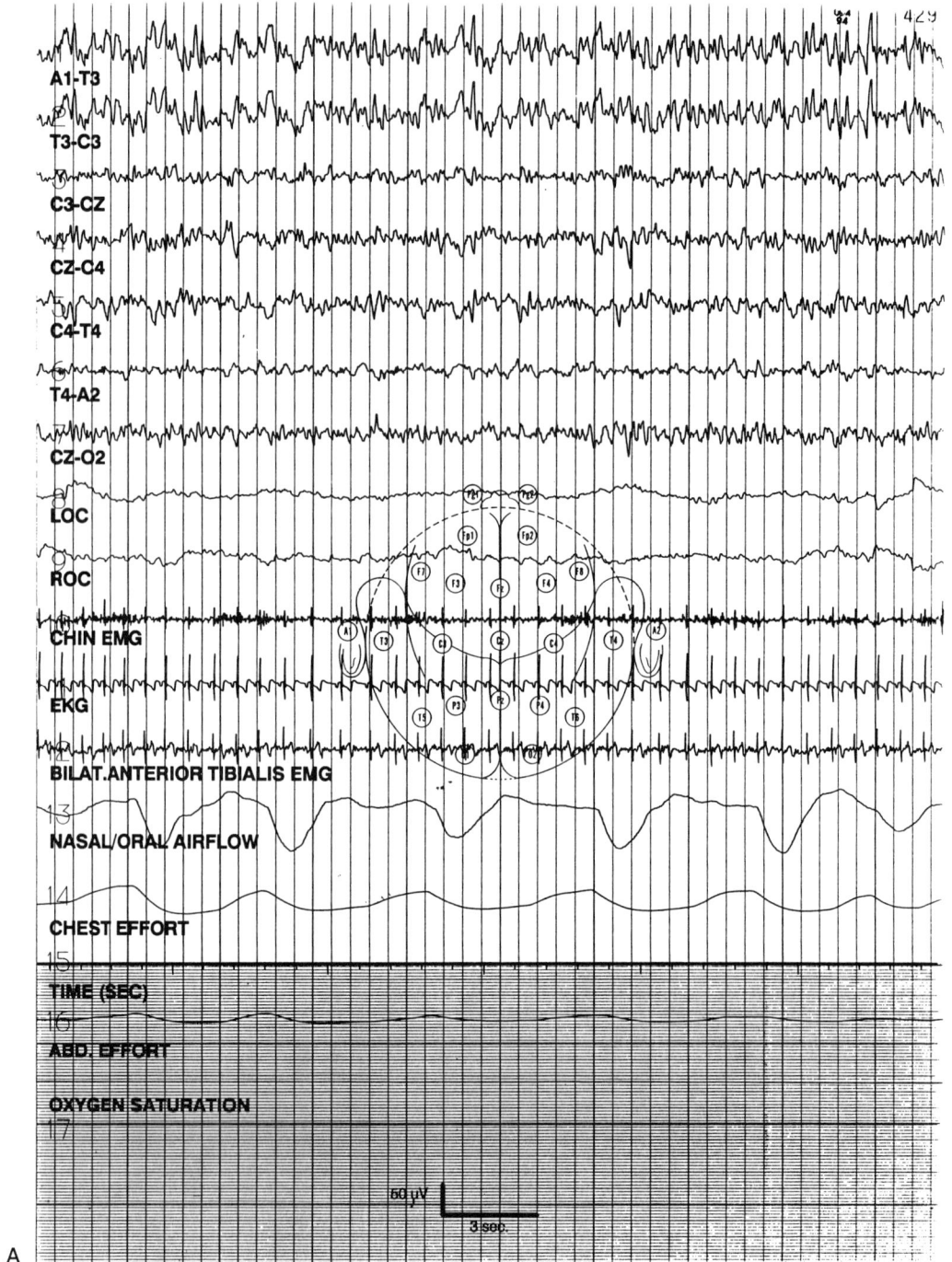

FIG. 11-16. A–B: REM sleep in a 5-year-old youngster. Further maturation of the EEG has occurred. There is some asymmetry in the EEG amplitude on the left side when compared to the right. Conjugate eye movements are present. Chin tone is low and glossopharyngeus ("snore") artifact is present. Cardiorespiratory instability can again be seen.

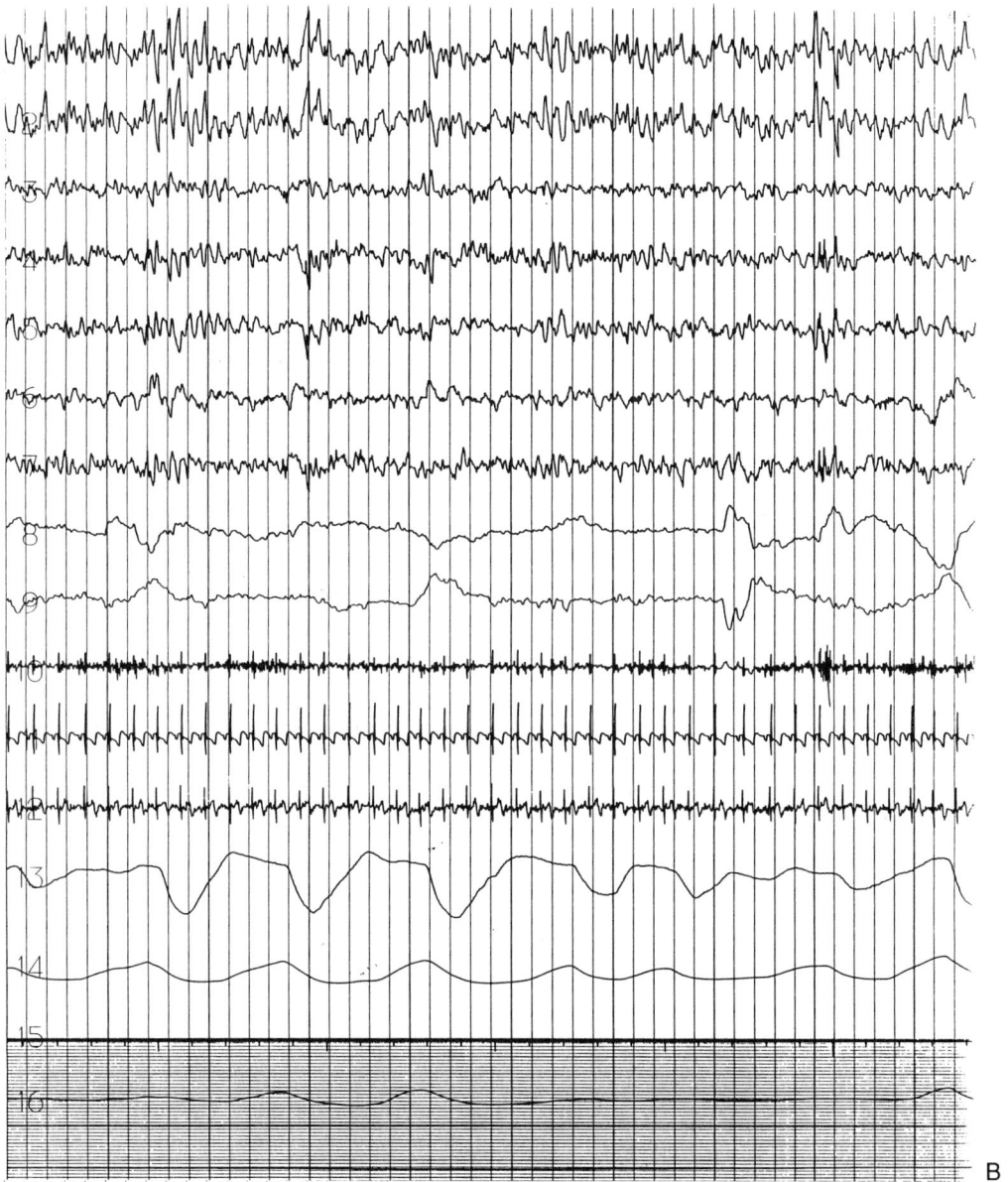

FIG. 11-16. *Continued.*

polysomnographically at different times. Blending of states is common, especially in younger toddlers and children. REM sleep can, therefore, be identified under a variety of circumstances.

Between 1 and 5 years of age, at least two of three standard criteria for identification of the REM state should be fulfilled. EEG should be preponderantly composed of notched theta activity. This activity should be distinctly different from the theta activity identified during wakefulness. Sleep spindles may or may not be present. Clearly identifiable K-complexes should be absent. EMG chin muscle tone should be significantly decreased. In younger toddlers and preschool children, however, phasic activity during REM sleep can be quite frequent and persist in much longer bursts of activity than in older children, adolescents, and adults. Limb movements and phasic limb activity is often quite pronounced in the younger child. Therefore, a REM-appearing EEG in the presence of intense phasic muscle activity and movement may not provide enough criteria for scoring of REM sleep, unless the muscle activity is clearly identifiable as bursts of phasic phenomena. EOG should reveal conjugate eye movements in bursts of saccades. These eye movements are often associated with phasic muscle activity, bursts of moderate voltage notched theta EEG activity, and respiratory changes.

Respiration

Respiration during REM sleep is typically very variable and irregular. Periods of tachypnea alternate with hyperpnea and hypopnea. Brief central apneas are normal during REM sleep. Mild oxygen desaturation may occur, but this change is minimal and occasional central hypopnea during REM sleep should be considered normal. EKG irregularity is also present and may be independent from the respiratory irregularity identified. EEG and respiratory characteristics and the most consistent physiologic changes of REM sleep, which occur during this developmental period and REM sleep, can be scored based on these criteria alone (Figs. 11-14–11-16).

REFERENCES

1. Sheldon SH, Spire JP, Levy HB. *Pediatric Sleep Medicine.* Philadelphia: WB Saunders; 1992.
2. Sheldon SH, Onal E, Lilie J, Spire JP. Sleep-related post-inspiratory upper-airway obstruction in children. *Sleep Res* 1993;22:270.
3. Hertz G, Cataletto M, Feinsilver SH, Angulo M. Sleep and breathing patterns in patients with Prader Willi syndrome (PWS): effects of age and gender. *Sleep* 1993;16:366–371.
4. Winter HS. Gastroesophageal reflux. In: Rudolph AM, Hoffman JIE, eds. *Pediatrics,* 18th ed. Norwalk, CT: Appleton Lange; 1987:906–908.
5. Sheldon SH, Irbe D, Applebaum J, Golbin, A, Levy HB, Spire JP. Sleep pressure in children with attentional deficits. *Sleep Res* 1991;20A:448.
6. Tirosh E, Sadeh A, Munvez R, Lavie P. Effects of methylphenidate on sleep in children with attention-deficit hyperactivity disorder: an activity monitor study. *Am J Dis Child* 1993;147:1313–1315.
7. Sheldon SH, Garay A, Jacobsen J. REM sleep motor disorder in children. *Sleep Res* 1994;23:173.
8. Rowe P, ed. *The Harriet Lane Handbook.* Chicago: Year Book; 1987:64.

12

Five to Ten Years

Maturation after 5 years of age progresses in a very stable and methodical manner. Development continues at a steady state until the onset of puberty. Within this age range, there is also a uniform continuation of maturation of sleep and sleep-wake cycles.

Between 5 and 6 years of age sleep generally consolidates into a single nocturnal sleep period. Diurnal naps are generally abandoned. Persistence of habitual lengthy napping after 6 years of age may suggest the presence of hypersomnia and/or sleep-related and/or nocturnal pathology. As middle childhood progresses, children become exquisitely alert during day-time hours. Children are probably most alert and awake than at any other time during the life cycle.

By the time middle childhood is reached, neuroanatomic development is generally complete. Neurophysiologic and functional development continues steadily. Socialization begins and cognitive development shifts from discovery learning to formal pedagogic methods. Where play had been the work of childhood prior to this developmental period, school assumes equal importance. The significance of sleep in the development of short-term and long-term memory and in the establishment and maintenance of these systems has yet to be completely uncovered.

It seems that sleep may affect learning and memory in several ways. First, evidence of a significant neurophysiologic role of sleep in the establishment and consolidation of memory has been identified (1–4). In order for foundations of long-term memory traces

TABLE 12-1. *Indications for polysomnography*

Most common indication	Indicated under certain circumstances	Potential indications
Obstructive sleep apnea syndrome	Unexplained attention deficits	Behavioral problems
Sleep-related seizures	Developmental delays	Unexplained school-learning problems
Uncontrolled diurnal seizures	Frequent sleepwalking	Possible PTSD
Frequent/injurious sleep-walking	Enuresis resistant to traditional treatment/ diurnal sleep-related symptoms	Unexplained sleep-maintenance insomnia
Rhythmic movement disorders		
S/P tonsillectomy/adenoi-dectomy	Nightmares with agitation and bed displacement	
Excessive day-time sleepiness	Unexplained CHF	
Unexplained drop attacks	Periodic/rhythmic limb movements	
Hypotonic syndromes		
Possible UARS		

within the brain to occur, appropriate percentages and cycling of REM sleep appear to be essential. Disruption or limitation of REM sleep may prove to have profound long-term consequences in vulnerable children. Second, cognitive development and learning depends (to a significant extent) upon alertness, attentiveness, and responsiveness during the learning situation. In short, *children need to be awake and alert during school hours.* Even moderate degrees of sleepiness can result in performance problems. Hyperactivity, attentional deficits, behavior problems, micro-sleep periods, easy distractibility, frustration, and other manifestations of increased sleep pressure can directly be caused by insufficient, inappropriate, and inconsistent sleep. Therefore, sleep seems to hold special significance both internally and externally in the biologic and cognitive development of the child.

MOST COMMON INDICATIONS FOR POLYSOMNOGRAPHY

Obstructive Sleep Apnea Syndrome

Still the most commonly accepted indication for polysomnography is suspected obstructive sleep apnea syndrome. Nocturnal symptoms in the 5- to 10-year-old age group are similar to those at other ages. Loud snoring is invariably present. The snoring may be interrupted by perceptible pauses and snorts. The pauses may or may not be associated with perceptible skin color changes (i.e., cyanosis). Sleep is most often described as restless and sleep-related enuresis is very common. Parents may notice gasping respirations, frequent nocturnal arousals and awakenings, and an inability to sleep in either a supine or prone position. Youngsters may prefer to sleep sitting upright. Although the hallmark of obstructive sleep apnea syndrome is sleep-related snoring, it is not invariably present and some youngsters may have significant occlusive upper-airway disease without the presence of significant snoring. Diurnal symptoms are almost always present. However, daytime symptoms are highly variable from child to child and may include hyperactivity, hyperactivity alternating with excessive somnolence, excessive day-time sleepiness and uncontrollable sleep attacks (e.g., frequently falling to sleep in school, at meals, talking on the phone). Attention span problems, staring spells, frequent day dreaming, school performance problems, learning difficulties, pathologic shyness, aggressiveness, memory deficits, and rapid mood swings are common. The most common cause of upper-airway obstruction in this age group is hypertrophic tonsils and adenoids. Polysomnography is indicated prior to surgery to provide information regarding severity, surgical and anesthesia risk, the likelihood of post-operative complications, and the potential for residual obstructive apnea after tonsillectomy and adenoidectomy. Comprehensive polysomnography can also provide important data regarding the presence of other sleep-related pathology that may contribute to or affect interpretation of historic and physical examination data.

Sleep-Related Seizures

It has been estimated that one quarter of all patients with epilepsy have seizures predominantly during sleep. During middle childhood, sleep-related seizures may present in a variety of ways, and manifestations can be quite variable. Any type of seizure can occur during sleep. Sleep is an important activator of potential epileptogenic EEG activity. Seizures may occur only diurnally, nocturnally, or occur at random. The more common types of seizures that are manifested during sleep include generalized tonic-clonic seizures, partial seizures with focal or partial motor symptomatology, and partial seizures with complex symptomatology. Benign focal epilepsy of childhood (rolandic epilepsy) tends to be manifested during sleep. Seizure episodes during sleep can result in complaints of frequent awakenings, subclinically disrupt sleep to a degree that results in excessive day-time sleepiness, and day-time symptoms can be exacerbated by treatment with anticonvulsants. Although sleep-related motor disorders such as somnambulism and sleep terrors rarely have an epileptic etiology, benign stereotypic activity associated with NREM partial arousal motor disorders may have remarkably similar features. Occasionally, sleep-related seizures can present with complaints referable to breathing difficulties. Laryngospasm, obstructive symptomatology, aspiration, and breath-holding which requires differentiation from other forms of sleep-disordered breathing may occur. Additionally, poor control of diurnal or random seizures may result from poor nocturnal control, especially if it is associated with less than optimal diurnal functioning. Polysomnography may assist in monitoring the control of seizures and medication efficacy, especially during night-time hours.

Frequent/Injurious Sleepwalking

Somnambulism can occur as soon as a child is developmentally capable of walking, however, it has its peak incidence between 4 and 8 years of age. Physical injury is fairly common, especially if agitation is present during the episode, attempts to "escape" occur, or the youngster walks into potentially hazardous situations. Somnambulistic attacks, however, are typically benign and resolve spontaneously over time. If frequent displacement from the bed occurs, the episodes are severe (occurring almost nightly or are associated with physical injury), medical management should be considered. If medication is to be prescribed, polysomnography is indicated to rule out other potentially treatable paroxysmal disorders. In addition, polysomnography can assist in identifying precipitating causes of partial arousals such as sleep-disordered breathing and periodic limb movement disorders.

Rhythmic Movement Disorders

Rhythmic movement disorders (RMD) are stereotypic behaviors involving large muscle groups, typically of the head and neck. Rhythmic movements generally occur immediately prior to sleep onset, during sleep-wake transitions, and can continue into light sleep. A wide variety of manifestations can occur. Polysomnography is generally indicated when the movements occur *only during sleep* and do not involve sleep-wake transition periods, are violent and result in injury, or only occur nightly (or almost nightly). Rhythmic movement disorders of sleep must be distinguished from other repetitive movements involving large and small muscle groups. It must also be differentiated from other less stereotypic activity such as periodic limb movement disorder. Diagnosis is generally based on history and physical examination, however, occasionally polysomnography is required to differentiate RMD from other repetitive activities associated with sleep (e.g., paroxysmal hypnogenic dystonia). It can also assist (although the need is relatively rare) in differentiation from other paroxysmal disorders, such as epilepsy.

Status Post Tonsillectomy/Adenoidectomy

Polysomnography after tonsillectomy and adenoidectomy for obstructive sleep apnea is often indicated. This is especially true if the pre-operative polysomnogram revealed an respiratory distress index (RDI) that is significantly elevated (5). It may also be advisable if profound oxygen desaturation and/or significant EKG changes associated with apneic events were documented prior to surgery. In addition, polysomnography may be useful in determining the presence of residual occlusive upper-airway disease when nocturnal symptoms have resolved, but diurnal symptoms persist after surgery.

Excessive Day-Time Sleepiness

Normative polysomnographic data regarding excessive day-time sleepiness (EDS) are available in the prepubertal age group. However, these data are based on limited numbers of subjects. Several manifestations of increased sleep pressure and excessive sleepiness seem to occur in this age group. First, excessive sleepiness may be extreme, result in uncontrollable sleep episodes and sleep attacks. Sleep occurs at unusual times such as at parties, during meals, and during school. In some children, intense sleepiness can be documented in the sleep laboratory and standard multiple sleep latency test criteria for EDS are present. Prepubertal youngsters may or may not have laboratory evidence of narcolepsy syndrome. In the presence of a history of cataplexy, diagnosis of narcolepsy syndrome is likely. When two or more sleep-onset REM periods are present and there is no evidence of other sleep-related pathology that could account for EDS, polysomnography should be repeated yearly throughout the stages of puberty. In the absence of cataplexy, it is difficult to differentiate narcolepsy syndrome from idiopathic CNS hypersomnia.

Youngsters in middle childhood who are diagnosed with obstructive sleep apnea syndrome experience EDS. It may be as severe as in youngsters with narcolepsy syndrome. More often the sleepiness is moderate and may alternate with periods of hyperactivity. Moderate degrees of sleepiness in middle childhood may be significantly more difficult to identify both clinically and in the laboratory (see Chapter 13). Standard criteria for EDS may not be met. Criteria for diagnosing increased sleep pressure may have to be modified.

Diurnal symptoms of increased sleep pressure and EDS are more commonly associated with hyperactivity, attention span problems, school learning difficulties, day dreaming, staring spells, pathologic shyness, unusual aggressiveness, rapid mood swings, easily frustrated, destructiveness, and/or behavioral problems.

Etiologies of EDS during middle childhood are varied, can be biologic or behavioral, and include, but are not limited to, narcolepsy syndrome, obstructive sleep apnea syndrome, periodic limb movement disorder, sleep-related seizures, sleep-related fragmentary myoclonus, environmental sleep disorder, insufficient sleep syndrome, and sleep-phase delay syndrome. Often, an exact cause cannot be identified and evaluation over time is necessary to observe and document the evolution of the pathophysiologic process.

Unexplained Drop Attacks

If after comprehensive work-up, an etiology for drop attacks (associated with sudden loss of muscle tone) cannot be ascertained, sleep laboratory evaluation may be helpful. If the drop attacks are manifestations of cataplexy, polysomnographic data will often be positive for narcolepsy syndrome. However, laboratory evidence of narcolepsy syndrome need not appear until puberty is nearly complete (Tanner 4 to Tanner 5).

Syndromes Associated with Muscular Hypotonia

Syndromes that are associated with skeletal muscle hypotonia in older children (e.g., Down syndrome, type II spinal muscular atrophy) are often associated with upper-airway obstruction and clinically significant obstructive sleep apnea. Anatomic abnormalities may contribute to the degree of sleep-disordered breathing, however, a lesser degree of anatomic occlusion may be more clinically significant in children with neuromuscular hypotonia than children with normal muscle tone. Nocturnal polysomnography is indicated to determine the effect of nocturnal sleep-related pathology to diurnal function or functional impairment.

Upper-Airway Resistance Syndrome

In the presence of sleep-related snoring associated with pauses and snorts, oxygen desaturation, periodic increases in negative intrathoracic pressure, persistent tachypnea, or persistent increase in expired CO_2, high upper-airway resistance syndrome (UARS) should be suspected. UARS may also be suspected based on clinical findings as well as polysomnographic evidence that might suggest increased upper-airway resistance. These characteristics include, but are not limited to paradoxic breathing, increased expired CO_2, biphasic abdominal respiratory efforts, snore artifact on EMG, frequent periodic electrocortical and/or movement arousal, and frequent periodic limb movements occurring *after* electrocortical arousal.

POLYSOMNOGRAPHY INDICATED UNDER CERTAIN CIRCUMSTANCES

Unexplained Attention Deficits

A wide variety of sleep-related disorders can be responsible for attentional deficits. Diagnoses range from pathophysiologic phenomena such as obstructive sleep apnea syndrome, periodic limb movement disorder, narcolepsy syndrome, and sleep-phase delay syndrome to behavioral abnormalities such as environmental sleep disorders, inappropriate sleep-onset association disorders, inappropriate caretaker expectations, anxiety-related sleep disorder, and irregular sleep-wake schedules. Careful history and physical examination can exclude many of these disorders, however, polysomnography would be required to differentiate between many of the pathophysiologic phenomena.

Developmental Delays

Initial assessment of developmental delays in this age group is first based on clinical evaluation. Etiologies are often identifiable by history alone. If delays are clinically prominent, comprehensive work-ups and evaluations have usually been conducted prior to 5 years of age. However, delays may be subtle and not identified until the youngster enters school. Children experiencing unexplained regression in development and/or failure to thrive after 5 years of age may benefit from polysomnographic evaluation. Assessment of state development and organization can be made, presence of other sleep-related pathology demonstrable (e.g., sleep-related seizures), and comparison to prior polysomnographic studies can yield important information in developmental assessment.

Frequent Sleepwalking

Frequent sleepwalking (displacement from bed which occurs almost nightly) may be associated with considerable risk of physical injury. In the presence of automatisms and/ or stereotypic behaviors, seizure disorder might be present. When clear dream mentation is present during somnambulistic attacks, REM motor disorder may be considered.

Enuresis Resistant to Traditional Treatment

Polysomnography is rarely indicated for evaluation of patients with sleep-related enuresis. Primary sleep-related enuresis is most commonly due to a maturational delay between bladder distension, uninhibited detrusor muscle contractions, spontaneous bladder emptying, and a high-arousal threshold. Pathologic causes of enuresis are more frequently present when the complaint is of secondary enuresis. Etiologies can be suggested by history and physical examination (e.g., chronic urinary tract infection, obstructive sleep apnea, diabetes mellitus). At times other laboratory evaluations are required that can include urinalysis, urine culture, electrolytes, BUN, and/or creatinine. Treatment regimens are generally empirical and instituted without the need for polysomnography. However, whenever treatment failures occur (in the presence of significant compliance) and/or when other nocturnal sleep-related or diurnal symptoms are present, polysomnography might be considered in the secondary or tertiary evaluation of patients with enuresis.

Enuresis has been documented as a common symptom associated with obstructive sleep apnea syndrome as well as NREM partial arousal motor parasomnias. It is not unusual for children with sleepwalking to urinate at unusual places around the house or to have a history of frequent bed wetting. Generalized tonic-clonic seizures can also be associated with urinary and/or fecal incontinence. If seizures are occurring only during sleep, enuresis may be the only manifestation identifiable by parents (who are typically sleeping during the ictal event).

Nightmares with Significant Agitation and Displacement from the Bed

Nightmares are the typical complaint whenever a child screams, cries, or presents with agitated symptoms during sleep. Dream mentation may be reported by the child. Nightmares can typically be diagnosed by clinical history. Anxiety dreams can occur any time of night, but tend to cluster during early morning hours. There is full awakening, and the waking episode tends to be prolonged (30 minutes or more). Agitation may occur after a nightmare, but the autonomic discharge tends to be rather mild. The youngsters are easily comforted by parents. In comparison, sleep terrors tend to occur early in the sleep-period time (during slow-wave sleep). A sleep terror is heralded by a piercing scream, intense autonomic discharge (diaphoresis, pupillary dilatation, tachycardia, and tachypnea), intense agitation, and the youngster tends to become worse upon parental intervention, often fighting and pushing away from the caretaker. They are typically short lived (lasting only a few minutes), the youngster rapidly returns to sleep, and there is amnesia for the event. At times sleep terrors can be frequent (occurring several times per night), prolonged (lasting for hours), and can be associated with displacement from the bed. When there is severe agitation and displacement from the bed, severe injury is common and can be potentially fatal. Children can jump out of windows, run through plate glass doors, or run out of the house and into the middle of busy streets. Medication may be required. Episodes must be differentiated from other treatable causes (e.g., sleep-related seizures, episodic nocturnal wanderings). Polysomnography can determine whether there are any sleep-related precipitating causes (e.g., obstructive sleep apnea, periodic limb movements). REM-sleep motor disorder has been reported in children (6) and polysomnography can provide useful information regarding the state in which the episodes occur. Treatment can be guided by polysomnographic findings. Patients with sleep terrors that are severe or episodes associated with displacement from the bed should undergo polysomnography. Certain paroxysmal disorders (e.g., temporal lobe seizures) may present with similar symptoms during early childhood and polysomnography can assist in evaluation of these patients.

Unexplained Congestive Heart Failure

Upper-airway obstruction may underlie congestive heart failure. Cor pulmonale can result from severe upper-airway obstruction during sleep. Congestive heart failure, in the presence of sleep disordered breathing, can be significantly improved by application of nasal CPAP.

Periodic/Rhythmic Limb Movements

Stereotypic behavior confined to the sleep period can be an indication for polysomnography. If frequent or severe, polysomnography should be conducted to rule out the presence of a paroxysmal disorder. Polysomnography should be considered when rhythmic movements are stereotypic, confined to a single side of the body, or occur solely during sleep. Conditions where rhythmic movement disorders are associated with sleep-wake transitions are less likely to require polysomnography.

POTENTIAL INDICATIONS FOR POLYSOMNOGRAPHY

Behavioral Disorders

Evaluation of behavioral abnormalities must begin with a thorough history and physical examination. A comprehensive sleep history is essential. If sleep-related symptoms suggest the presence of a physiologic sleep abnormality, polysomnography may be indicated. Sleep-related disorders contributing to or underlying behavioral abnormalities may range from environmental sleep disorders to circadian rhythm abnormalities and sleep-disordered breathing.

Unexplained School Learning Problems

Unexplained school learning difficulties may occasionally have their origins during sleep. Children must be awake and alert during the day to afford themselves of full educational value of the school experience. Attention span problems, hyperactivity (especially if it alternates with sleepiness), unexplained staring spells, unusual aggressiveness or shyness, and frequently falling to sleep in school might suggest the presence of a sleep disorder contributing to, or underlying the school learning problem.

Post-Traumatic Stress Disorder and Other Anxiety-Related Sleep Disorders

Evaluation and diagnosis of clinically significant anxiety-related sleep disorders are quite difficult and based on modification and extrapolation of adult data. As yet, no physiologic markers exist to identify children suffering from post-traumatic stress disorder (PTSD) or other anxiety-related sleep disorders. Only recently have polysomnographic data become available in adults with PTSD (7).

Clinical history is most important in making the initial assessment. Complaints of nightmares are frequent in many youngsters who have suffered from physical and sexual child abuse (8). Polysomnographic data from youngsters with a diagnosis of PTSD seem to show similar characteristics to adults with PTSD. These characteristics consist of frequent major body movements, considerable fragmentation of the continuity of REM sleep, and occasional increase in chin muscle tone during REM sleep.

Unexplained Sleep-Maintenance Insomnia

Sleep-maintenance insomnia in youngsters between 5 and 10 years of age is generally not a primary indication for polysomnography. Behavioral and environmental etiologies are much more common than physiologic abnormalities. However, if there is an isolated sleep-maintenance insomnia with frequent nocturnal wakings without apparent causes after initial evaluation, polysomnography may be indicated. Some common causes may include, but are not limited to obstructive sleep apneas, high upper-airway resistance, periodic limb movement disorder, sleep-related seizure disorders.

TECHNICAL CONSIDERATIONS AND TECHNIQUES

Preparation

Patient preparation during middle childhood is considerably easier than during previous developmental periods. As with all other age groups, patient preparation is the most important consideration in obtaining an accurate and reproducible polysomnographic study. Significant fears of strange places and fear of strangers is less common, but fear of the unknown can present at any age. Careful introduction to personnel and to the laboratory by a visit prior to the study and demonstration of the sensors and electrodes prior to set-up can greatly assist in improving compliance. Increased compliance improves the technical quality of the investigation.

Parents are encouraged to remain with their children during the course of the study. However, for older children and those who are developmentally capable of staying in the laboratory alone, the presence of the parents is sometimes made optional.

At the time the appointment for the study is scheduled, the parents are provided an information sheet that describes the laboratory and study and alerts the parents/caretakers to specific procedures (Fig. 12-1).

Patients and parents are encouraged to arrive at the laboratory at 2000. Arriving early provides the youngster time to assimilate to the environment and to be oriented to the procedure by technical staff. Similar to younger children, the set-up room should be separate from the patient's sleeping/monitoring room. This permits the sleeping environment to appear as home-like and safe for the youngster as possible. Decorations in the monitoring rooms should be developmentally appropriate. Hospital room appearance should be avoided as much as possible.

Only occasionally is parental assistance required for set-up. Parental presence, however, is recommended unless the parents become a distraction for the older youngster.

Preparation can be comfortably done with the child sitting in a chair. During this developmental period, providing the child with *some control* over the procedure can be often helpful in obtaining compliance. We, therefore, recommend permitting the child the choice of which electrodes or sensors are to be applied *first* and in what order they wish the monitoring devices to be attached. In younger children, it is advisable to apply the least intrusive or frightening electrodes first. The most difficult applications may have to wait until the child has achieved slow-wave sleep.

As with all other age groups, the electrode site should be meticulously prepared prior to electrode application. Head wrapping is generally not necessary in youngsters in this age group. Application of all electrodes can generally be completed prior to lights-out.

Length of the Study

During this developmental period (as with others) the timing and length of the study should reflect the youngsters habitual sleep-period time. Although greater than 400 minutes of sleep is ideal, this is not always possible and modifications need to be taken into account during interpretation. Parents may have to awaken early to prepare for work. Youngsters need to wake to prepare for school. Accurate interpretation of the structure of sleep across the sleep period and assessment of appropriateness of stage percentages depend upon knowledge of the child's habitual sleep-period time. For example, a late time of lights-out and early morning termination of the study in order for the parent to get to work on time may result in slow-wave sleep occupying a much greater than expected percentage of the sleep period. In addition, REM sleep may be significantly decreased under these circumstances. If a major portion of the final REM-sleep period is missed, determination of the severity of certain sleep-related pathologies (e.g., obstructive sleep apnea syndrome) may not be appreciated.

Recommended Equipment

Standard polysomnographic equipment is recommended. Electrodes and sensors should be appropriately sized and individualized for each child. Additional recording equipment and choice of montage should be determined by the needs of the patient. Equipment for measurement of esophageal pH, estimation of intrathoracic pressure, audio and video recording, EMG of other non-traditional muscle groups, surface laryngeal microphones, and CPAP equipment should be available. Fluoroscopy and indwelling fiberoptic video recordings are utilized in some laboratories, but are not traditionally included in the standard pediatric sleep center/laboratory equipment. Use of these techniques are generally reserved for specific situations and are often done with the patient hospitalized, rather than in the out-patient pediatric sleep laboratory.

Center for Pediatric Sleep Medicine

Stephen H. Sheldon, D.O., A.B.S.M., F.A.A.P.
Director, Sleep Medicine Services
Clinical Associate Professor, University of Chicago

PATIENT: _____   **APPOINTMENT DATE:** _____

PATIENT INSTRUCTION SHEET FOR A SLEEP STUDY

A Sleep Study is a very simple procedure. A number of "sensors" are attached to different parts of your child's body (for example, the head, chest, legs) to monitor the changes which occur when your child is sleeping. The sensors are attached with special skin paste and tape. No needles are used and there is no pain associated with a sleep study. Typically, you will need to spend only one night in the sleep laboratory. All you and your child have to do is go to bed in the usual way at night. Surprisingly, most people find that the sensors do not interfere with sleep. This is exactly what we want because we want to assess your child's natural sleep pattern. The time and effort of a sleep study is well worth it, because we learn a great deal about a person's sleep difficulties from this procedure. The sleep study is often essential in order to make an accurate diagnosis and develop an effective treatment plan.

YOU SHOULD ARRIVE AT THE HOSPITAL AT APPROXIMATELY 8:00 P.M. Go to the hospital's Information Desk in the Main Lobby and tell the receptionist that you are at the hospital for a SLEEP STUDY. They will phone the **Sleep Laboratory (hospital extension 4625)** and the technician will come down to meet you and bring you to the laboratory.

The Sleep Laboratory is located on the fourth floor of the North Building of the hospital. Take the "E" elevators. The laboratory resembles a small hotel room rather than a hospital room. It contains a bed, color television, and other furniture to make you and your child as comfortable as possible. Adjacent to the laboratory is a washroom with shower facilities. You and your child will spend approximately eleven (11) hours in the sleep laboratory (for example, 8:00 p.m. to 7:00 a.m.). If you need to get to work early in the morning or if your child needs to wake up earlier to get ready for school, please let the technician know what time you would like to wake up, and she/he will wake you at that time. IF YOU WOULD LIKE TO VISIT THE LABORATORY BEFORE YOU SPEND THE NIGHT, WE WILL BE HAPPY TO GIVE YOUR A SPECIAL TOUR.

We require a parent or caretaker to say overnight with their child in the laboratory so she/he feels as secure and comfortable as possible. The parent will sleep in the room with their child on a "fouton" (a small sofa that converts into a bed).

For your comfort and for your child's comfort, you should bring regular bed clothes (preferably two-piece pajamas), personal toilet items (such as toothpaste, deodorant, etc.), and a change of clothes for the following day. Meals are not provided in the laboratory. There is a cafeteria in the building where you can purchase food. Towels and bedding will be provided. Please feel free to bring a special blanket, doll, teddy bear, or favorite toy which will aid in making your child as comfortable as possible. You may also want to bring a relaxing game or bedtime book.

Sleep Medicine Center, Grant Hospital of Chicago, 550 West Webster Avenue, Chicago, Illinois 60614, (312)883-3836
ACCREDITED, AMERICAN SLEEP DISORDERS ASSOCIATION

A   Sleep Medicine Associates, 2156 S. Western Avenue, Chicago, Illinois 60608, (312)579-1450

FIG. 12-1. A–B: Polysomnogram information sheet for parents.

A few preparations must be made in order to insure the best results possible from the sleep study. They are the following:

1. Please bathe your child and wash her/his hair before coming to the laboratory. **DO NO PUT OIL, STYLING GEL, HAIR SPRAY, OR ANY OTHER MATERIAL IN YOUR CHILD'S HAIR PRIOR TO THE STUDY.** These types of grooming aids interfere with the sensors placed on the scalp.

2. After 3:00 p.m. on the day of the test, do not give your child any tea, soda, pop, or candy which contains caffeine (for example, chocolate).

3. Give your child any medication that she/he would normally take unless you have been specifically instructed not to. No medications will be dispensed by the technician at any time.

4. Prepare a list of all medications your child has taken during the past two weeks.

You will need to bring your insurance claim form and/or your health insurance card and register in Room 101 prior to the study. Most insurance companies cover a portion, if not all, of the payment for this test. You should contact your insurance representative prior to the sleep study to determine the extent of coverage of your specific policy. If you have any questions, or need assistance in dealing with your insurance company concerning this test, please feel free to contact us at the Center prior to the study.

IF YOU CANNOT MAKE THE STUDY OR IF YOU NEED TO CANCEL/RESCHEDULE THE APPOINTMENT, IT IS VERY IMPORTANT THAT YOU NOTIFY US AT LEAST 48-HOURS IN ADVANCE. MANY OTHER PATIENTS ARE IN NEED OF SLEEP STUDIES. NOTIFYING US THAT YOU CANNOT KEEP THE APPOINTMENT WELL AHEAD OF TIME WILL GIVE US AN OPPORTUNITY TO SCHEDULE OTHER CHILDREN FOR THAT TIME.

After the sleep evaluation is completed, the record of your child's sleep will be scored and interpreted by a physician on the Sleep Disorders Center Staff. The information will then be used to make a diagnosis and recommend treatment. The final report will then be sent to your doctor within 2 to 3 days. If you would like a copy of the report, please bring a stamped, self-addressed envelope with you on the night of the study. When the report is finalized, a copy will be mailed to you.

If you have any questions, call us at (312)883-3836. We look forward to seeing you and helping you with your child's sleep problem.

Stephen H. Sheldon, D.O., A.B.S.M., F.A.A.P.
Director, Sleep Disorders Center

Sleep Medicine Center, Grant Hospital of Chicago, 550 West Webster Avenue, Chicago, Illinois 60614, (312)883-3836
ACCREDITED, AMERICAN SLEEP DISORDERS ASSOCIATION

Sleep Medicine Associates, 2156 S. Western Avenue, Chicago, Illinois 60608, (312)579-1450

B

FIG. 12-1. *Continued.*

Technical Considerations

EEG

Bipolar, transcoronal montage is the standard EEG recording in our laboratories. It can provide useful information regarding symmetry and background activity, and screen for the presence of epileptiform discharges better than the traditional referential polysomnogram EEG montage. The EEG montage may be modified for repeat studies or when additional recording channels are required for specific patient situations, accordingly. The more complete the EEG recording montage, the greater the information affordable from the polysomnogram. In screening for sleep-related seizures or in evaluation of patients with parasomnias, a bipolar parasagittal montage is recommended.

Other Physiologic Parameters

A minimum number of EEGs, EOGs, EMGs, EKGs, nasal/oral airflows, chest and abdominal efforts, and oxygen saturations by pulse oximetry must be recorded in order to obtain a reliable and comprehensive polysomnogram. Limited channel studies and routine use of unattended studies have not yet been validated in children and their effectiveness and sensitivity seems to be questionable at the present time. Other physiologic parameters to be recorded should be based upon the patient's specific needs (e.g., $TcPO_2$, $TcPCO_2$, growth hormone determinations, enuresis monitors).

Machine Calibrations

Standard machine calibrations should be conducted before the study begins. Pen alignment should be checked, validated, and corrected (if needed). High-frequency filters, low-frequency filters (time constants), and line filter (60 Hz) are calibrated with 20, 50, and 100 μV square pulses. Paper speeds are verified. Pulse oximeter should be calibrated and the scale recorded on the tracing. Capnograph should also be calibrated with known concentrations of CO_2.

Patient Calibrations

Children are capable of following directions and patient calibrations are similar to those described for adults. Prior to lights-out, impedance of all recording electrodes should be checked. Impedance should be below 5,000 ohms in order to provide the most reliable signal. When impedance is greater than 5,000 ohms, the electrode should be repaired. Disruption of the recording to repair electrodes after the study has begun should be minimized. Technician observations are still extremely important in assessing electrophysiologic parameters. The technician should record the patient's ability to comply with instructions, whether the patient is awake and moving or quiet with eyes open or closed, squirming, and other behavioral observations needed for interpretation of the recording. Video synchronization and split-screen recording is very helpful. Standard instructions are identical to adults and include: eyes open, eyes closed; look left, look right, up, down; blink 5 times; flex right then left leg; grit teeth, and hold breath. Identification of the direction of pen deflection corresponding to inspiration and expiration is important. Polarity should be adjusted so that the pen deflections are *in phase* when the chest and abdominal efforts are in phase. The polarity of the EKG recording channel is not critical, but EKG convention places pen deflection of positive potentials upward.

Initial Polygraph Settings

Initial amplifier settings should be standard and according to individual laboratory protocol. Adjustments of gain and filter settings must be clearly documented. If deviation from the standard protocol is required, changes may be made to obtain the highest quality, reliable recording. Once completed and a high-quality signal is obtained, settings should not be modified for the remainder of the study (unless very poor-quality signal is being recorded which requires modification. Any changes in amplifier settings must be clearly documented on the record. Changes in gain and filter setting should be minimal during the course of the study and should be reserved only to obtain an interpretable signal and to eliminate obscuring artifacts. Flexibility is present during paperless/digital recording systems. However, EEG resolution is not as great as with analog (paper) recordings.

EVALUATION AND SCORING OF POLYSOMNOGRAMS OF CHILDREN ONE TO FIVE YEARS OF AGE

Behavioral Observations

As with all other age groups, frequent documentation of patients' behaviors during the course of polysomnography is essential for accurate interpretation. Although state determination is less difficult polysomnographically during middle childhood, movements, activities, and possible causes for sleep-related behaviors greatly assists the evaluation of both state and pathophysiologic processes. Technicians' notations are an important part of the polysomnographic study.

Wake

EEG of wakefulness during this developmental period continues maturing until adult characteristics are completely achieved. With the eyes open, there is low-voltage, mixed-frequency background activity. Movement artifact is common. With the eyes closed, well-formed alpha activity predominates. Most youngsters have well-formed alpha activity by 8 years of age. Amplitude of alpha activity gradually increases during middle childhood. There also may be asymmetry of the amplitude of alpha activity (lower on the left when compared with the right). This asymmetry is generally more pronounced in children than in adults. Bilateral low-amplitude alpha activity or absence of alpha activity after 8 years should be considered abnormal. *Chin muscle EMG* shows significant tone and jaw movements are common. *EOG* reveals clear saccadic/conjugate eye movements when the eyes are open and when closed. Blink artifact is common. *EKG* reveals a sinus rhythm and normal respiratory variation in heart rate may be present. *Respiration* can be regular during periods of quiescence and quite irregular with breath holding and respiratory pauses during movements. *Oxygen saturation* remains stable.

Transitional Sleep/Stage 1

Transition from wake to sleep becomes more clear. *EEG* alpha rhythm becomes diffuse and is gradually replaced by relatively low-voltage, mixed-frequency EEG activity. Sleep onset may be heralded by the presence of micro-sleep periods that become more frequent and then coalesce when sleep consolidates. Voltage often increase as transition into sleep occurs and mixed-frequency activity between 2 and 7 Hz appears with amplitudes that may range from 50 μV to bursts of 200-μV activity. Stage 1 sleep tends to be brief. Other characteristics of EEG sleep are conspicuously absent. *EOG* reveals a gradual disappearance of conjugate eye movements, which are replaced by slow and rolling eye movements. These slow eye movements may be brief and most prominent during the early portions of this transitional/stage 1 sleep. *EMG* remains tonic, but can be slightly below that of relaxed wakefulness. *EKG* remains regular and heart rate slows slightly. *Respiration* becomes regular and steady. Occasionally, transitional apneas and/or hypopneas occur. If isolated, these apneas seem to be of limited clinical significance. *Oxygen saturation* remains stable and the baseline is generally above 95% (depending upon the oximeter utilized).

NREM Sleep

NREM sleep during this developmental period is distinct and states are easily demonstrable. *Stage 2* sleep is defined by a background *EEG* rhythm of relatively low voltage and mixed-frequency activity, *and* the presence of sleep spindles and K-complexes. Sleep spindles are well-formed waxing and waning wave forms of about 12–14 Hz lasting at least 0.5 seconds in duration. K-complexes clearly stand out from background activity as high-voltage, negative sharp waves generally concentrated about the vertex that is followed by a positive component and lasts greater than 0.5 seconds. Sleep spindles often immediately follow K-complexes, but do not constitute part of the wave form. K-complexes occur either spontaneously or in response to a sudden external stimulus.

According to Rechtschaffen and Kales (9), sleep spindles and K-complexes are transient phenomena and there may be relatively long periods that intervene without the occurrence of stage change. If less than 3 minutes of record that would ordinarily meet the requirements for stage 1 intervene between sleep spindles and/or K-complexes, these intervening epochs are scored as stage 2 (if there is no indication of movement arousal or pronounced increase in muscle tone during the interval in question). If the interval without sleep spindles or K-complexes last 3 minutes or more, the interval is scored as stage 1, even if it contains no movement arousal. If movement arousal or increase in muscle tone does occur during the interval in question, the prior proportion of the record should be scored as stage 2. The proportion of the record that follows should be scored as stage 1 until the next sleep spindle or K-complex occurs, provided that the epoch requirements and criteria for stage 1 are otherwise met. This 3-minute criterion was arbitrarily selected. It was based on anecdotal *adult* data that inter-spindle intervals of that length might occur without a stage change although such occasions would be rare.

Slow-wave sleep (SWS) is often separated into two stages based upon the percentage of slow-wave EEG activity present during any given 30-second epoch. Physiologically, stages 3 and 4 are similar and can be considered together as SWS. For the purpose of definition, "stage 3" is characterized by high-voltage (greater than 75 μV) *EEG* activity of 2 Hz or less comprising at least 20%, but not more than 50% of the 30-second epoch.

Slow-wave activity should be differentiated from K-complexes. K-complexes generally stand out from background activity. Slow waves tend to be less distinct, although differentiation is sometimes difficult. "Stage 4" is characterized by high-voltage (greater than 75 μV) EEG activity of 2 Hz or less comprising greater than 50% of any given 30-second epoch. Sleep spindles may or may not be present during stage 3 and stage 4.

The *EOG* during stage 2 sleep reveals the absence of conjugate eye movements. Depending upon the amplifier sensitivity setting, frontal EEG activity may be seen. Pen deflections are also seen concurrently with K-complexes. EOG artifact should not be confused with conjugate rapid eye movements that result in simultaneous *opposite* pen deflections. Because of the continuous high-voltage slow-wave activity during slow-wave sleep, frontal EEG artifact is common. Although skeletal muscle tone may diminish slightly during NREM sleep, *chin muscle EMG* remains tonic in all NREM-sleep stages. *EKG* remains stable and *respiration* is impressively monotonous. *Oxygen saturation* also remains quite stable during NREM sleep.

REM Sleep

REM sleep is defined by relatively low-voltage, mixed frequency *EEG* activity that is remarkably similar to stage 1 sleep. Several important distinctions are present. Bursts of vertex sharp waves are not present during REM sleep, the EEG frequency is slightly slower in REM when compared to stage 1, and bursts of "saw-tooth waves" appear. Saw-tooth waves are generally concentrated over the vertex, about 4–6 Hz in frequency, and appear "notched." Except for the first REM episode of the sleep period and during brief times of transition to REM from other sleep states, K-complexes and sleep spindles are absent. Scoring of REM sleep in the presence of sleep spindles can be difficult. Rechtschaffen and Kales (9) suggest scoring these situations in the following manner: any section of record contiguous with stage REM in which the EEG shows a relatively low-voltage, mixed-frequency pattern is scored REM regardless of the presence of eye movements, providing there are no intervening movement arousals and the EMG tone remains at the level seen in unambiguous REM sleep; and any section of record of relatively low-voltage, mixed-frequency EEG activity between two sleep spindles or K-complexes should be considered stage 2 regardless of EMG level as long as there are no conjugate eye movements or movement arousals during the interval and if the interval is less than 3 minutes long.

REM sleep is also defined by the presence of rapid conjugate eye movements. Rapid eye movements frequently occur in association with bursts of saw-tooth waves. *Tonic REM* sleep occurs when scoring criteria for REM sleep are met, but there are no clear conjugate eye movements. This is particularly true in REM episodes during the early portions of the sleep period. There is some preliminary evidence that the angular velocity of extra-ocular movements during REM sleep is quite slow and eye movements can be sparse in some children with reading disabilities (10). In these cases, if all other criteria are met for REM sleep, the epochs should be classified as REM sleep.

Chin muscle EMG reaches its lowest level of activity during REM sleep. There are no clear criteria regarding the decrease in amplitude of EMG activity required for REM. However, stage REM should not be scored in the presence of relatively elevated tonic chin muscle EMG activity. For each child in any given recording session, EMG reveals enough variation to make relative comparisons. During stage REM the EMG is not higher than the level during the preceding sleep stage and it almost always reaches its lowest

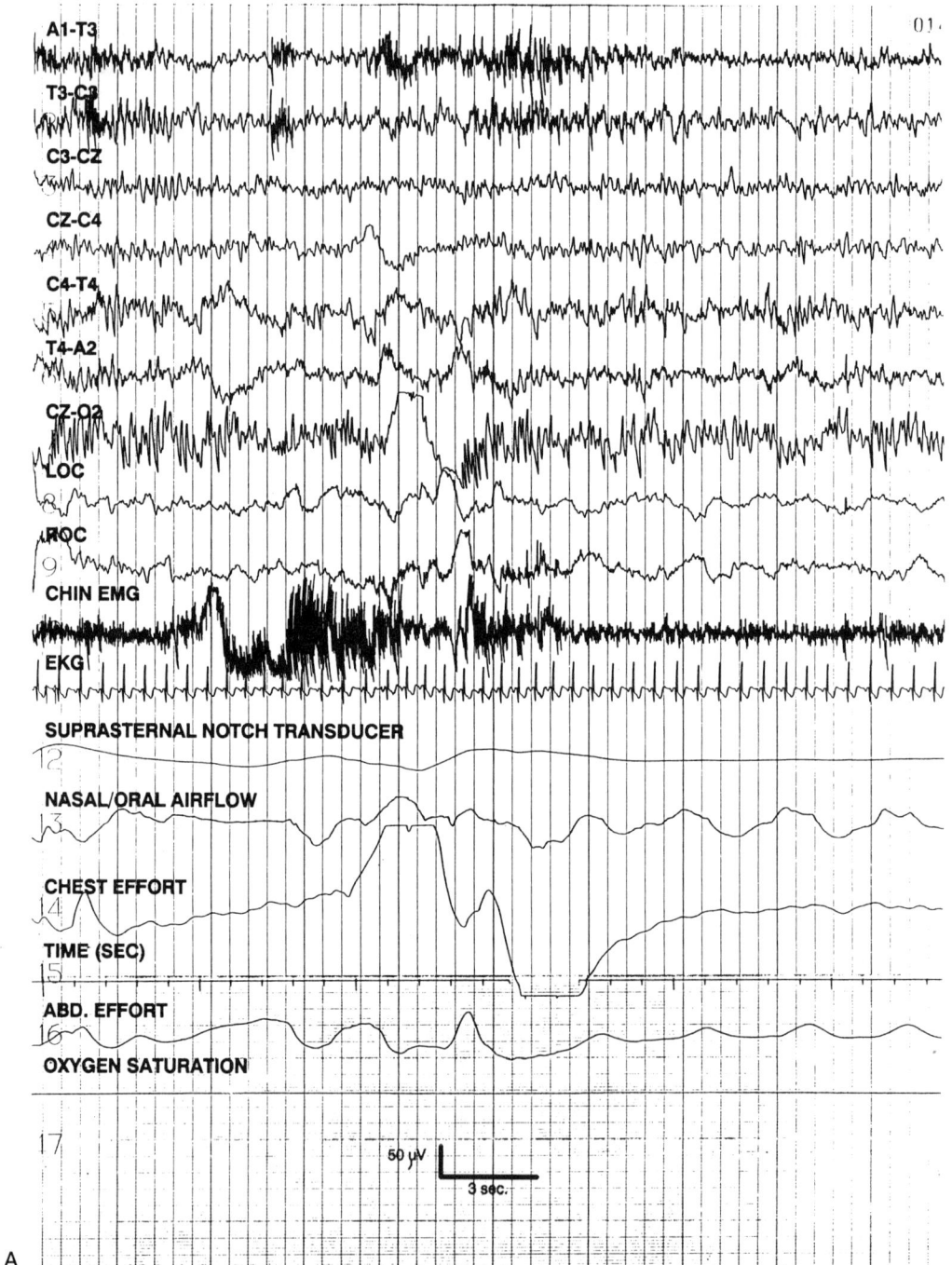

FIG. 12-2. A–B: Active wake in a 7-year-old youngster. Note the significant movement artifacts, well-formed alpha activity posteriorly with the patient's eyes closed, and activation of the EEG with eyes open.

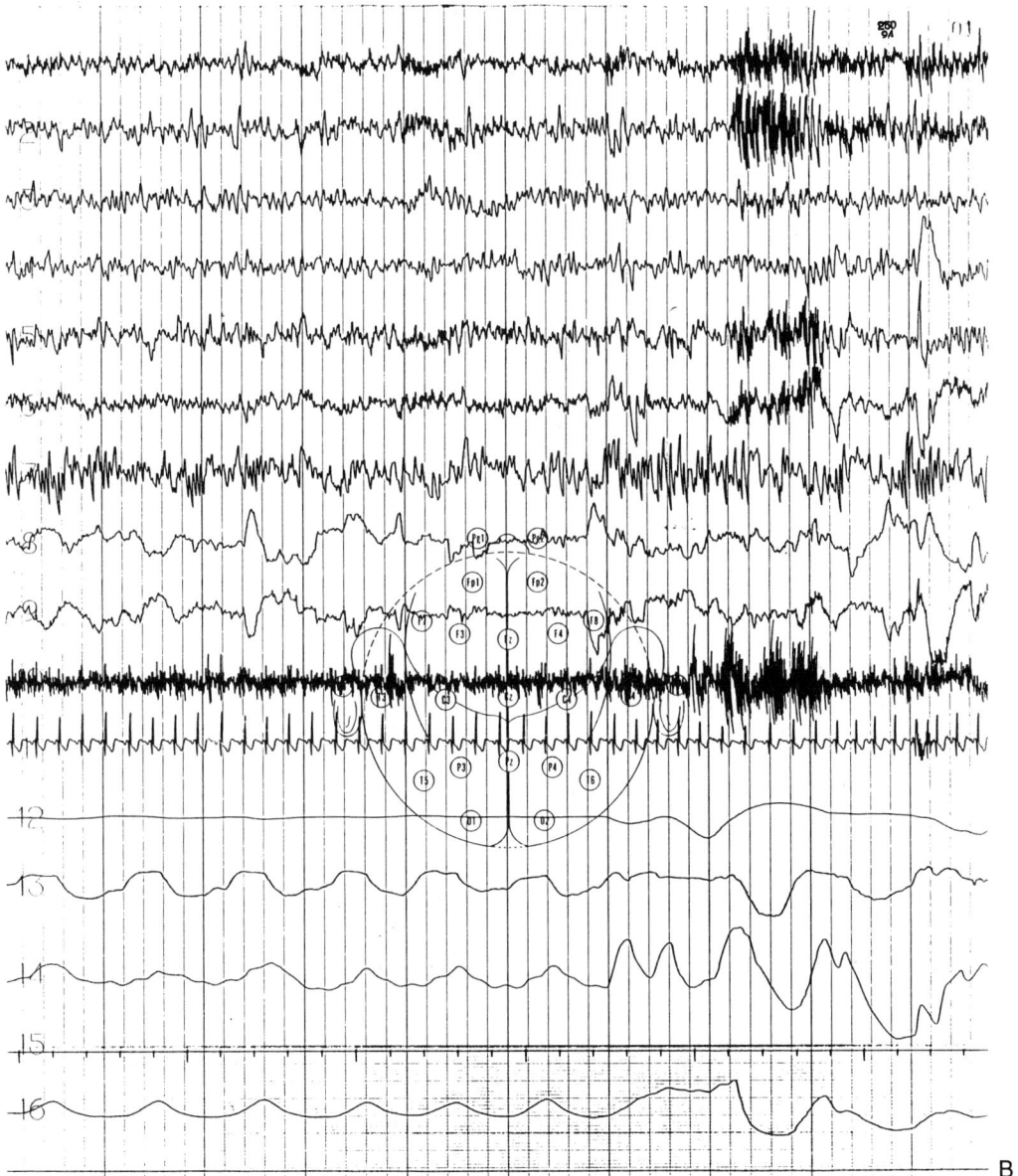

FIG. 12-2. *Continued.*

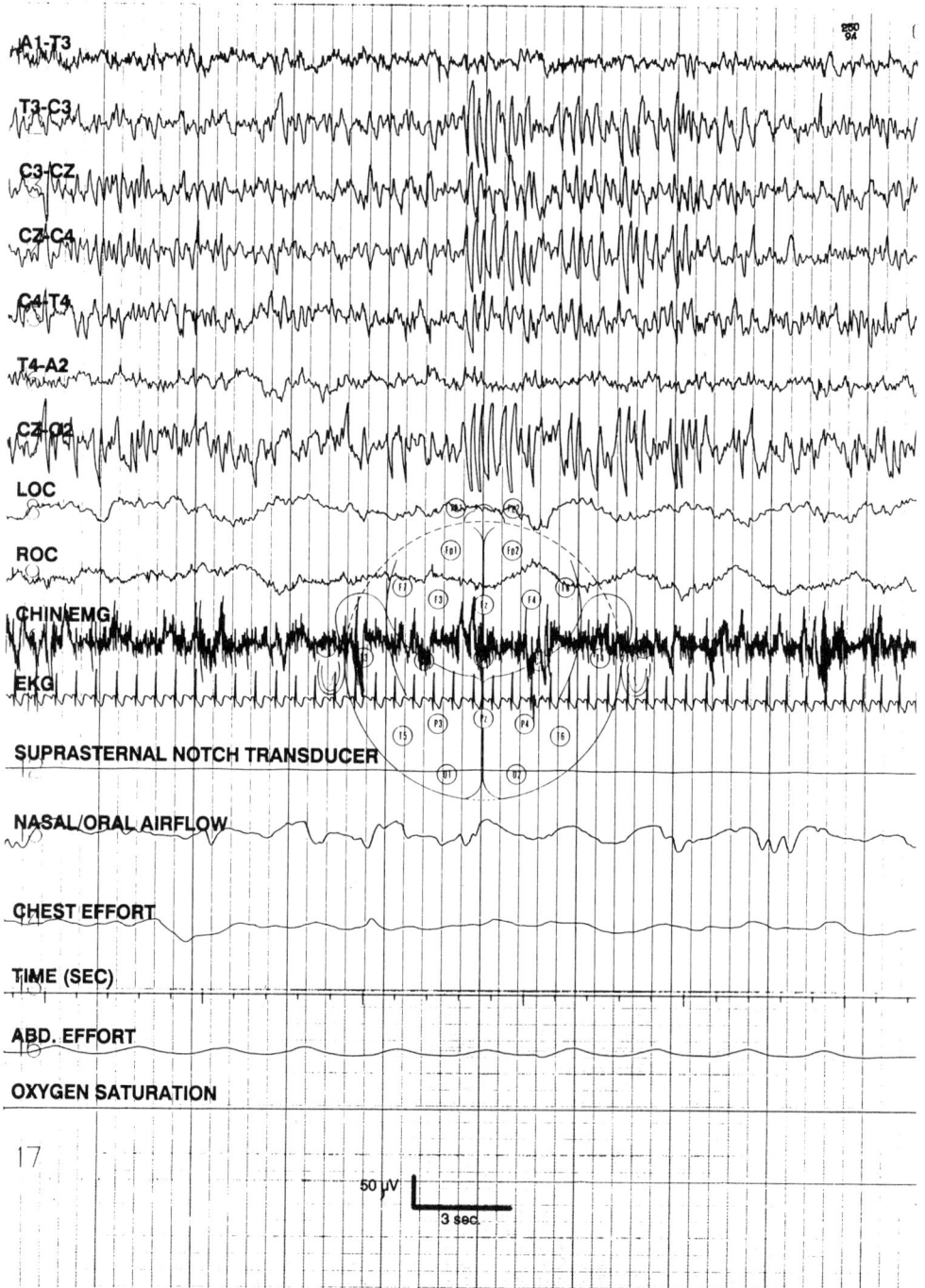

FIG. 12-3. A–B: NREM stage 1 in a 7-year-old youngster. Note bursts of hypersynchronous theta activity (hypnogogic hypersynchrony) originating from the vertex. Also note the sharp vertex waves.

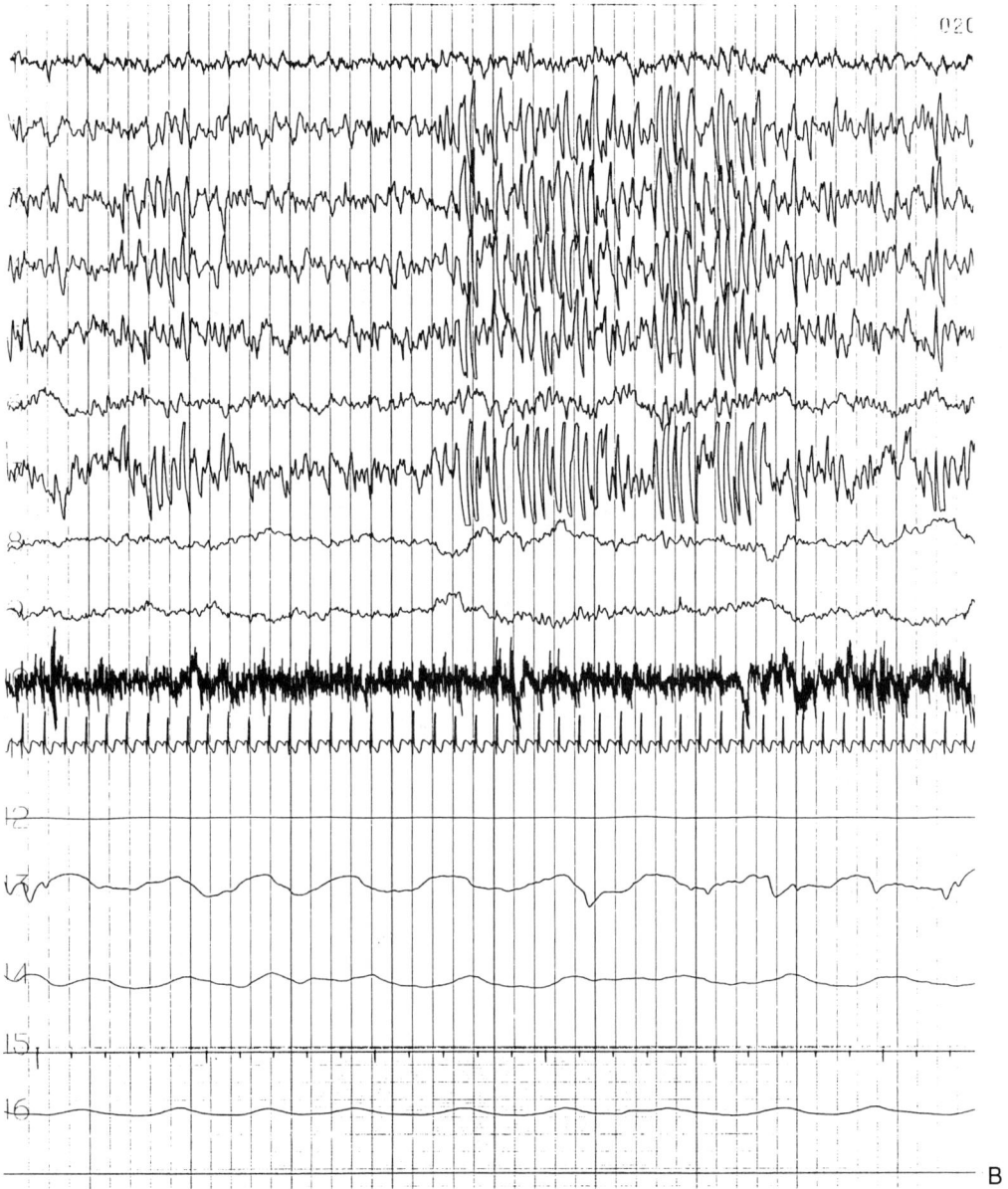

FIG. 12-3. *Continued.*

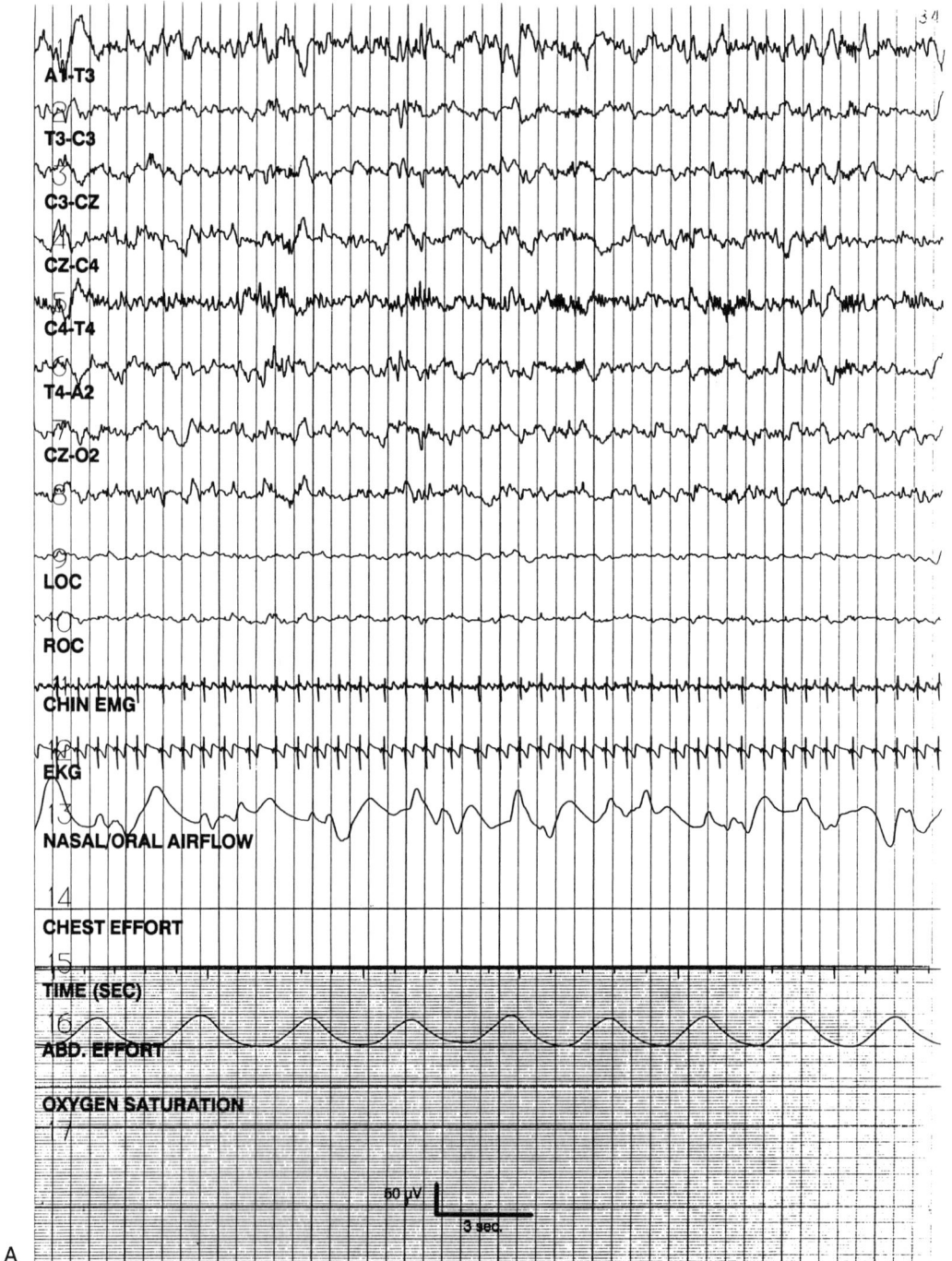

FIG. 12-4. A–B: NREM stage 2 in a 7-year-old youngster. There is a relatively low-voltage, mixed-frequency background rhythm associated with well-formed and symmetric sleep spindles with a frequency of about 12–14 Hz.

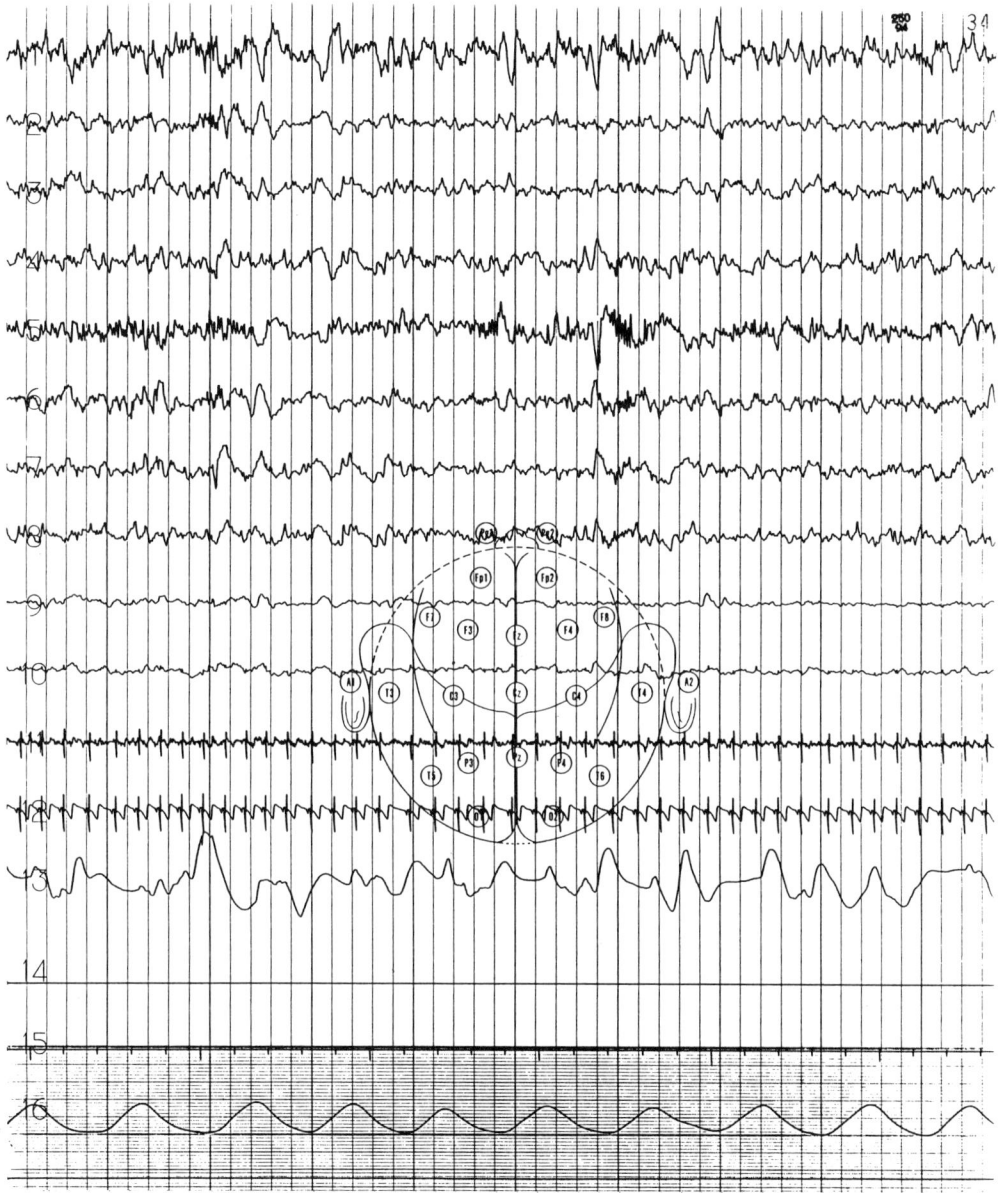

FIG. 12-4. *Continued.*

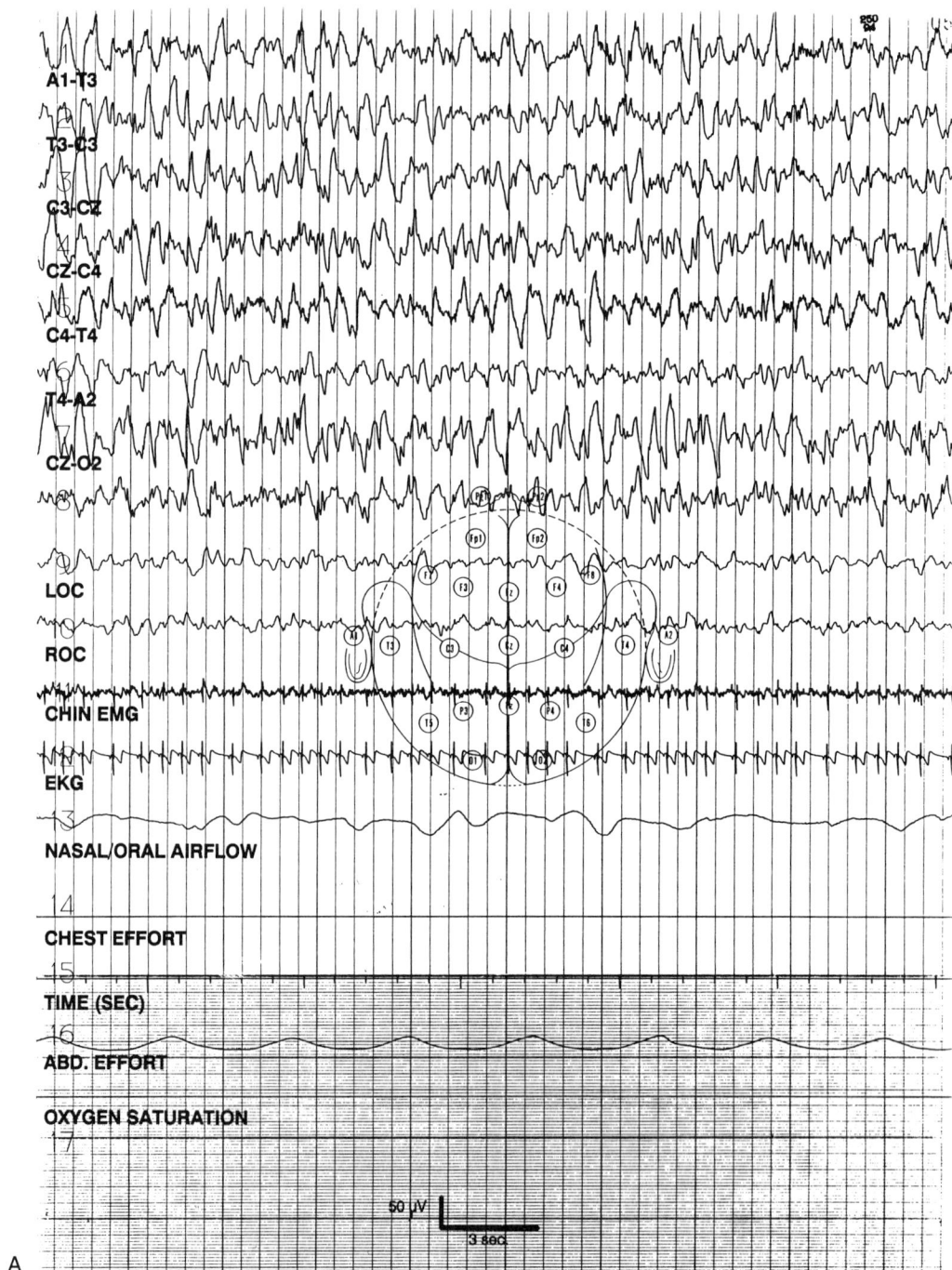

FIG. 12-5. A–B: Slow-wave sleep in a 7-year-old youngster. High-voltage slow waves predominate. Note the sinus arrhythmia in the EKG. Respiration is regular.

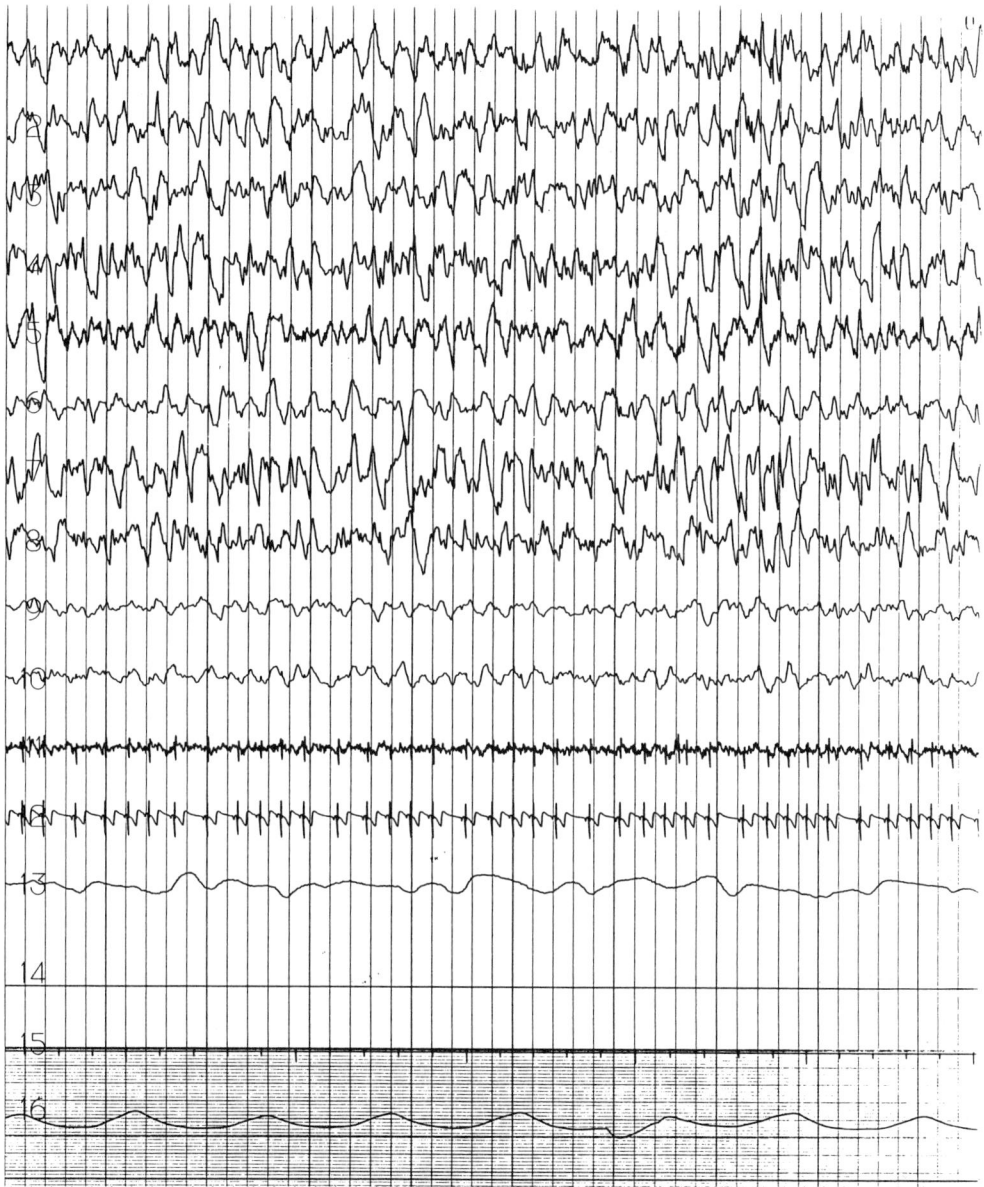

FIG. 12-5. *Continued.*

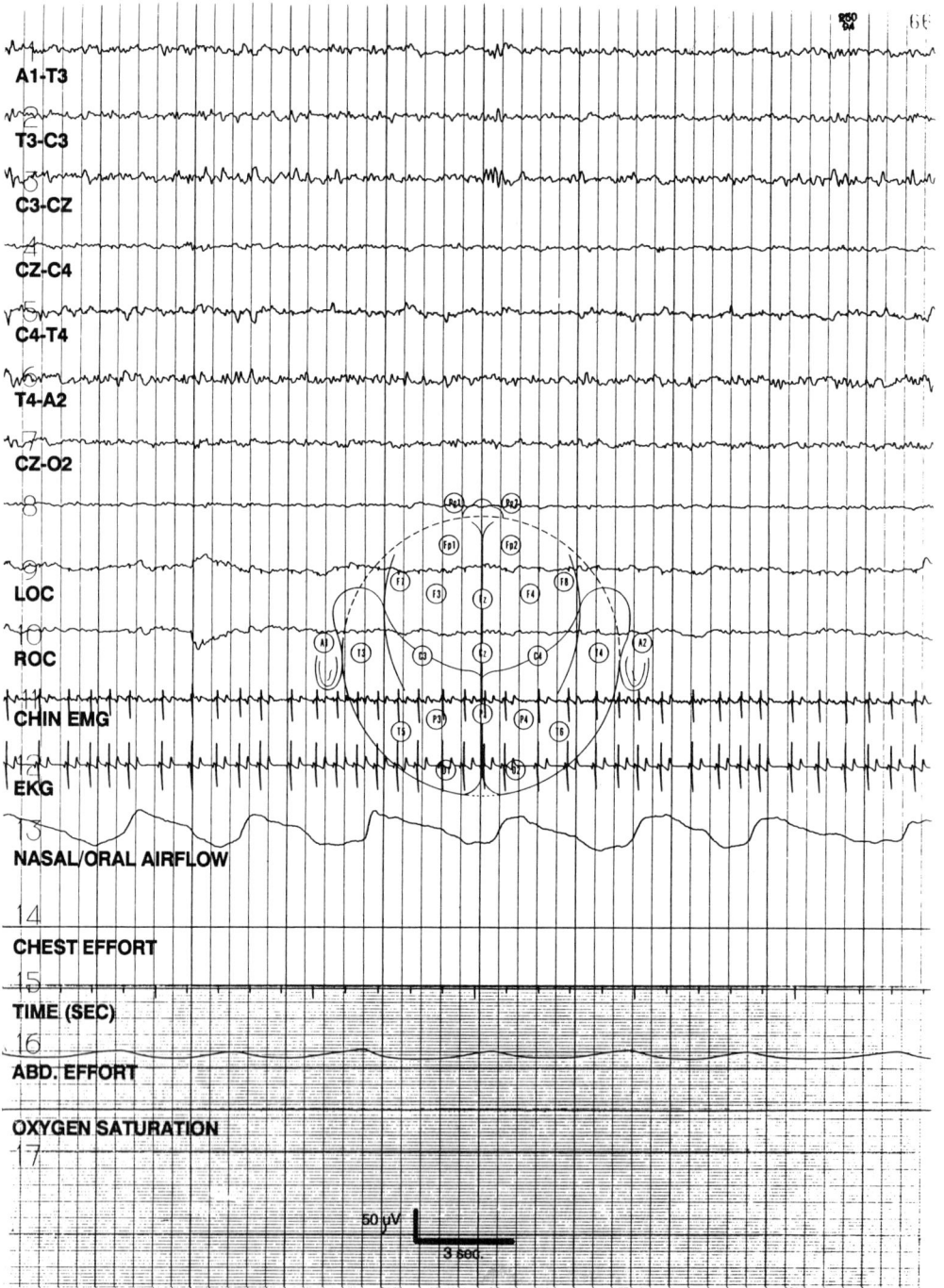

FIG. 12-6. A–B: Stage REM in a 7-year-old youngster. Note the cardiorespiratory instability and respiratory variation in the R-R interval in the EKG.

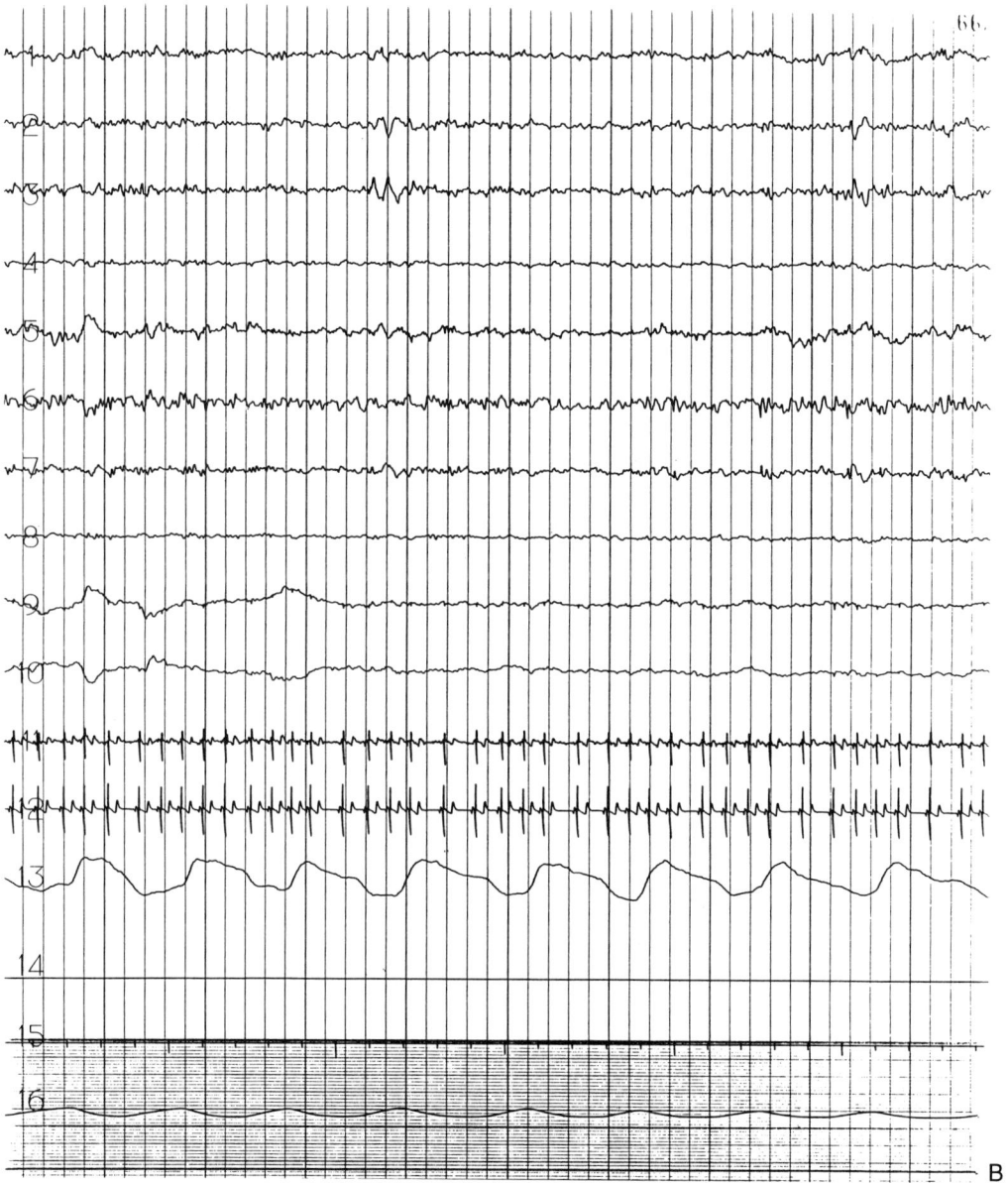

FIG. 12-6. *Continued.*

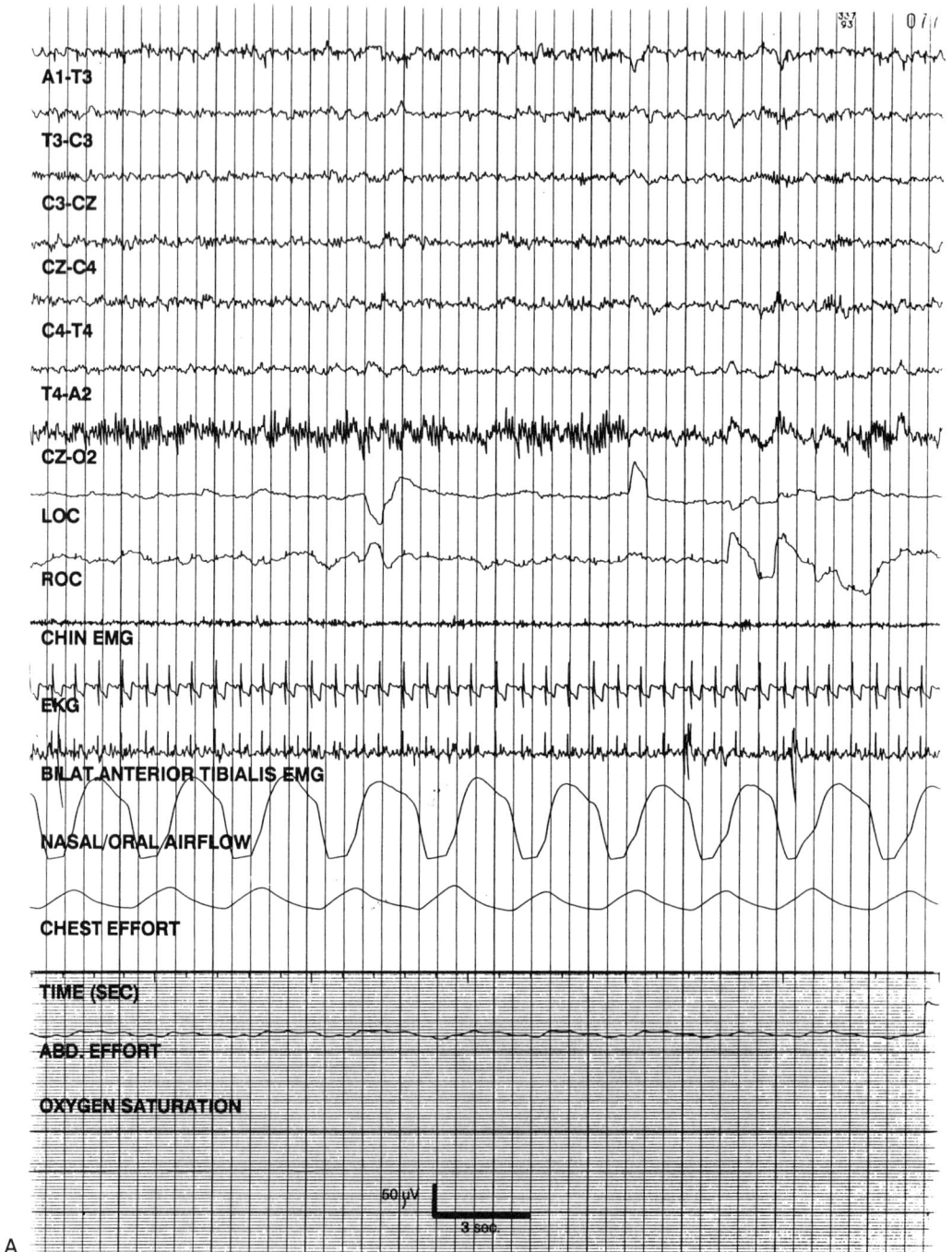

FIG. 12-7. A–B: Relaxed wakefulness in a 10-year-old youngster. Note the well-formed alpha activity predominantly over the posterior region of the head. In addition, disappearance of the alpha activity and driving of the EEG with eye opening. Minimal 8- to 12-Hz, synchronous activity can be seen in the other EEG channels.

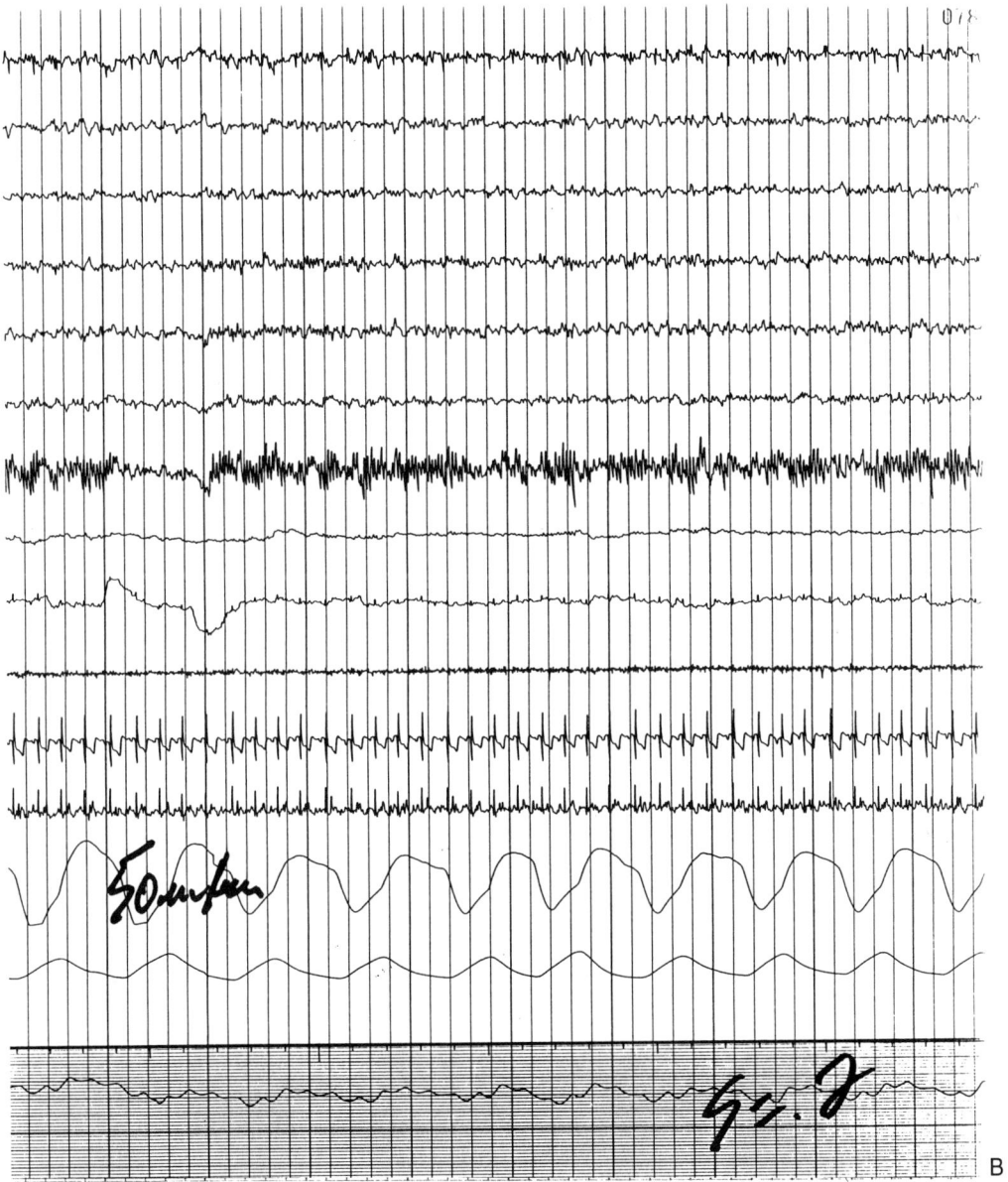

FIG. 12-7. *Continued.*

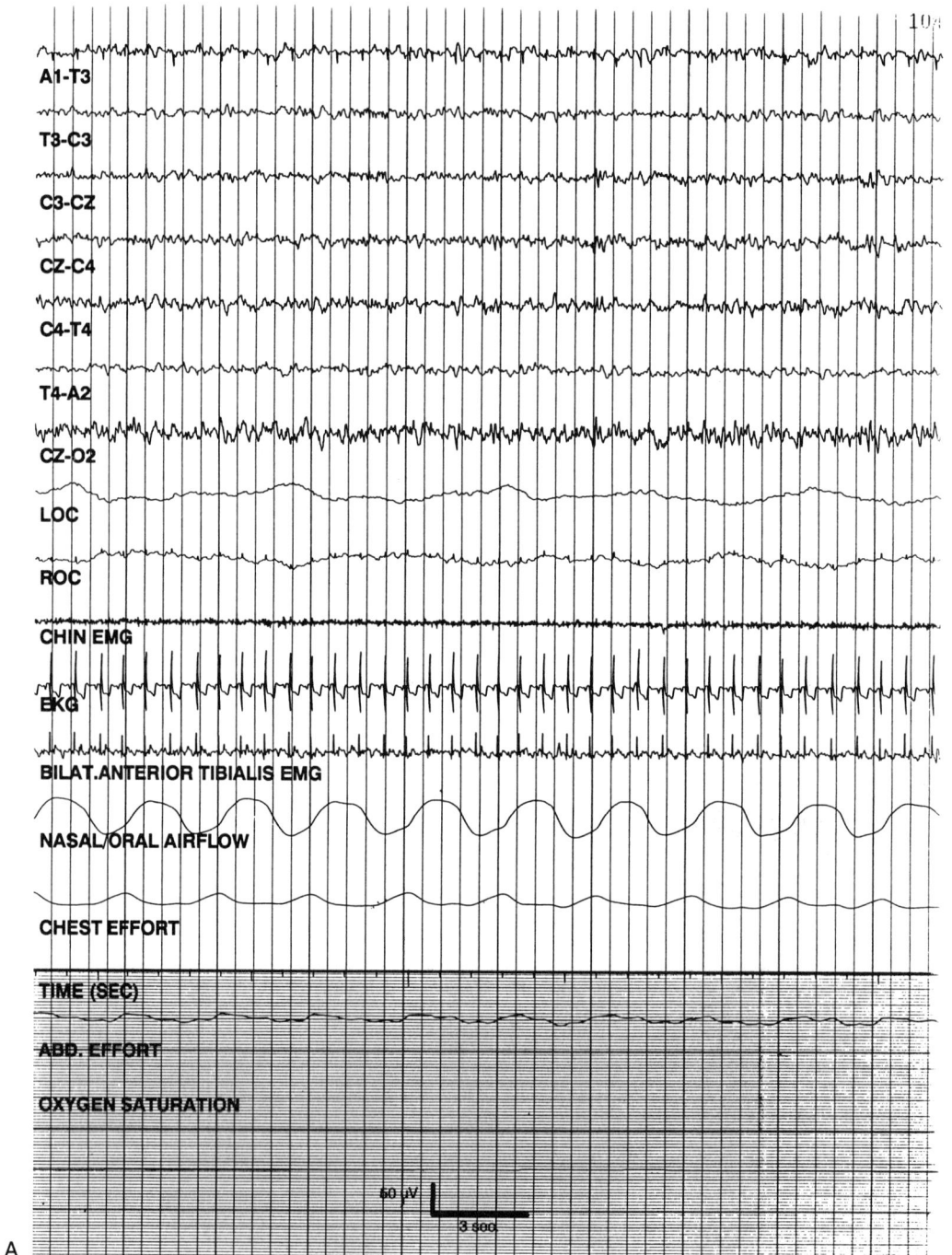

FIG. 12-8. A–B: NREM stage 1 sleep in a 10-year-old youngster. Alpha activity has dropped out of the EEG and is replaced with a relatively low-voltage, mixed-frequency pattern. Slow, rolling eye movements are clearly present. Chin EMG is tonic and respiratory variation can be seen in the EKG. Breathing is quite regular.

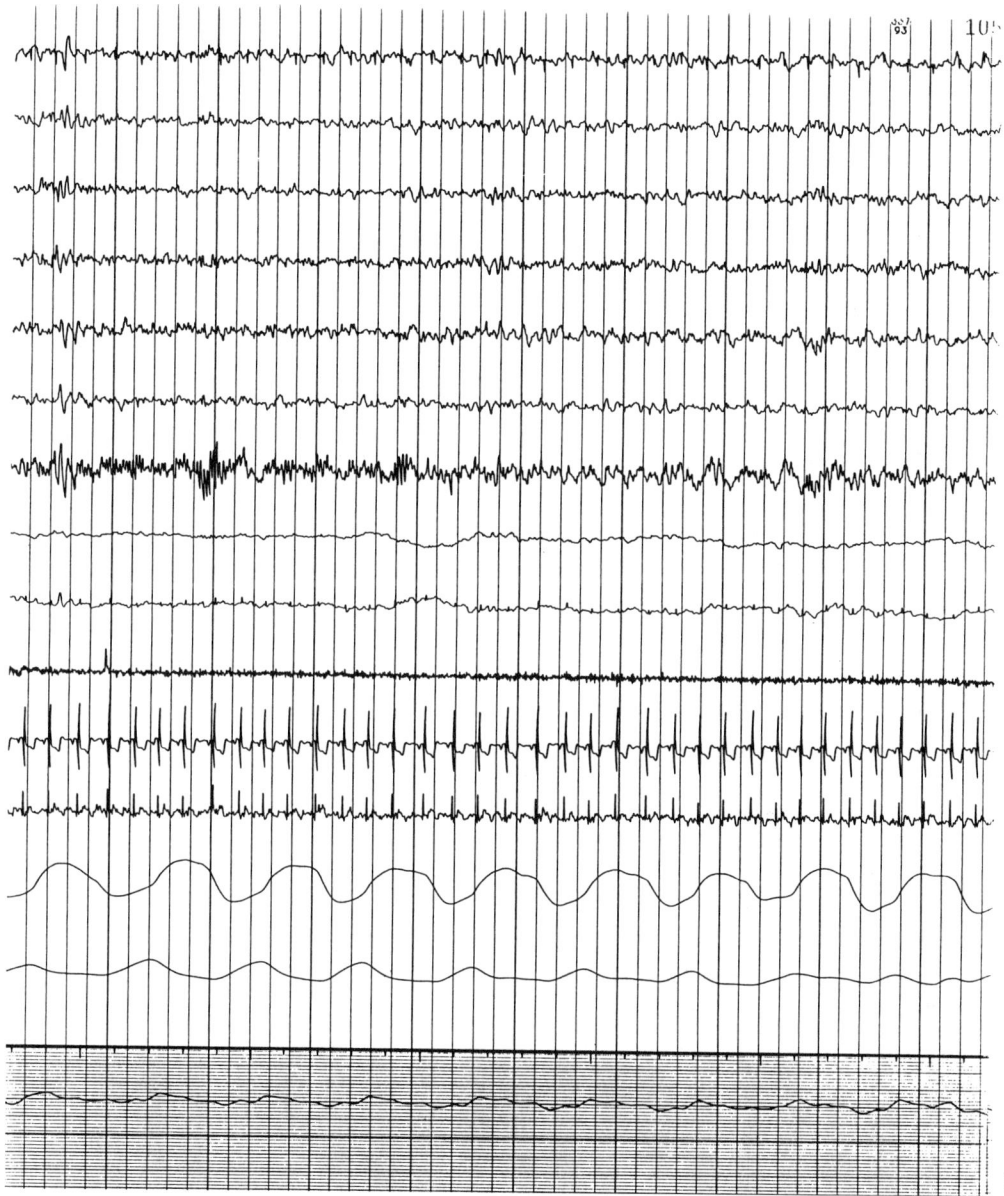

FIG. 12-8. *Continued.*

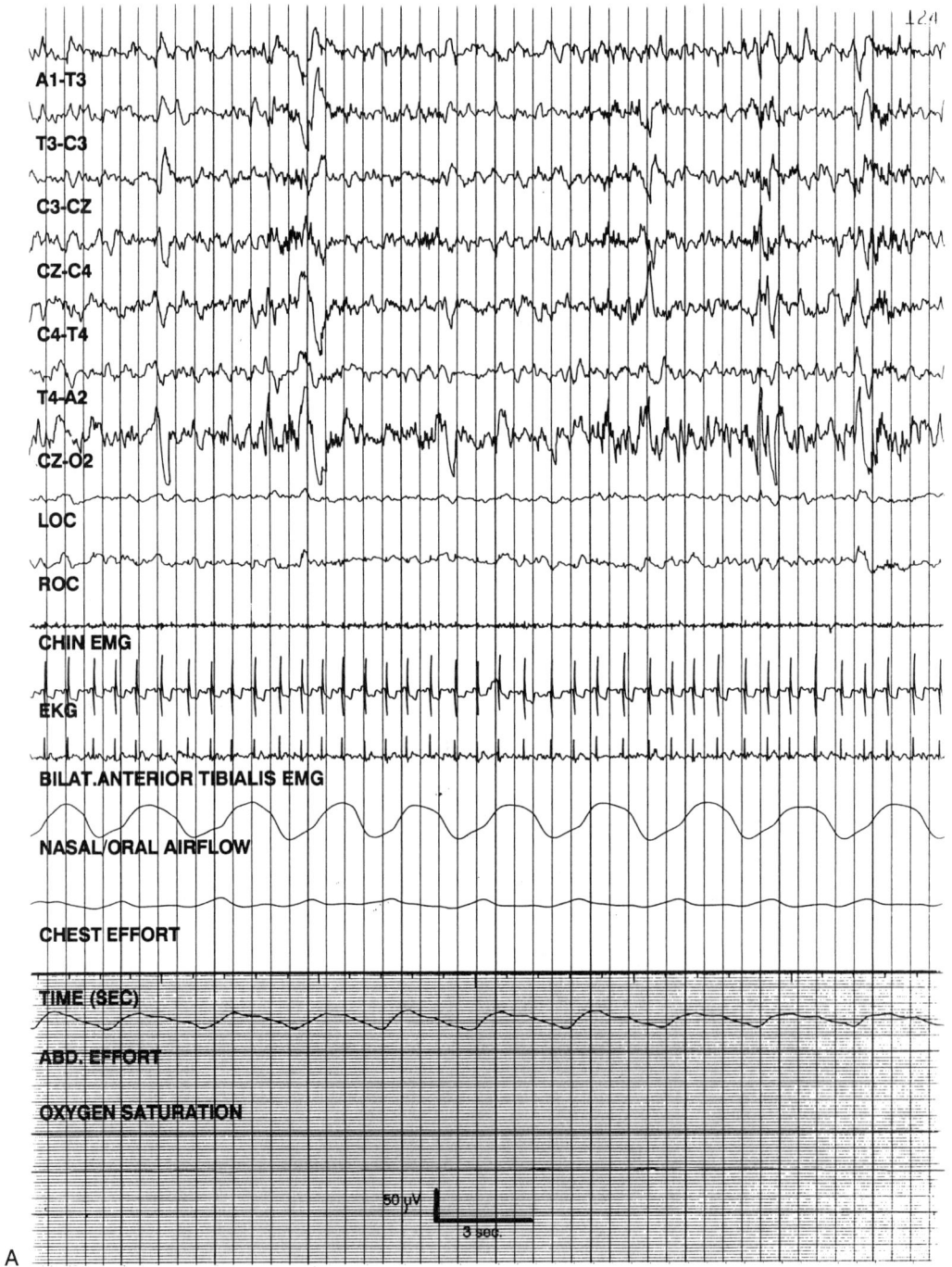

FIG. 12-9. A–B: NREM stage 2 in a 10-year-old youngster. K-complexes and symmetric sleep spindles clearly stand out from the background EEG activity.

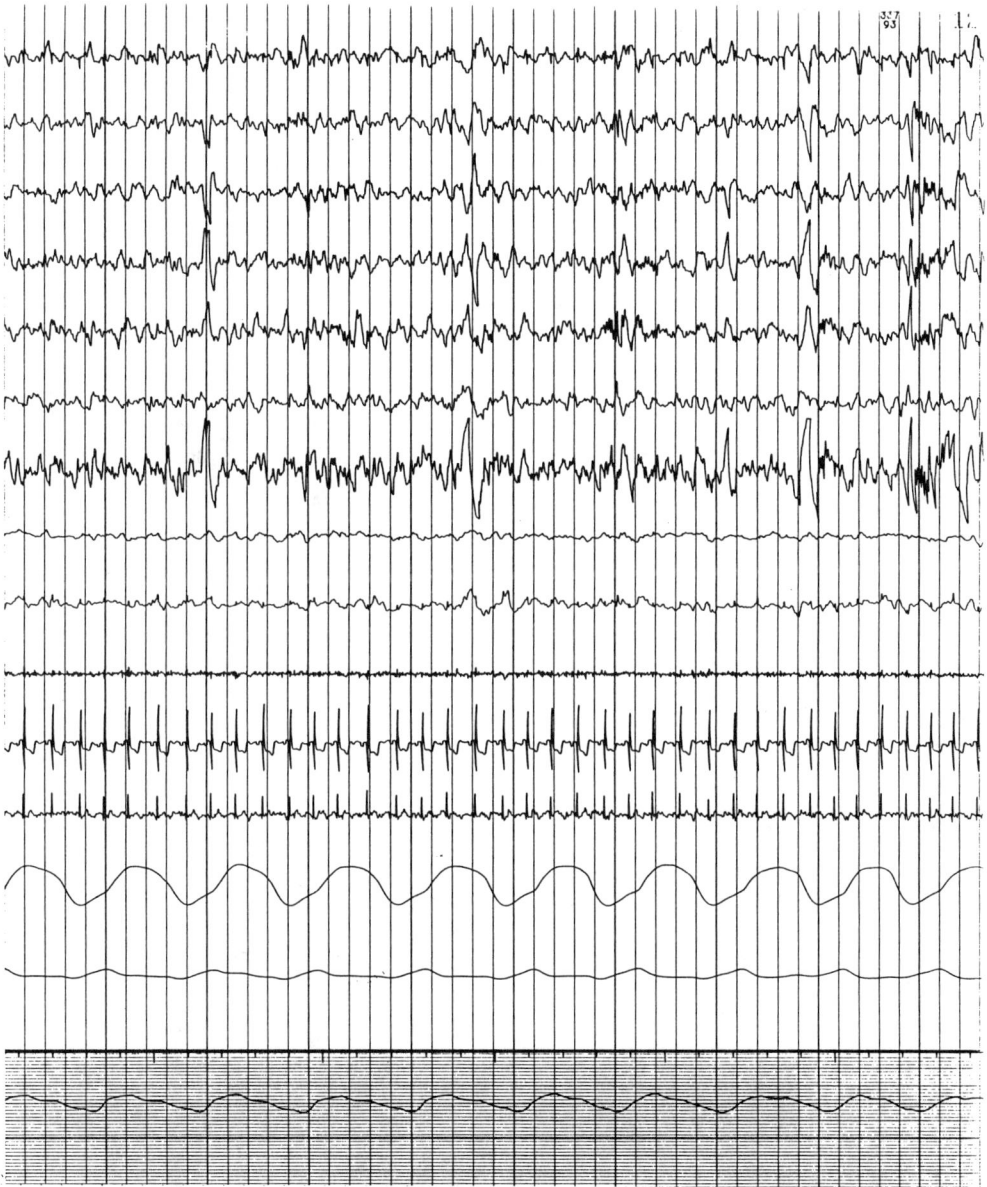

FIG. 12-9. *Continued.*

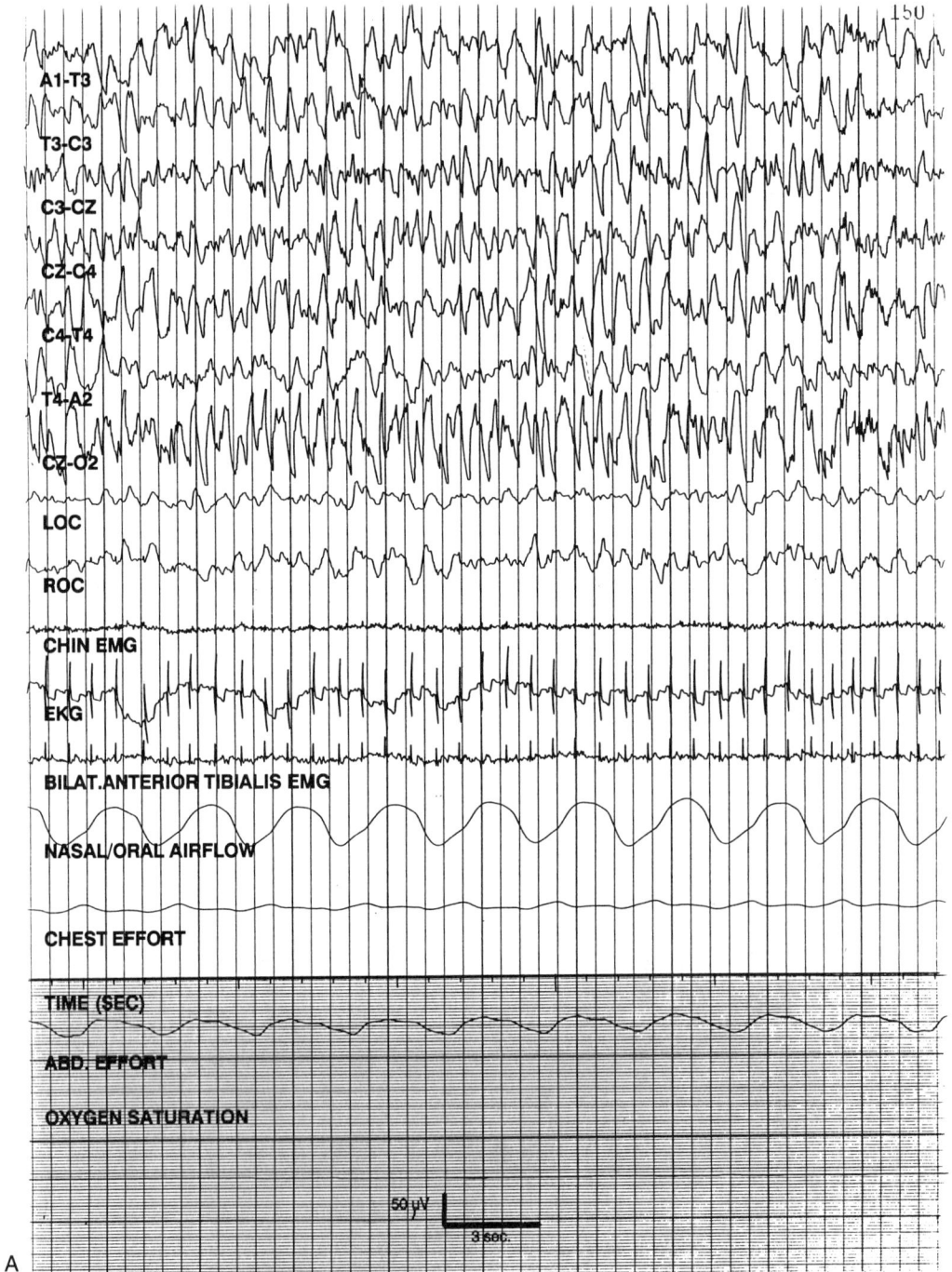

FIG. 12-10. A–B: NREM slow-wave sleep in a 10-year-old youngster. Note sleep spindles in the EEG and sweat artifact in the EKG lead.

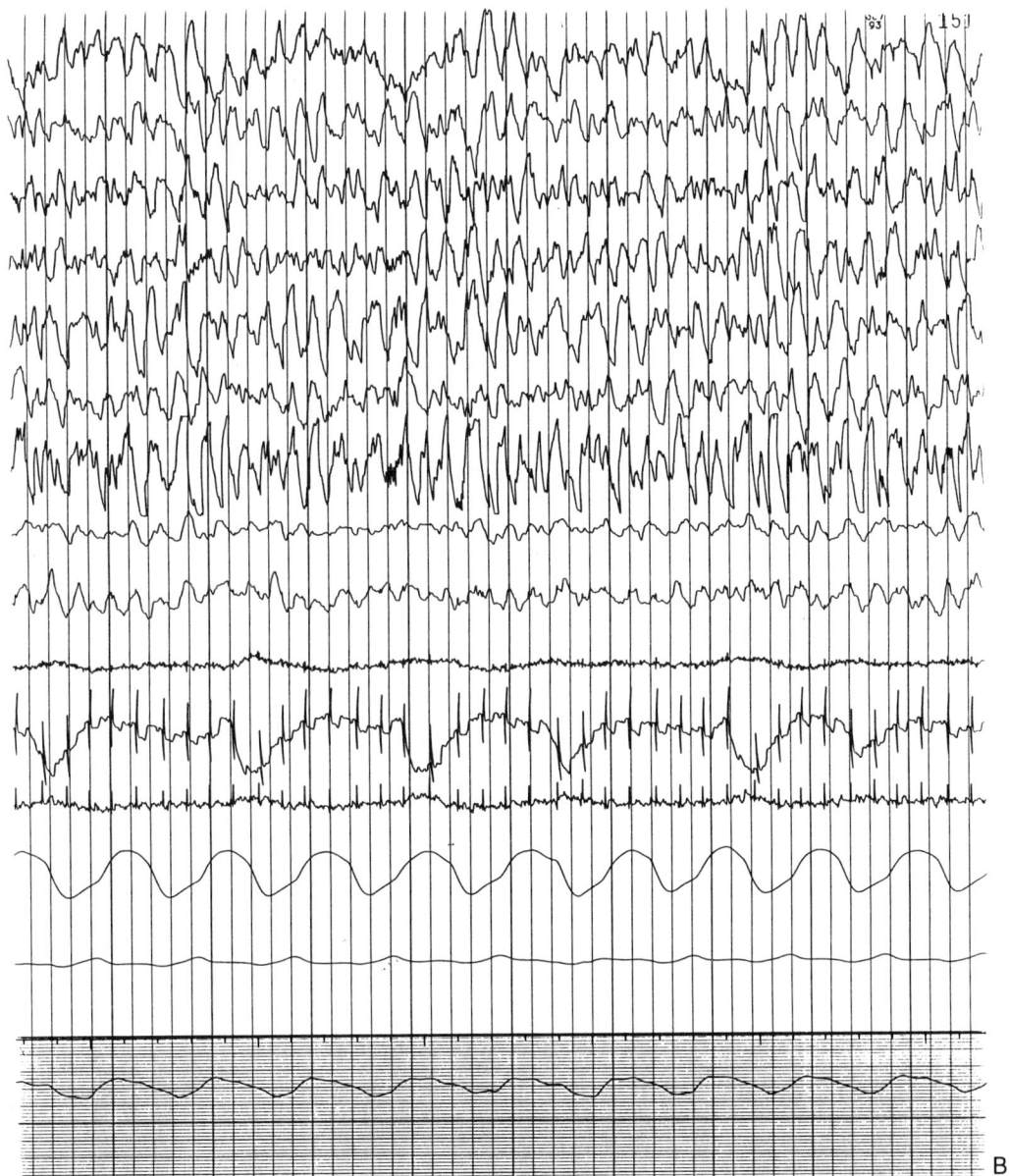

FIG. 12-10. *Continued.*

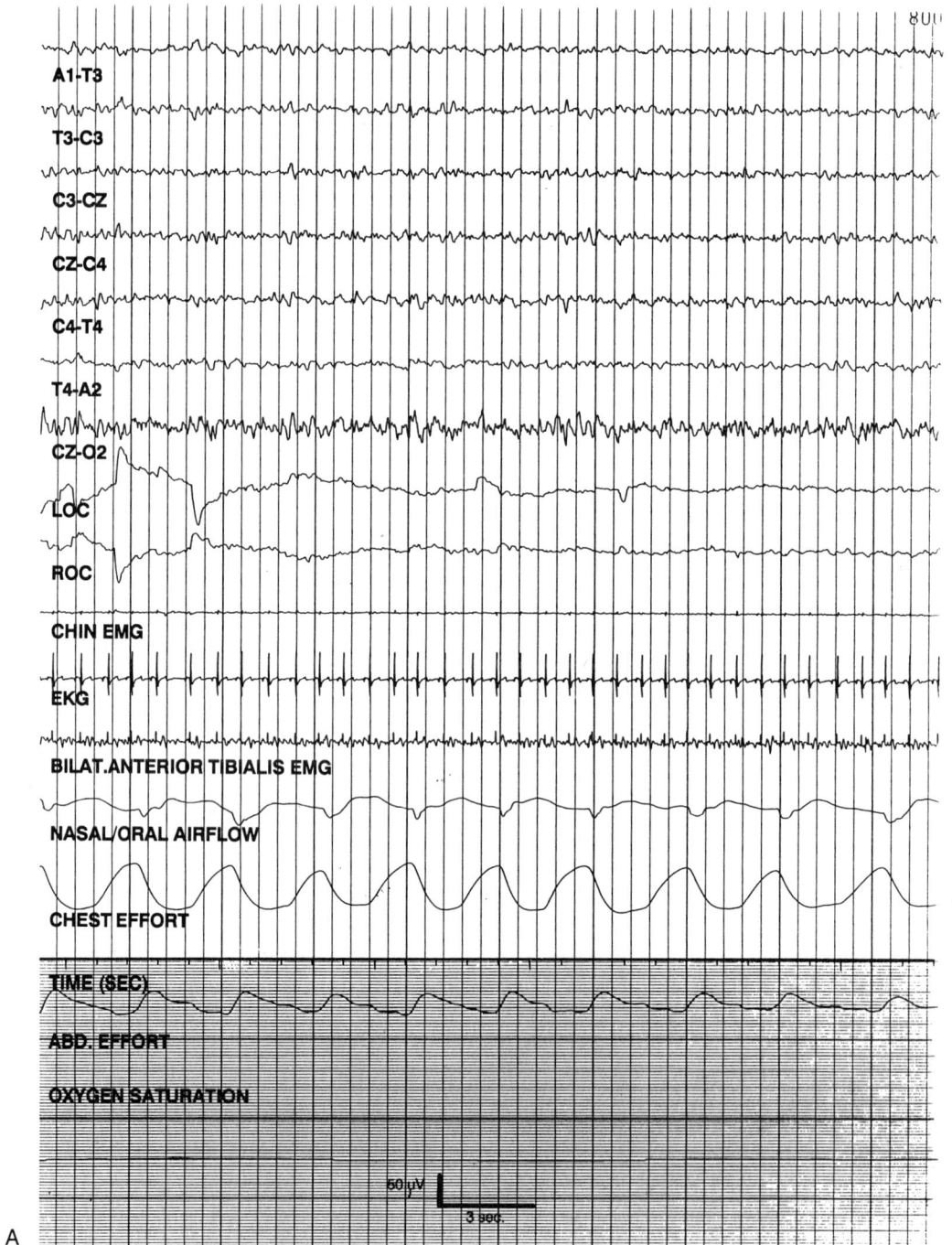

FIG. 12-11. A–B: Stage REM sleep in a 10-year-old youngster. Note the relatively low-voltage, mixed-frequency EEG background, saw-tooth waves, dense eye movements, low chin muscle tone, and considerable respiratory variability.

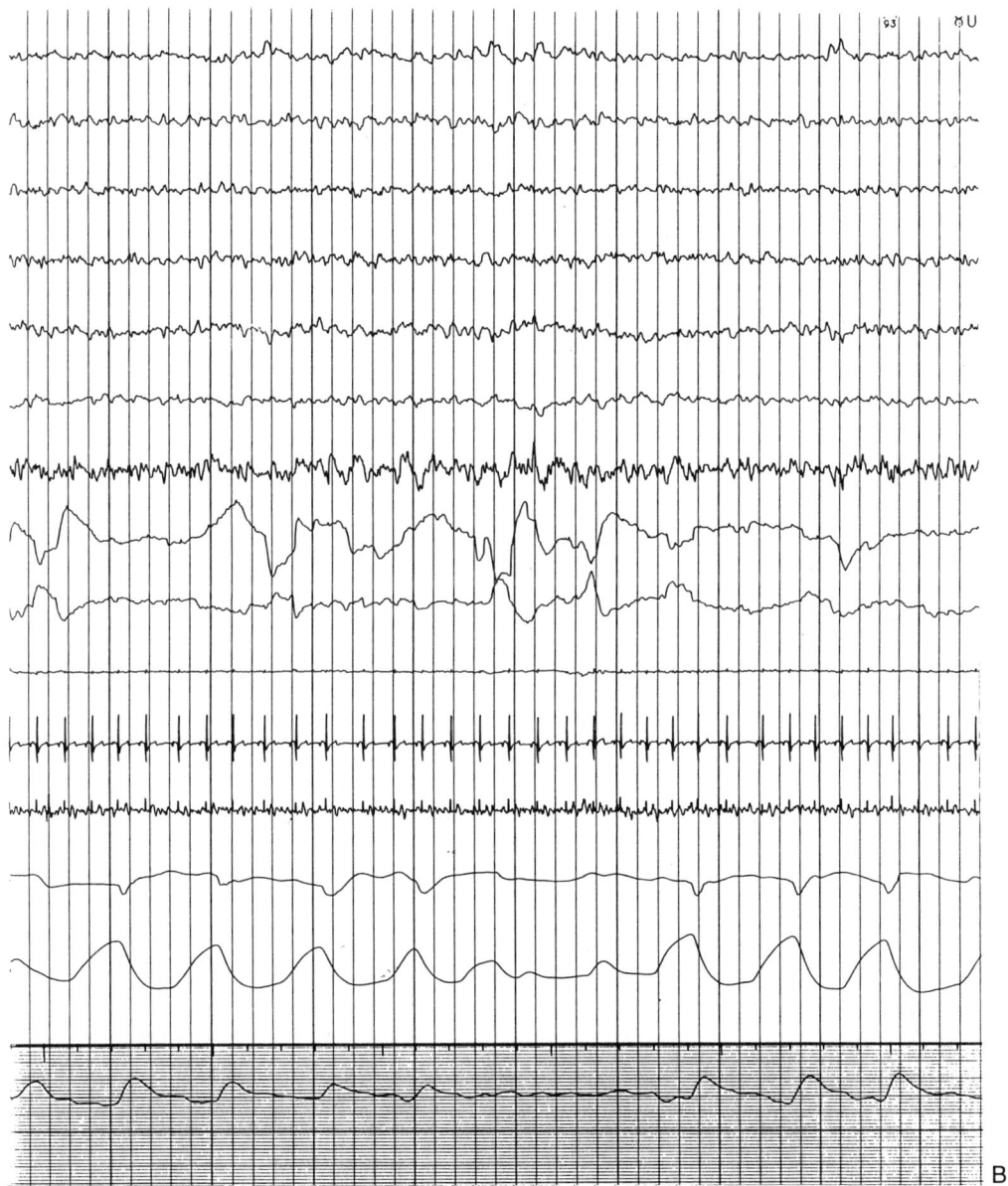

FIG. 12-11. *Continued.*

amplitude during REM sleep. These low levels may occur during other sleep stages, however, they are uniformly reached during unambiguous REM. Transient phasic bursts of chin muscle activity is common during REM sleep and the presence of phasic muscle activity can assist in state identification.

Although a normal sinus rhythm continues, *EKG* rhythm can vary during REM sleep. This may be partly due to significant respiratory variability seen during REM sleep. *Respiration* is unstable with periods of relative (or absolute) tachypnea, bradypnea, hyperpnea, hypopnea, and brief apnea. Because of a decrease in responsiveness of baroreceptor and chemoreceptors during REM sleep (when compared to NREM sleep and wakefulness), oxygen saturation can fall slightly during this time, especially during periods of normal REM-related hypopnea. Differentiation from abnormal falls in oxygen saturation is sometimes difficult. Pathologic decrease in oxygen saturation due to upper-airway obstruction during REM sleep is generally periodic and associated with a greater degree of desaturation, EKG changes, and/or arousal when compared to NREM sleep.

Movement Time, Movement Arousals, and Electrocortical Arousals

Movement time is used to designate epochs where greater than 50% of the 30-second epoch of EEG and EOG are obscured by movement/muscle artifact. If less than 50% of the epoch is obscured, the epoch should be scored as the predominant sleep state. In general, movement time is not scored as sleep or wake. According to Rechtschaffen and Kales, "not enough is known about the behavioral correlates of movement time to classify it unambiguously as either sleep or wakefulness."

Discrete *body movements* also occur, but are brief and muscle movement artifact obscures less than half of the epoch. Technician notations regarding the characteristics of the movement can be quite helpful in interpretation of the significance of these movements. Body movements should be considered specific physiologic events that occur during both sleep and movement time.

A *movement arousal* is defined as any increase in EMG activity on any polygraph channel that is accompanied by a change in pattern on any other channel. Movement arousal need only indicate increase in muscle activity and does not require the presence of substantial or observable body movement. There are several reasons for describing movement arousals. They may represent significant disruption in the continuity of sleep and have specific clinical significance and they can aid in the scoring of stages by signaling the possibility of a stage change.

Electrocortical arousals are defined by EEG criteria alone: the sudden appearance of a slow wave (or K-complex) followed by at least 3 seconds of EEG activity that is faster than the background state-related EEG activity (and is not a sleep spindle). Extreme spindles occur in some children and can last longer than 3 seconds, but should not be considered electrocortical arousals. There may or may not be a movement arousal associated with the electrocortical arousal (Figs. 12-2–12-11).

REFERENCES

1. Wilson MA, McNaughton BL. Reactivation of hippocampal ensemble memories during sleep. *Science* 1994;265:676–679.
2. Karni A, Tanne D, Rubenstein BS, Askenasy JJM, Sagi D. Dependence on REM sleep of overnight improvement of a perceptual skill. *Science* 1994;265:679–682.

3. Paul K, Dittrichova J. Sleep patterns following learning in infants. In: Levin P, Koella U, eds. *Sleep: 1974.* Basel: S Karger; 1975:388.
4. Feinberg I. Eye movement activity during sleep and intellectual function in mental retardation. *Science* 1968;159:1256.
5. Eliaschar I, Lavie P, Halperin E, Gordon C, Alroy G. Sleep apneic episodes as indications for adenotonsillectomy. *Arch Otolaryngol* 1980;106:492.
6. Sheldon SH, Garay A, Jacobsen J. REM sleep motor disorder in children. *Sleep Res* 1994;23:173.
7. Ross RJ, Ball WA, Dinges DF, et al. Motor dysfunction during sleep in post-traumatic stress disorder. *Sleep* 1994;17:723–732.
8. Sheldon SH, Ahart S, Levy HB. Sleep patterns in abused and neglected children. *Sleep Res* 1991;20:333.
9. Rechtschaffen A, Kales A, eds. *A Manual of Standardized Terminology, Techniques and Scoring System for Sleep Stages of Human Subjects.* Los Angeles: UCLA Brain Information Service, NINDS Neurological Information Network; 1968.
10. Sheldon SH, Spire JP, Levy HB. REM sleep eye movements in reading disabled children. *Sleep Res* 1990;19:128.

13

Testing Excessive Day-time Sleepiness

THE MULTIPLE SLEEP LATENCY TEST (MSLT)

The MSLT (1–3) was developed in an attempt to provide objective information regarding degrees of day-time sleepiness in human subjects. It consists of identification and measurement of (i) the "censored" mean sleep-onset latency, and (ii) the presence of sleep-onset REM periods (SOREMPs).

The MSLT is a measure of sleepiness/alertness. The more prolonged the latency to sleep onset, the more alert the individual. Conversely, the shorter the sleep-onset latency, the sleepier and less alert the individual (4).

REM sleep tends to vary with body temperature rhythm and reaches its maximum frequency when the body temperature rhythm reaches its nadir (5). Except during early infancy, it is rare for sleep to be entered through REM or to occur during diurnal naps. However, REM sleep occurs during day-time hours with: narcolepsy syndrome, rebound from extreme sleep deprivation, and rebound from selective REM deprivation.

Mean sleep-onset latencies on MSLTs can vary considerably and may be related to the amount of sleep obtained on one or several nights preceding testing, age and maturation of the patient, sleep continuity, time of day, and the presence of drugs/medications. Typically, mean sleep-onset latencies on MSLTs less than 5 minutes is considered pathologic sleepiness. Pathologic sleep-onset latencies are associated with performance decrements and unintentional sleep episodes.

In order to adequately assess MSLT data, comprehensive polysomnography is required on the night prior to MSLT testing. Specific sleep-related abnormalities that disrupt the continuity of sleep can be identified. An adequate total sleep time prior to the MSLT can also be objectively assured. A 1- to 2- week sleep log prior to the MSLT can provide information regarding habitual sleep-wake cycles since the MSLT results may be influenced by sleep habits up to 7 nights prior to testing.

The clinical history should be carefully searched for the presence of drugs or medications that could bias the MSLT results. A urine drug screen may sometimes be helpful, especially if the history is unreliable. If not medically contraindicated, medications that could affect the results of the MSLT should be discontinued at least 2 weeks prior to the study.

Standard MSLT Protocol

MSLT protocol (1) requires five test naps attempted at 2-hour intervals across the day. Prior to the onset of each nap, the patient should be asked whether they require to void. This will prevent disruption of the onset of naps and delay in the time of lights-out. The first nap begins 1.5 to 3 hours after the time of morning sleep offset. The patient is encouraged to dress in loose fitting, comfortable street clothes and is placed in a quiet, dark, temperature-controlled room. This is typically the same room in which the nocturnal recording had taken place, but can be a different room in the laboratory. Machine and patient calibrations are performed prior to beginning the nap trial in a similar manner to nocturnal polysomnography. Lights are then turned out and the patient is instructed to lie quietly, close their eyes, and to try to sleep (or to not resist falling asleep). Identical instructions are given immediately prior to each nap trial. Nap periods are ended after 20 minutes if objective polygraphic evidence of sleep has not occurred (it is utilization of a sleep-onset latency of 20 minutes in naps where sleep onset has not occurred in the calculation of the mean sleep-onset latency that transforms the results into a *censored* mean, rather than a true mean). Naps may also be ended after the appearance of three consecutive 30-second epochs of stage 1 sleep, or one 30-second epoch of any other sleep stage. If the presence of SOREMPs is an issue, the nap is ended 15 minutes after the first identifiable epoch of sleep.

Sleep-onset latency is defined as the time from lights-out to when sleep occupies greater than 50% of any 30-second epoch. REM latency is measured from sleep onset to the onset of the first epoch of REM sleep. For each nap, the sleep-onset latency is calculated. An average is computed for all naps across the day's testing.

If the censored mean sleep-onset latency is less than 5 minutes, pathologic sleepiness is present. An average sleep-onset latency of this magnitude is associated with impaired performance, significant attentional problems, and uncontrollable sleep episodes. In the adult patient, a censored mean sleep-onset latency on MSLT of between 10 and 20 minutes is considered normal. Latencies between 5 and 10 minutes are questionable.

Since REM sleep rarely occurs during day-time naps, the presence of two or more SOREMPs on a five-nap MSLT is consistent with and characteristic of narcolepsy syndrome. SOREMPs are exceptionally rare in normal individuals. They are occasionally recorded in patients with sleep apnea syndrome or during rebound from significant sleep deprivation. In these patients, the presence of REM sleep during day-time naps reflects a chronic pattern of disturbed or fragmented sleep. However, two or more REM periods may indicate the coexistence of narcolepsy and sleep apnea syndrome, especially if symptoms of cataplexy are present.

Patterns of day-time alertness and degrees of day-time sleepiness appear to be dependent upon age. A high level of alertness seen in middle childhood gives way to augmentation of day-time sleepiness during pubertal development, even in the presence of a constant total sleep time (4). Slow-wave sleep decreased significantly in a linear fashion across maturational groups, with a near 35% decline from Tanner 1 to Tanner 5. In a parallel manner, day-time alertness, as measured by the MSLT, declined at mid-puberty (Tanner 3) and remained at the reduced level, *despite the fact that total sleep time remained constant* (6).

Short censored sleep-onset latencies are quite rare in middle childhood and normative data are not available in early childhood. During middle childhood, normal children *rarely* fall asleep during testing, and those who do fall asleep generally have censored mean sleep-onset latencies greater than 16 to 18 minutes. Indeed, children between 6 and 10 years of age are very alert, probably the most alert of any age group. Several normative studies of sleep in the preadolescent child have been published (7–10) and Carskadon and Dement have performed studies on patients during middle childhood (11). The most notable feature of the MSLT data was that during middle childhood, *subjects rarely fell asleep. Sleep was seen within the 20-minute test period on fewer than one fourth of the tests*. In those tests where sleep was noted, the children *never* fell asleep in less than 15 minutes. Children during middle childhood who do have significant sleep tendency on the MSLT, most likely are indeed excessively sleepy during the day-time, regardless of day-time symptomatology.

Clinical Modifications of Standard MSLT Protocol

In many clinical situations, it may be unwise to apply strictly adolescent and adult protocols and assessment criteria to performance and interpretation of MSLTs in younger children. Because of the paucity of normative data, the MSLT is infrequently done in youngsters below the age of 6 years. Children over 6 years of age, however, can be tested in the laboratory. Several modifications of the standard protocol and methods of interpretation have been proposed (12).

First, the study is typically done in the room that was used for nocturnal monitoring. The youngster will be most comfortable in "their" room, minimizing environmental bias. Second, the montage is modified from the nocturnal polysomnogram, eliminating some sensors that may be more intrusive than others (e.g., nasal/oral thermistor). In our laboratories we record four referential EEG channels during MSLT testing, two central and two occipital (C3-A2, C4-A1, O1-A2, and O2-A1). This montage permits accurate identification of sleep onset and affords adequate back-up channels in the event that electrodes become displaced during the course of a nap study. In addition, we limit the montage to recording of EEG, EOG, submental EMG, and EKG. Third, prior to onset of the nap attempt, the youngster is asked if she needs to void and is given the opportunity. Electrodes are checked and re-gelled. Machine calibrations are conducted, *but patient calibrations are not performed.* Patient calibrations during the MSLT seems to result in a stimulating effect. The youngsters enjoy speaking with the technician over the intercom and become excited during the exercise. Patient calibration prior to each nap provides no additional information that is helpful in interpretation and has the potential to bias nap parameters. Fourth, the youngster is awakened at the habitual time of morning sleep offset on school days and the first nap begins 2 hours after this time. Subsequent naps are attempted 1 hour and 40 minutes after termination of the previous nap. It is essential to keep the youngster awake between nap attempts. We also try to have the youngster perform school-like activities and/or homework during the inter-nap intervals. Since performance and behavior at school is often at question, having the day structured similar to that of a typical school day is desirable.

Interpretation of the MSLT nap results is also slightly modified. If MSLT criteria for these youngsters meet adult criteria, diagnosis is clear. Because of the natural history of narcolepsy syndrome and the many sleep-related disorders that can result in varying degrees of day-time sleepiness, classical adult criteria for excessive day-time sleepiness are often not met, *even in the presence of increased sleep pressure.* Therefore, supplemental criteria is necessary to clinically assess diurnal naps. In addition to traditional criteria such as mean sleep-onset latency, presence of SOREMPs, and REM latency, further parameters evaluated include:

1. Number of sleep onsets across the five naps;
2. Number of micro-sleep periods of 6 seconds or longer in naps where sleep onset does not occur or sleep-onset latency is prolonged;
3. Modification of the definition of excessive sleepiness as delineated by the censored mean sleep-onset latency; and
4. Identification of the number of individual nap studies where sleep-onset latency is considered profoundly short, even using adult criteria.

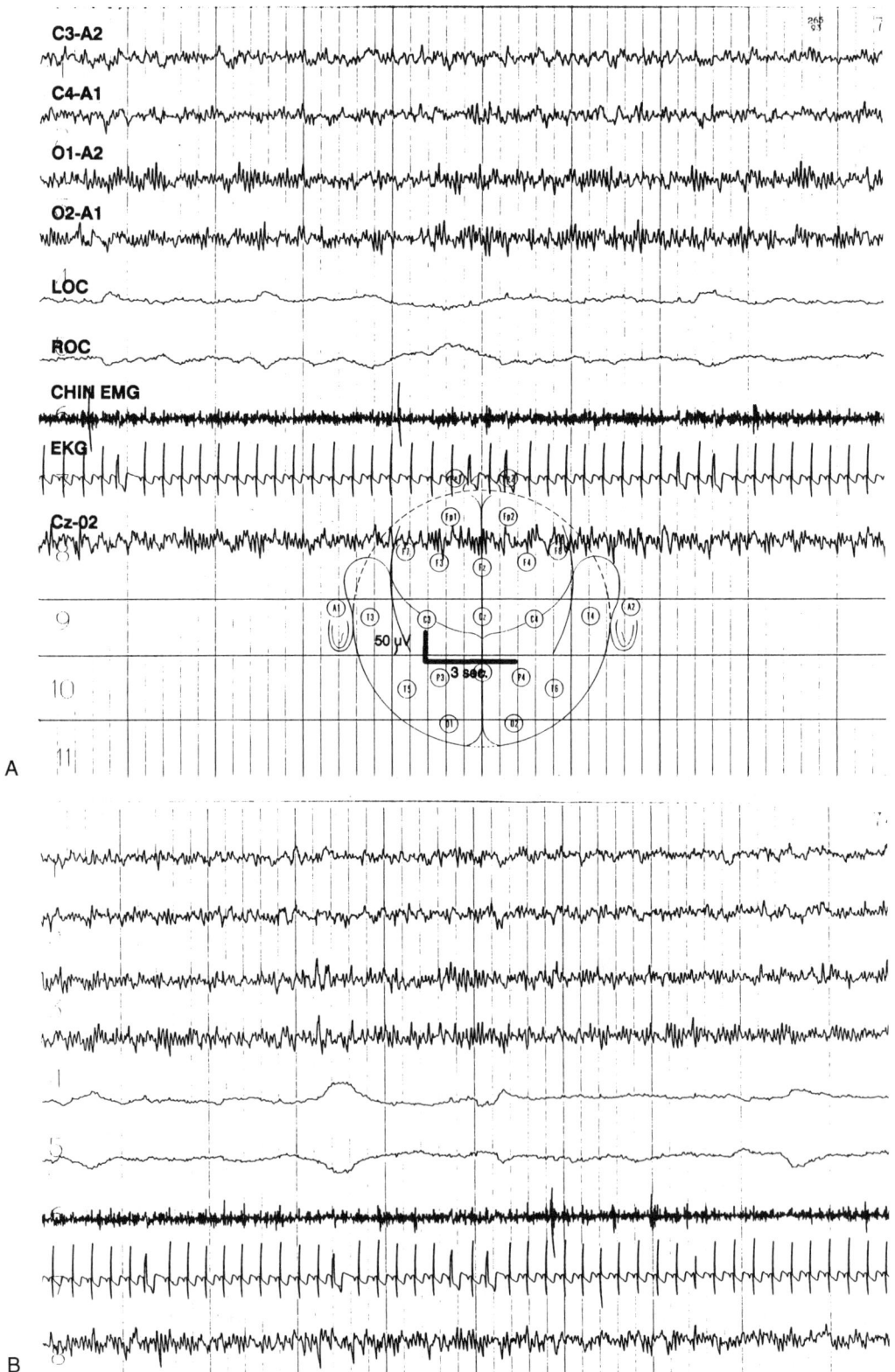

FIG. 13-1. A–D: Sleep-onset. Note dissipation of alpha activity and replacement of the alpha activity with a relatively low-voltage, mixed-frequency background EEG rhythm. A K-complex can be identified in epoch 13–1D.

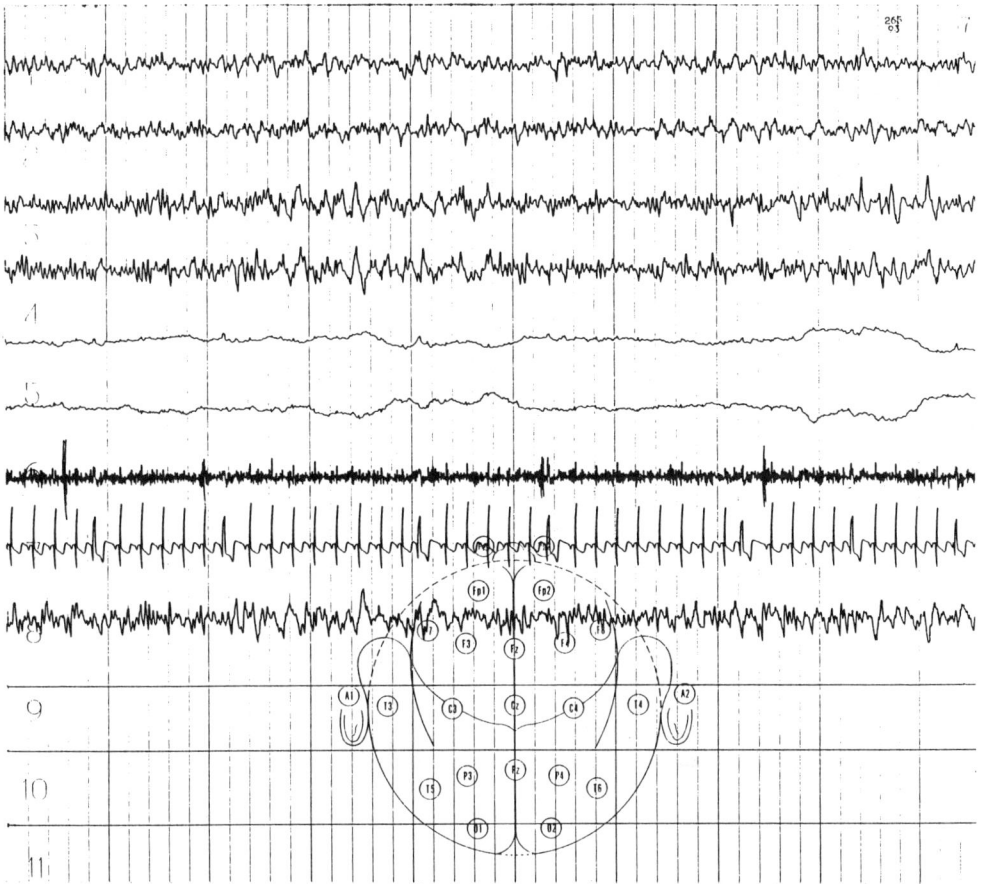

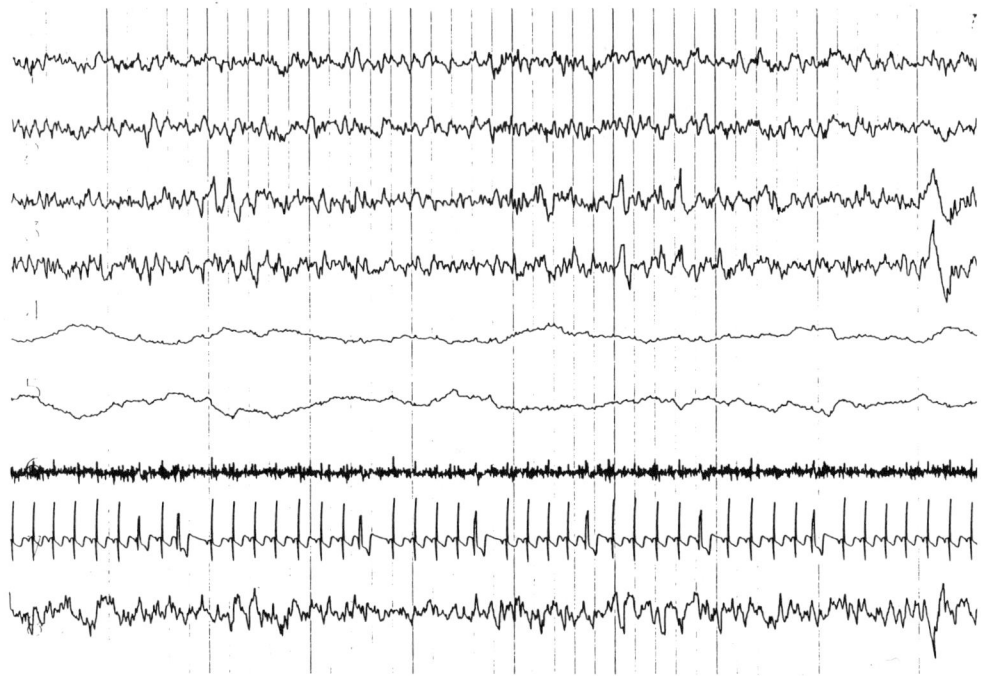

FIG. 13-1. *Continued.*

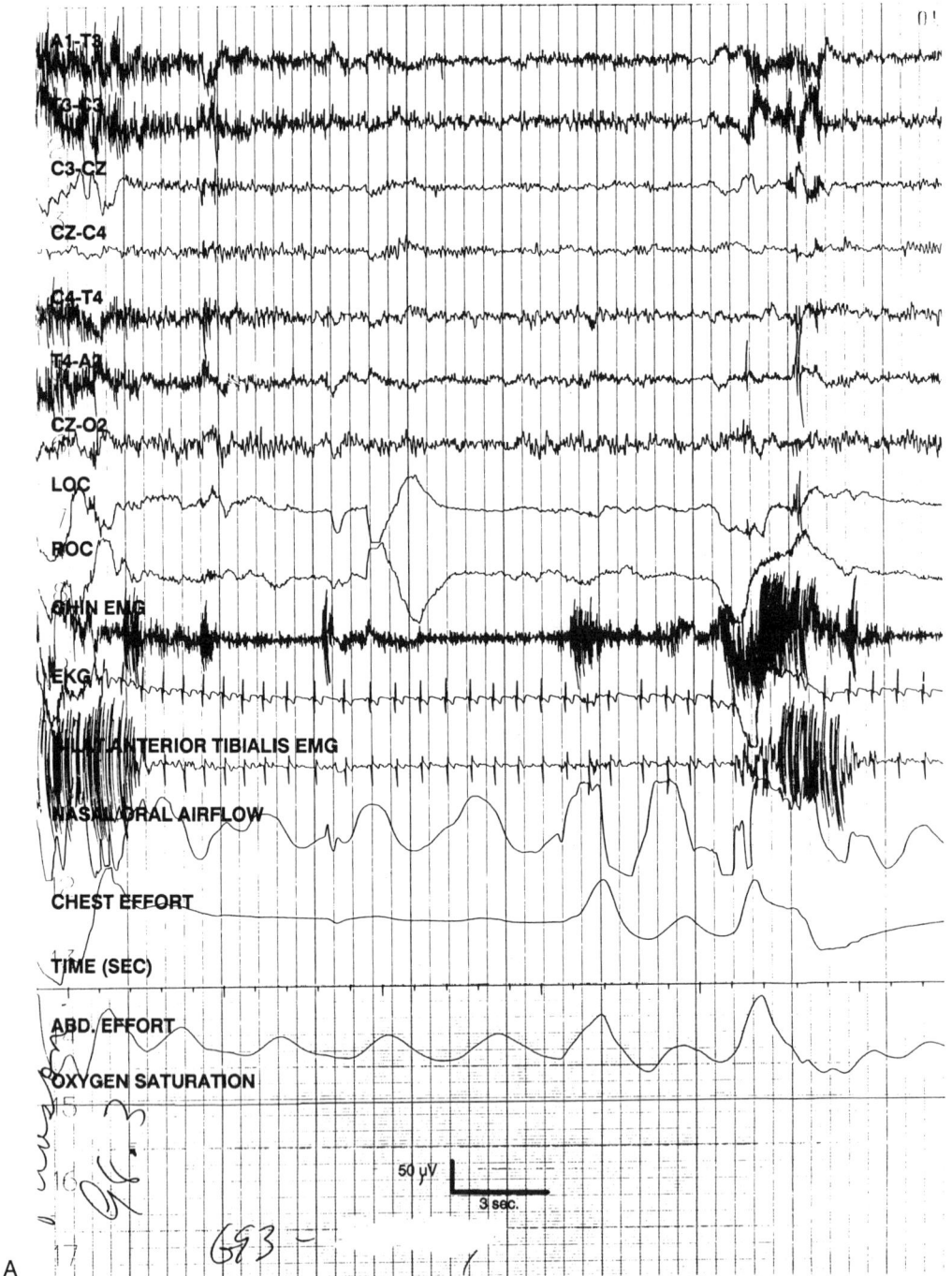

FIG. 13-2. A–E: Sleep-onset REM period in a 10-year-old patient with narcolepsy syndrome. Note the decrease in chin muscle tone and phasic twitches, appearance of a relatively low-voltage, mixed-frequency background EEG rhythm, saw-tooth waves, and rapid eye movements.

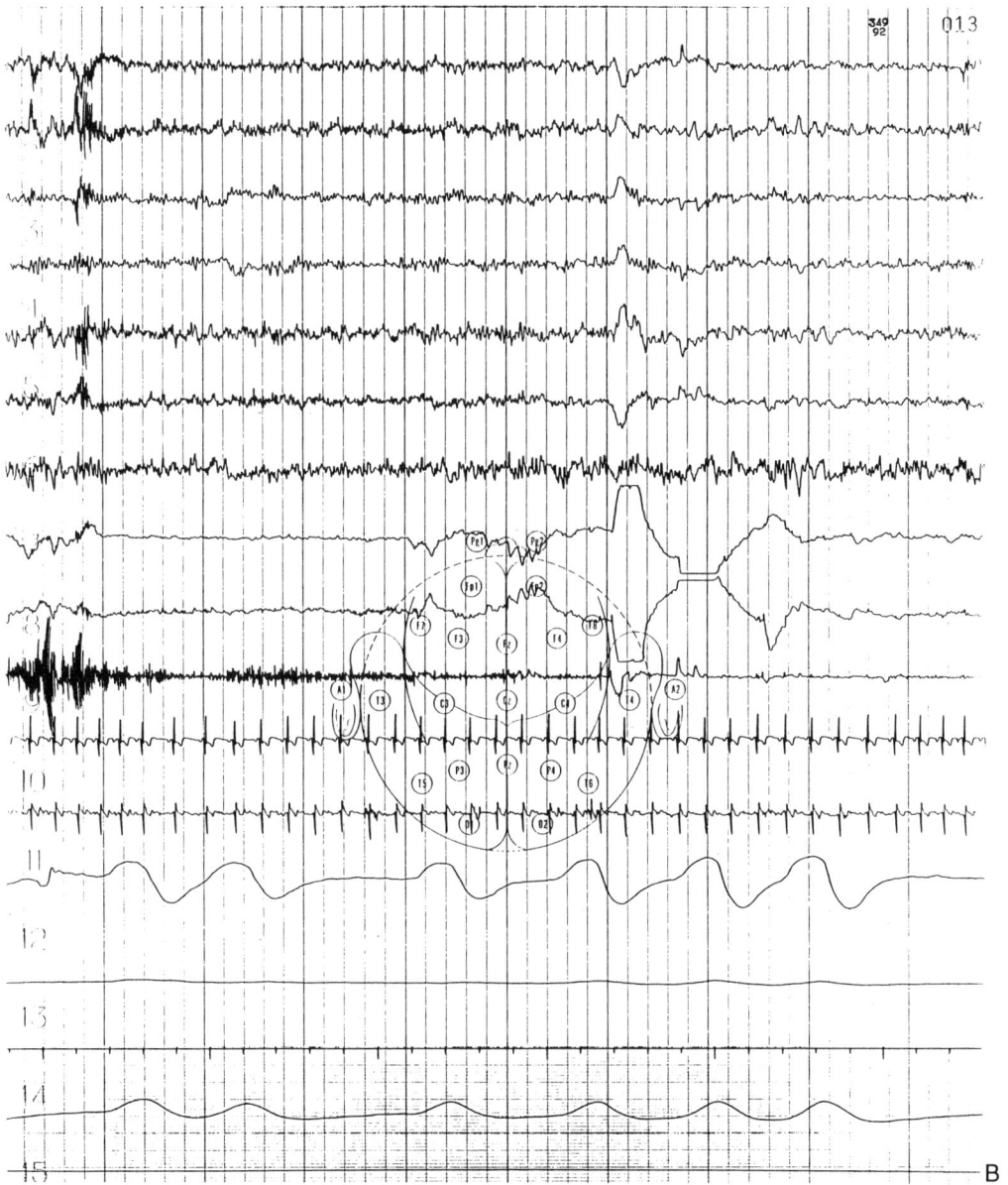

FIG. 13-2. *Continued.*

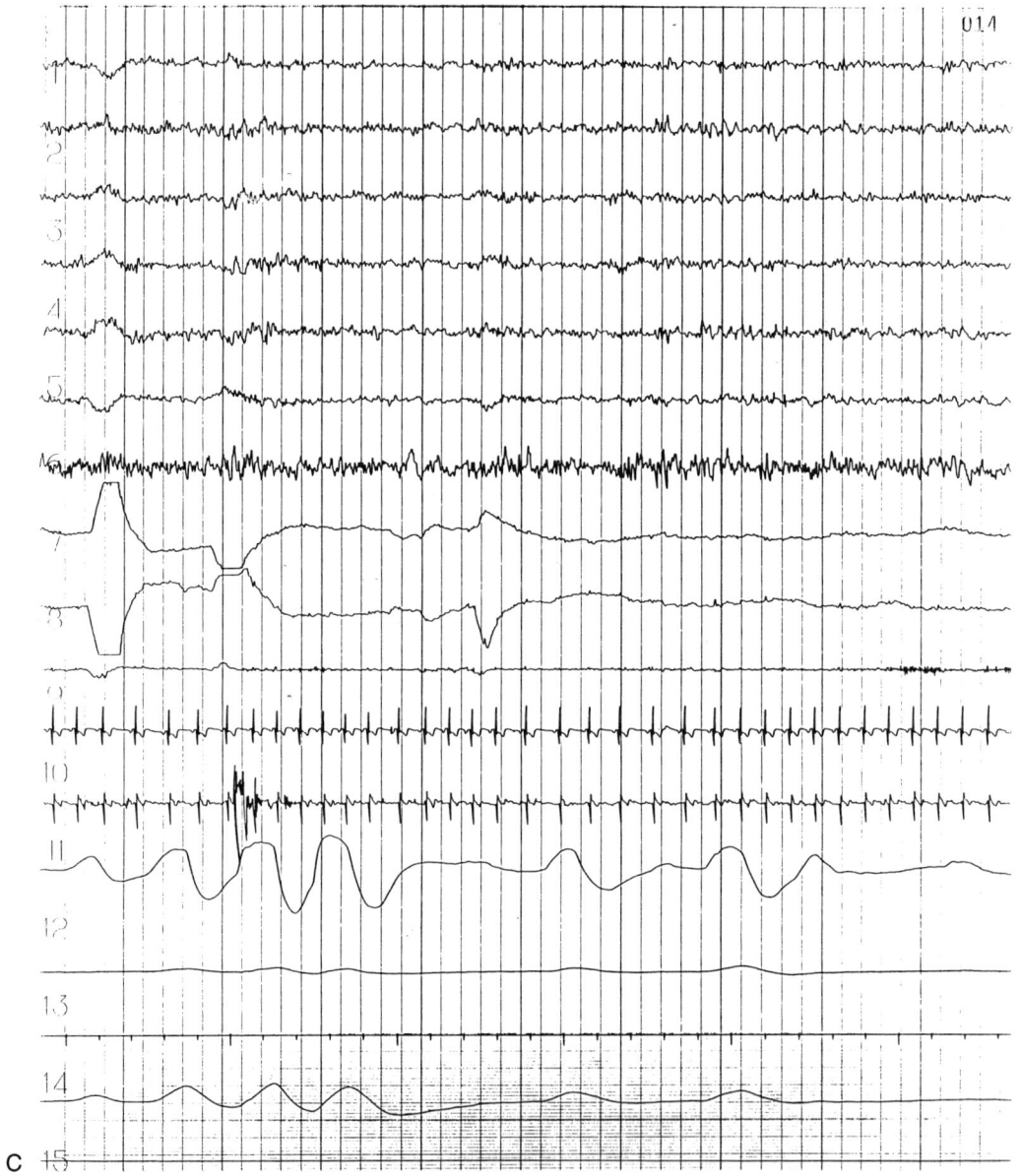

FIG. 13-2. *Continued.*

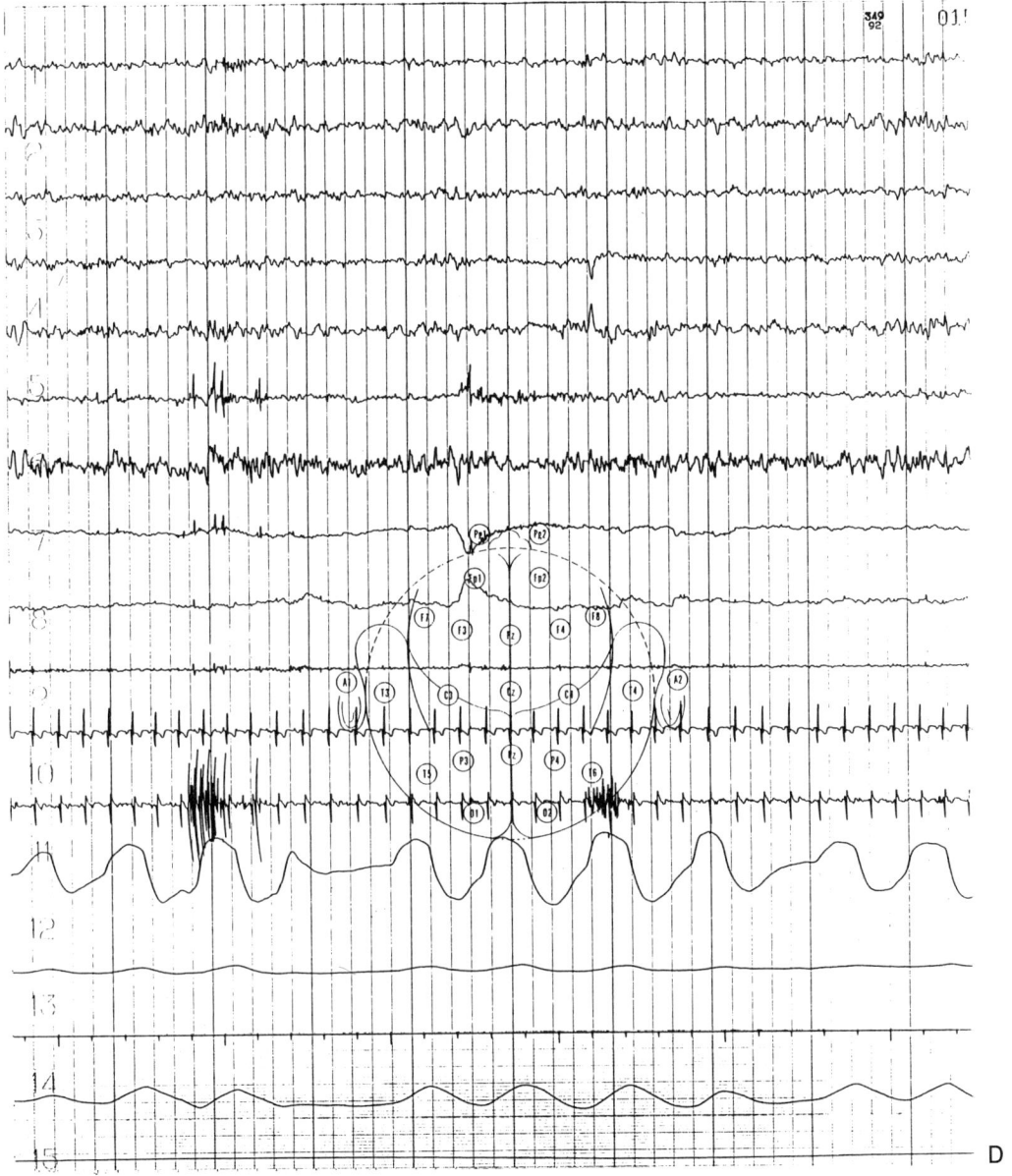

FIG. 13-2. *Continued.*

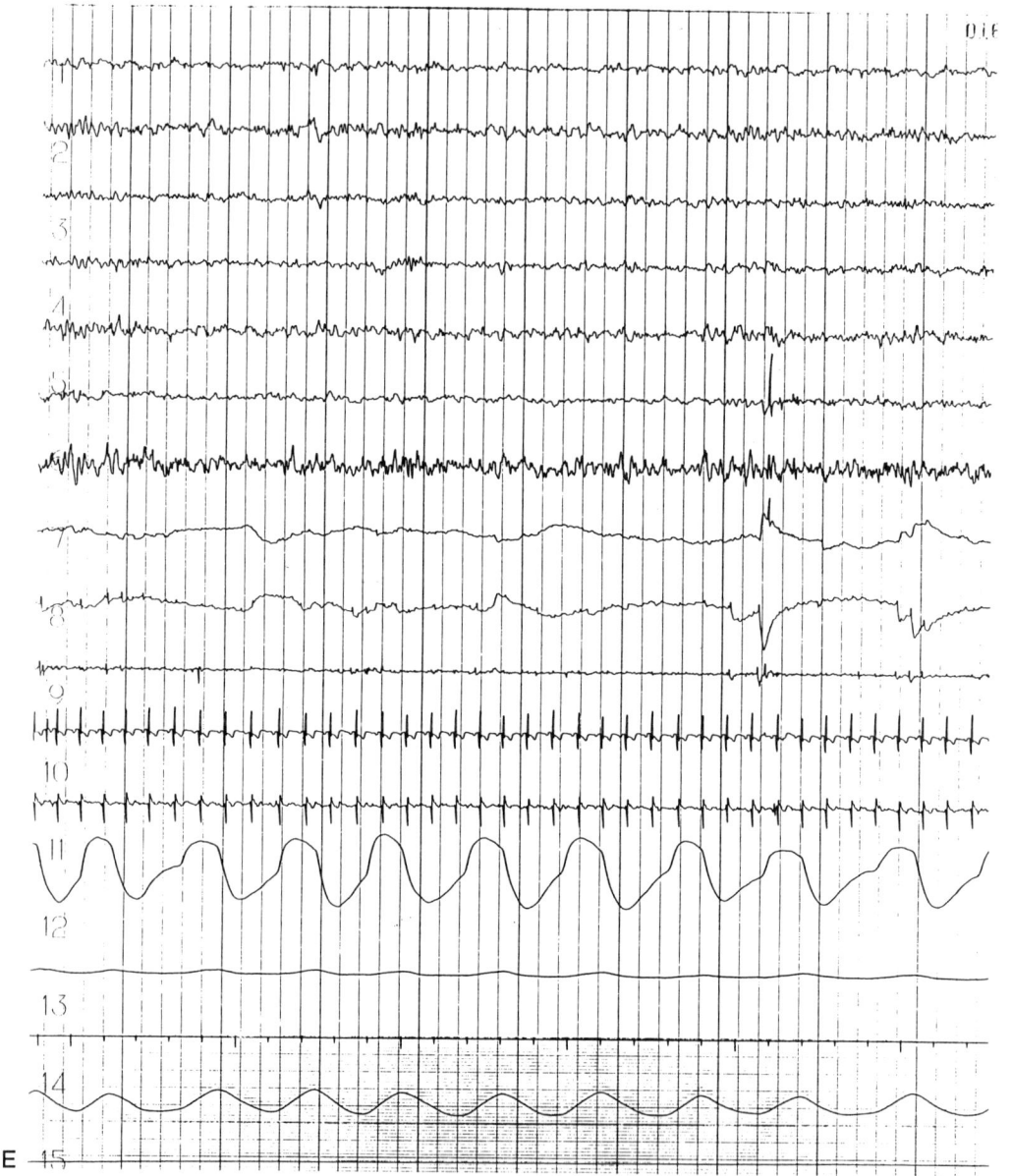

FIG. 13-2. *Continued.*

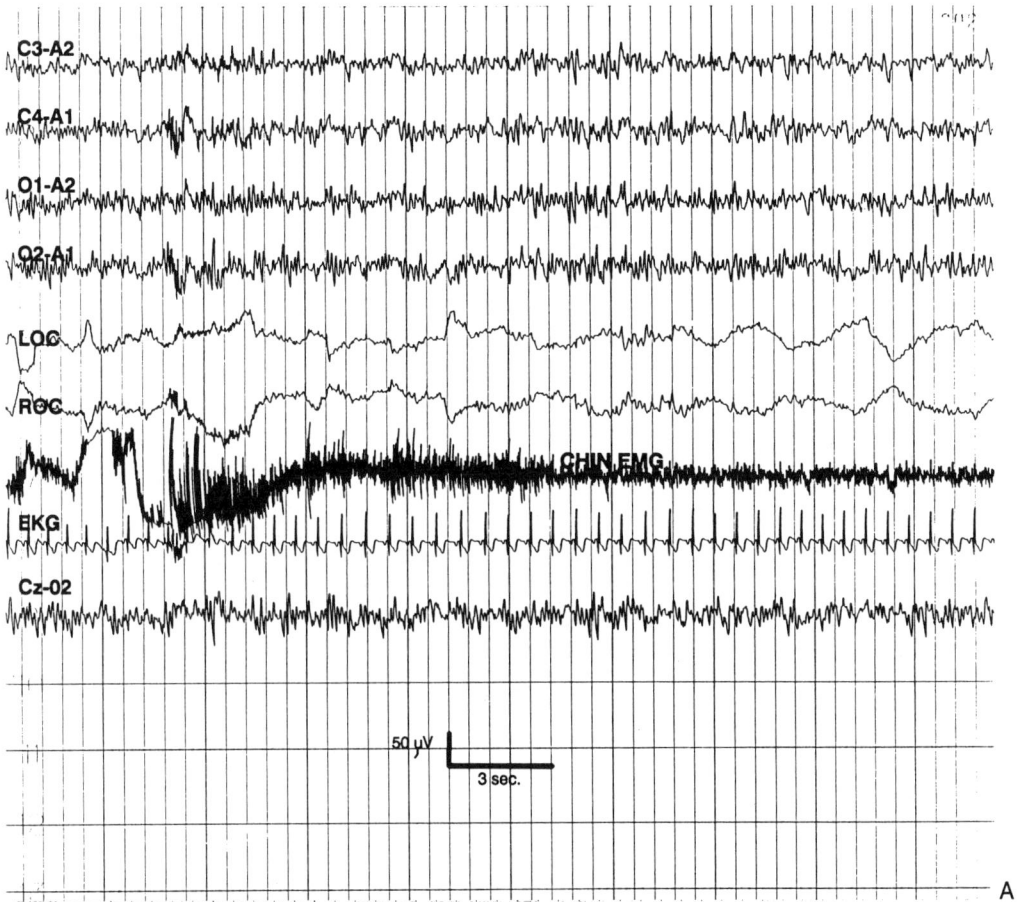

FIG. 13-3. A–C: Micro-sleep periods. A and B show micro-sleep periods of approximately 30 seconds; and C shows a micro-sleep period of about 6 seconds.

Clodoré and coworkers have suggested that the number of sleep onsets in a five- nap MSLT is a more sensitive indicator of excessive sleepiness than the mean sleep-onset latency (because of artificial censoring of the mean) (13). Children who suffer from attentional deficits due to sleepiness and who improve on stimulant medication fall to sleep on three or more MSLT naps (12). Excluding the first morning nap, most will have at least one (and usually more than one) of these naps with a sleep-onset latency within the pathologic range (less than 5 minutes), even though sleep onset may not occur on the other naps.

Micro-sleep periods occur when they are at least 6 seconds long, but less than 30 seconds, and the polysomnographic recording reveals *all* of the following criteria:

1. Absence of alpha activity and/or driving of the EEG by eye opening and the presence of relatively low-voltage, mixed-frequency activity;
2. Absence of conjugate eye movements and/or blink artifact on EOG, with or without the presence of slow, rolling eye movements;
3. Muscle tone at or below waking levels and absence of any movement artifact.

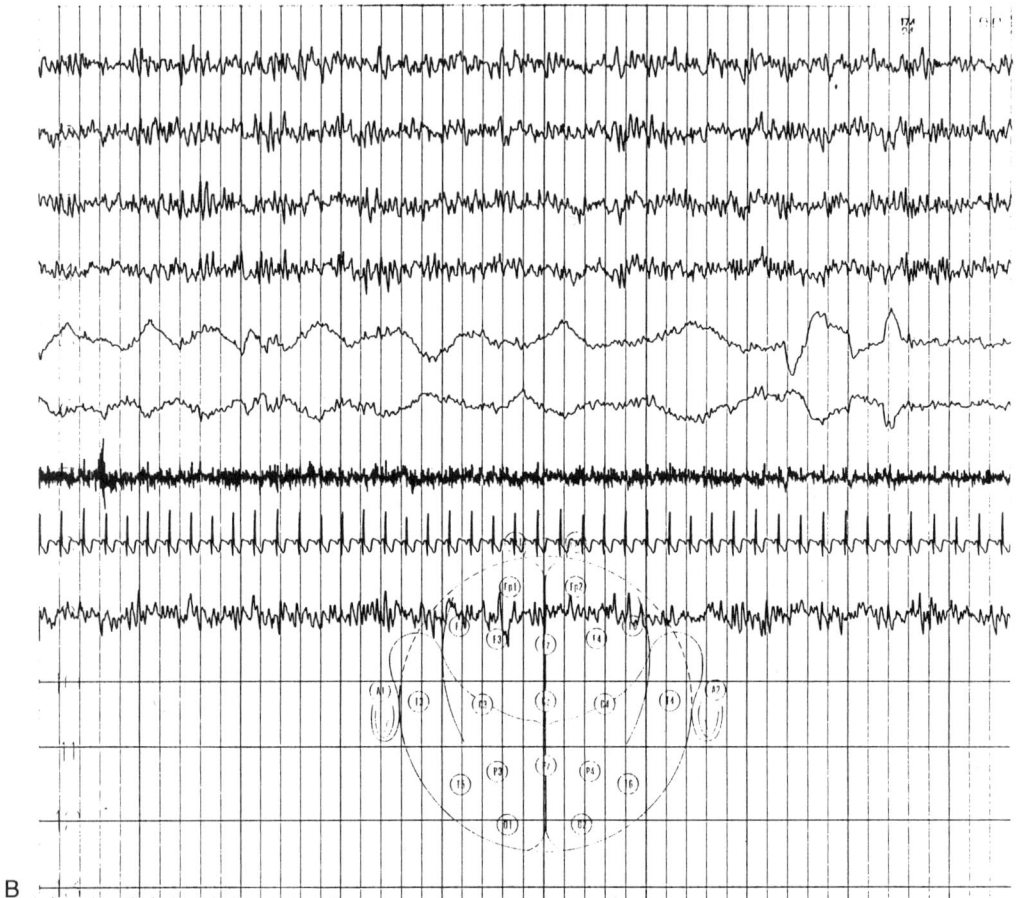

FIG. 13-3. *Continued.*

The frequency and average length of micro-sleep periods are calculated for each nap. Regression analysis reveals that the frequency of micro-sleep shows a highly significant positive relationship to the length of sleep-onset latency (i.e., the longer the sleep-onset latency, the greater the frequency of micro-sleep in these children. The length of micro-sleep periods also increases when consolidation of sleep occurs. Indeed, it is common to see increasing frequency and length of micro-sleep just prior to sleep onset.

Censored mean sleep-onset latency in children is generally long, almost always greater than 16 minutes in normal individuals, and characteristically greater than 18 minutes. Children with moderately increased day-time sleepiness and day-time symptoms often reveal MSLT censored mean sleep-onset latencies between 10 and 16 minutes. At least one, and often two or more of the naps have sleep-onset latencies less than 5 minutes. If naps without sleep onset are excluded from calculation of the mean, the sleep-onset latency across the three or more naps with sleep onsets is often in the pathologic range. Although clear conclusions cannot be made from these comparisons due to differences in methodology, the implications are intriguing and worthy of further investigation.

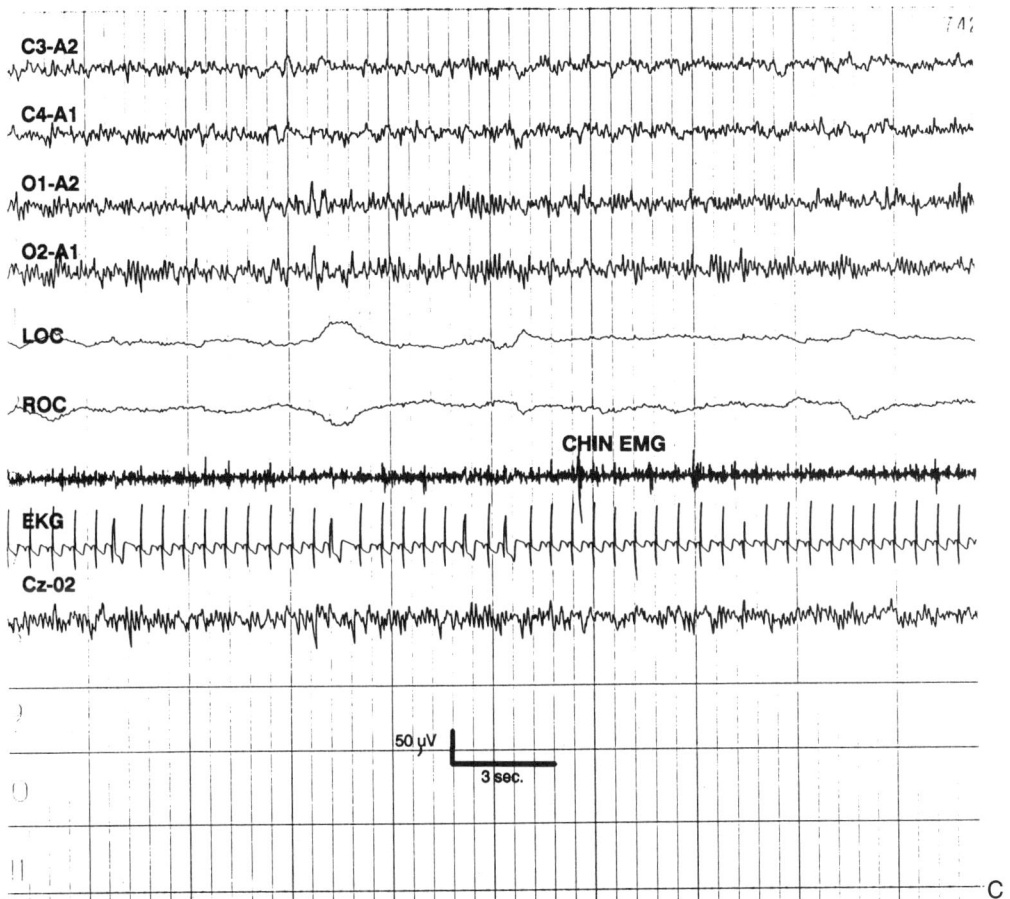

FIG. 13-3. *Continued.* Micro-sleep period of about 6 seconds. Note the brief disappearance of alpha activity, replacement with relatively low-voltage, mixed-frequency activity, and slow, rolling eye movements without consolidation of sleep.

Although these studies require replication and large numbers of children must be analyzed in order to arrive at normative data, additional parameters have greatly assisted in identification of children during middle childhood who are suffering from moderate degrees of sleepiness that significantly affect performance and behavior (Figs. 13-1–13-3).

REFERENCES

1. Carskadon MA, Dement WC, Mitler MM, et al. Guidelines for the multiple sleep latency test (MSLT): a standard measure of sleepiness. *Sleep* 1986;9:519–524.
2. Carskadon MA, Dement WC. The multiple sleep latency test: what does it measure? *Sleep* 1982;5: S67–S72.
3. Carskadon MA, Dement WC. Sleep tendency: an objective measure of sleep loss. *Sleep Res* 1977;6:200.
4. Sheldon SH, Spire JP, Levy HB. *Pediatric Sleep Medicine.* Philadelphia: WB Saunders; 1992.
5. Carskadon MA, Dement WC. Sleepiness in the normal adolescent. In: Guilleminault C, ed. *Sleep and Its Disorders in Children.* New York: Raven Press; 1987:53–66.
6. Carskadon MA, Harvey K, Duke P, et al. Pubertal changes in day-time sleepiness. *Sleep* 1980;2:453–460.
7. Feinberg I. Changes in sleep cycle patterns with age. *J Psychiatr Res* 1974;10:283–306.

8. Coble PA, Kupfer DJ, Taska LS, Kane J. EEG sleep of normal healthy children. Part I. Findings using standard measurement methods. *Sleep* 1984;7:289–303.
9. Ross JJ, Agnew HW Jr, Williams RL, Webb WB. Sleep patterns in preadolescent children: an EEG-EOG study. *Pediatrics* 1968;42:324–335.
10. Williams RL, Karacan I, Hursch CJ. *Electroencephalography (EEG) of Human Sleep: Clinical Applications.* New York: Wiley; 1974.
11. Carskadon MA, Dement WC. The multiple sleep latency test: What does it measure? *Sleep* 1982;5: S67–S72.
12. Sheldon SH, Irbe D, Applebaum J, Golbin A, Levy HB, Spire JP. Sleep pressure in children with attentional deficits. *Sleep Res* 1991;20A:448.
13. Clodoré M, Benoit O, Foret J, Bouard G. The multiple sleep latency test: individual variability and time of day effect in normal young adults. *Sleep* 1990;13:385–394.

Subject Index

ISBN 0-397-51628-2